THE
POCKET
RAD
TECH

THE POCKET RAD TECH

MARY J. HAGLER, MHA, BA, RT(R)(N)
Professor of Allied Health
Bakersfield College
Bakersfield, California

Photography by

Cheryl Mestmaker and Judy Alfter

W.B. SAUNDERS COMPANY
A Division of Harcourt Brace & Company
Philadelphia   London   Toronto   Montreal   Sydney   Tokyo

W.B. SAUNDERS COMPANY
A Division of
Harcourt Brace & Company

The Curtis Center
Independence Square West
Philadelphia, Pennsylvania 19106

Library of Congress Cataloging-in-Publication Data

Hagler, Mary J.

The pocket rad tech / Mary J. Hagler.

p. cm.

ISBN 0–7216–3981–X

1. Radiography, Medical—Positioning—Handbooks,
   manuals, etc.   I. Title.   [DNLM: 1. Technology,
   Radiologic—methods—handbooks. WM 39 H145p]

RC78.4H34 1993   616.07′5721—dc20

DNLM/DLC   91–46874

THE POCKET RAD TECH   ISBN 0–7216–3981–X

Printed in the United States of America.

Last digit is the print number: 9   8   7   6   5   4   3

Dedicated to
Bernette and Riley J., Betty Jo, and Riley R. Goedeke,
and to my stepfather, Ralph Schanz.
And to Betsy, who helped me survive the process
of writing this book.
And to Uncle Bill, who had faith in me.

Preface

The Pocket RAD TECH has been developed to accommodate radiologic technologists of various backgrounds. For the student technologist, this text is a quick reference for use in radiography laboratories and at clinical sites during training. For technologists who are recent graduates, *The Pocket RAD TECH* is a refresher for not-yet-familiar radiographic routines. For the experienced technologist, it is a quick reference for use during the course of a day's work that includes a few not-so-routine routines.

As most technologists are aware, the conditions of patients and types of radiographic examinations vary greatly from clinical site to clinical site. When a technologist does not practice certain x-ray studies on a continuing basis, his or her performance of radiographic routines becomes less efficient and a review of previously learned radiographic procedures is in order. It is very common for experienced technologists to seek different employment, make significant career advancements, and end up restudying various sections of their old textbooks for review (that is, if the textbooks are still accessible). This text attempts to bridge the gap for staff technologists in varying clinical environments as well as for student technologists in radiography laboratories and clinical training who desire a comprehensive, quick review of basic radiographic positions. Many radiographic texts differ in the suggested protocol for a certain position (for example, the various methods described for the anteroposterior [AP] skull). In order to accommodate regional differences, *The Pocket RAD TECH* attempts to include many, if not all, variations described in the most popular radiographic anatomy and positioning textbooks. You, the reader, will have to decide which CR placement or body position is appropriate for your situation.

The table of contents included in this text serves as a reference list of your department's routines. Simply check those projections or positions that apply, add any positions that may not be included, and you have an itemized list of your department's standardized x-ray routines.

Each projection or position in the text will be coded with an icon representing the position of the patient identification (ID) blocker on the x-ray cassette. Typically, the ID blocker placement has been contingent on the shape of the anatomy of interest, departmental policies, patient body habitus, and individual variances in positioning. The icon code represented in this text is simply a recommendation for those needing guidance and not necessarily a definitive solution for everyone in all instances. You must decide each ID blocker position on an individual basis. For that purpose, a blank icon is provided for convenience in coding the blocker position relative to your own situation (i.e., the blocker configuration differs on your film cassette) or if your faculty standardizes their placement. Encircle the appropriate icon or use the blank to encode blocker positions for your facility. An example of such blocker variation is a situation in which one radiologist likes to have technologists take all overhead upper gastrointestinal films with the blocker in one set location and does not have the technologists use lead markers. The blockers, in this case, are used as anatomical markers in lieu of lead markers. The provision of blank icons recognizes that there are many other factors that influence the final position of a film ID blocker. (See Chapter 10 in regard to marking radiographs and using blocker position to verify anatomical right and/or left.) As a general rule, anatomical markers are placed on the lateral aspect of long bones and joints, and blockers are placed toward the x-ray tube for those positions requiring a tube angle.

Of note are the sections entitled *Common Error*. This section depicts errors that commonly force a repeat of the position. It is hoped that this will alert students and technologists to common pitfalls of radiographic positioning or technique formulation and will lower the number of repeated examinations. Suggestions for special patient handling, radiation safety or standards of practice are included under the heading of *Notes*. Additional explanations or clarifications are included under the heading of *Comments*.

An abbreviated table for recording techniques is included in Appendix C for the radiologic technologist. Not only may the obvious kilovoltage peak (KV), milliamperage (MA), and seconds (S) of techniques be recorded, the caliper measurement used in technique chart assessment may be recorded as well. The use of a grid and its ratio, table Bucky, and tabletop can be indicated. Distance from tube to image receptor is a major consideration in correct technique formulation. The abbreviation SID (source-to-image distance) instead of focal-film distance (FFD) is used here. A record of the use of differing intensifying screens (or none at all) is also provided. Body habitus can also be assessed and recorded. The following abbreviations are used: hypersthenic (hyper), sthenic (s), hyposthenic (hypo), and asthenic (a). For those technologists using general body size assessments, the abbreviations XS (extra small), S (small), M (medium), L (large), XL (extra large), and XXL (extra, extra large, e.g., a right guard for the San Francisco 49ers football team) may be indicated for technique assessment. All of the aforementioned criteria are major factors in the formulation of technique. Radiographic techniques will vary from facility to facility and may even vary from radiographic room to radiographic room. Because of space limitation you might record a technique that is representative of the average body size, the sthenic body habitus. By establishing this baseline, you can then increase or decrease from this value accordingly for larger or smaller body sizes and densities. Pediatric techniques should be formulated separately. A conversion chart for milliamperage-seconds (mAs) is included in Appendix A.

There exist many ways to achieve the same end. Radiography is no exception. Often there will be different angles and different baselines used in order to achieve a similar (if not the exact) demonstration of radiographic anatomy. I have tried to include all of the most common variations and to footnote them for the reader's convenience. Each technologist should confer with his or her supervisor or department manager in order to standardize radiographic procedures within the facility. Appendix B is provided for the technologists' use in recording positions and projections that are not included in this text, but that may be used at individual health care facilities. Appendix C is provided for the technologists' use in recording additional techniques.

A review of body landmarks is provided in Chapter 1 for radiography students. Guidelines for how to find landmarks are included (to a very sick patient, gentle hands are healing hands!). Portable radiographic exams force you to be innovative. Often there are structural constraints such as traction bars, respirators, and other equipment in the way, as well as limits to patient range of motion. These cases are reviewed in Chapter 8. Cranial radiography and side best demonstrated are summarized in Chapters 11 and 12, respectively, for those angst-ridden students awaiting their boards.

The following are some of the basic practices that *must* be observed in the course of an x-ray examination: correct patient/procedure identification; practical consideration given to the patient for his or her comfort; adherence to standards of practice such as (but not limited to) patient confidentiality, good patient care, comprehensive but appropriate exams and ethical conduct within the practice of radiography; correct collimation; correct techniques; the minimalization of repeats; proper film, screen, and grid combinations used in order to achieve optimal radiographs while minimizing patients' radiation doses; and observation of protocols in radiation protection for patient and technologist.

In the effort to simplify and condense information (but not to diminish the importance of these areas), the practice of radiography for technique formulation, film processing, accessory equipment use (phototiming, grid selection, etc.), fluoroscopy, and other specialty examinations will not be comprehensively covered in this text. For referencing information about these, consult the Bibliography included at the end of this text.

The standards, code of ethics, and scope of practice of radiography are espoused by the American Society of Radiologic Technologists and the American Registry of Radiologic Technologists. For a complete review of the standards, code of ethics, and scope of practice for the radiologic technologist in the United States, contact these organizations. For a review of the international standards and scope of practice, contact the International Society of Radiologic Technologists and Technicians.

This book is also dedicated to those student technologists and staff technologists ever striving to refresh and keep abreast of what no longer is sharpened by continued use, but who remain skillful and competent because of their desire to learn and relearn the radiographic arts.

MARY J. HAGLER, MHA, BA, RT(R)(N)

Acknowledgments

My gratitude to those who shared their valuable skills, effort, equipment, and expertise with me in the development, production, and design of this book. I profoundly thank the photographers, Cheryl Mestmaker and Judy Alfter, for their good humor, exceptional skills, and patience, and the models, Frances M. Barton, Lisa Baruian, Jackie Betancourt, Jasmine Burnett, Donald Cooper, Dottina Dixon, DeSheala Dixon, Janet Gonzales, Susan Hill, Chris Hughey, Anita McBride, Katie McBride, Lynette Moses, Brianne Moses, Elizabeth Peterson, and Martha Tarin, for their Zeus-like patience and cold tolerance. Great appreciation is extended to those facilities that allowed my trusty crew (and later dusty crew) of film archivists, Lori Netherton, Martha Tarin, and Maureen Wade, into the bowels (so to speak) of their facilities: Bob Balow of Kern Radiology Medical Group, Inc.; Lucky Sells, formerly of Kern Medical Center; and Glen Hawkins, formerly of San Joaquin Community Hospital and now of Fuji Medical Systems. To good friend and talented (although she wouldn't admit to it) radiologic technologist, Marga, my gratitude for her patience in sorting through stacks of expired x-rays packratted away at my house. To Rose, thanks for being my friend. Many thanks to those facilities' personnel and their patience with our photography crew for on-the-scene shoots: Kern Radiology Imaging, Bakersfield Memorial Hospital, and Mercy Hospital. John McHargue and Sherri Hartwell's time and effort to arrange the use of a room and the portable radiographic unit at Mercy Hospital were greatly appreciated. Thanks to Lynette Moses for her assistance in staging the x-ray films and to Debbie Fieber and others for the scrupulous third, fourth, and fifth looks. My wholehearted thanks to the research assistance and graphics development help of Merita (Paki) Scanlan. Thanks to my colleagues at Bakersfield College and to Shirley Pike, department assistant, for her help in all those last minute requests of mine. Thanks to radiography students (Class of '92) Lorena Mendez, Robert Merryman, Danya Heibert, Tere Abney, and Maureen Wade and others for contributing their x-ray films.

Much appreciation to Carlos Rangel for his assistance and recommendations regarding chiropractic radiographic procedures.

My gratitude to Glen Hawkins and Fuji Medical Systems, U.S.A., Inc., and Dennis Kampa and General Electric Medical Systems for their assistance in providing access to and equipment for the photography shoots. Finally, and most appreciatively, my thanks to Lisa Biello, Editor-in-Chief of Health Related Professions at W. B. Saunders Company, Linda R. Garber, Production Manager, and Lucille Cater, Marketing staff, who went out of their way to make sure my questions, concerns, and angst were addressed.

This text was made possible because of the ease of operation of Apple's Mac SE computer and the availability of my Lizard Lazerprinter (no more midnight runs to the local, full-service copy shop!).

MARY J. HAGLER, MHA, BA, RT(R)(N)

Contents

Suggested routine projections are in **boldface** type; place checks in boxes that indicate the routine projections used in your current workplace. If **boldface** type is *not* indicated within a routine, it means that the routine varies greatly from clinical site to clinical site, and thus a definitive recommendation is not possible.

Introduction

The following sequence of events in performing radiographic studies will be repeated hundreds of times during your career. The importance of the exact replication of these events is not as important as the fact that your actions should be appropriate and equitable to *all* of your patients. Later, as you become more knowledgeable and skillful, you will develop your own methodology that will meet your needs and your facility's needs perhaps better than the one listed here. This is not intended to be a comprehensive record of events, but one which you can alter or add to as you and your patient's own needs dictate. Feel free to use this list and add to it as your needs indicate. If you are currently working with radiography students, posting the recommended steps to taking a radiograph particular to your clinical facility would be a great help.

STEP ONE

Receive patient's radiography orders and admitting diagnosis. Set up the room for the procedure with the patient's transportation mode in mind (ambulatory, wheelchair, gurney, or bed). Have the chest board and tube in alignment or the tube aligned near the table. Ensure a clean x-ray table. Markers needed for that particular study should be ready for use. Have contrast medium, venipuncture setup, etc., ready if appropriate. Have the appropriate film cassettes particular to the study ready for use.

STEP TWO

Verify the patient's identity (usually by wrist ID bracelet or explicit verbal confirmation). Put the patient at ease by explaining who you are and what you are going to do. For female patients, ascertain if there is a possibility of pregnancy. If there is, delay the exam until you confer with the radiologist or patient's physician. (Check your department policy.)

STEP THREE

Assess the patient's condition. Find out if there are multiple injuries or pre-existing disabilities. Find out why the patient is having this test by asking, or by reading the chart if the patient is not able to communicate (be familiar with patient chart organization so you may access this information quickly).

STEP FOUR

Escort the patient into the x-ray room if not already there. Never leave a patient standing while you rearrange the room or leave the room. Always stay close to the patient until he or she is seated or recumbent. Your decision to later leave the patient while you develop or assess x-rays depends on the information you have gathered up to this point from the interaction you have allowed yourself to have with the patient. Can you make the correct decisions either based on the information you have elicited or the information gained by observation? Should you leave the patient? Is the patient pale and/or is the skin damp? Did he or she understand your explanations or instructions? Do you have enough information or did you observe long enough in order to make a correct decision on these issues?

STEP FIVE

Set a basic technique. Select the appropriate film size and place in table Bucky, tabletop, or chest film holder if you haven't done so in setting up the room. Mark the film. (If you form the habit of tying together the two motions of film placement and marking the film, you will not forget to mark the film.) Move the Bucky tray and/or center the film to the area of interest.

STEP SIX

In order to alleviate the patient's apprehension, let the patient know what you are doing as you go along. For pediatric patients, always explain first or demonstrate before you actually do anything. From now on when you have to move the tube, use individual locks for individual movements (for example, longitudinal). This will allow the tube to remain centered to the center of the x-ray table or film while you adjust the tube's position. If you have a floating tabletop, move it instead of the tube and patient.

STEP SEVEN

Place the patient in the appropriate position. Adjust the area of interest by moving the patient's area of interest to the center of the table, chest film holder, or tabletop film cassette. Make sure the patient isn't tender or sore at the site you will have to palpate for body landmarks. Center the tube to the film at the correct SID.

STEP EIGHT

Fine tune your positioning. Recheck that the area of interest is centered and completely on the film, that the collimation includes the area of interest but does not exceed the film size, that the side is correctly marked, and that the film is centered to the CR. If using the Bucky, make sure that the tray is pushed in all the way.

STEP NINE

After positioning the patient, you should have an opportunity to assess body habitus. Reassess your technique choice as you return to the console and make any changes as appropriate. Make sure the Bucky is activated if in use. Give the patient final instructions as to respiration or holding still. While viewing through a leaded glass window, observe the patient's response and then make the exposure. Have the patient resume respiration again and relax.

If more positions are required for the examination, go to Step Ten. If not, make the patient comfortable and explain that you are leaving the room momentarily to process and evaluate the films.

STEP TEN

While at the console, set the technique for the next exposure. Inform the patient of the next stage of the exam. Verbally instruct the patient to move into the next position of the exam while adjusting the film. Place a fresh film in the film holder while removing the exposed film. Place an anatomical marker on the film. Store the exposed film away from any supplies of fresh film cassettes. (Many techs place unexposed films upright and exposed films transversely, or sideways. Obviously, this does not work for square films.) Return to Step Six.

CHAPTER

Body Landmarks and Cranial Baselines

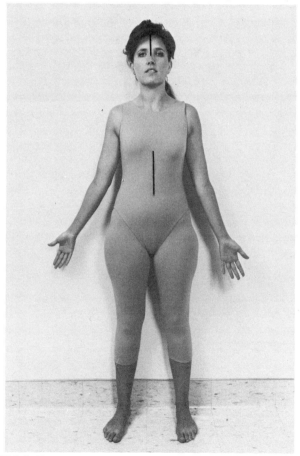

FIGURE 1–1. The anatomical position. Facing forward, arms and legs are extended, with palms of hands forward. The midsagittal plane (*line*) separates the body and skull into equal right and left halves.

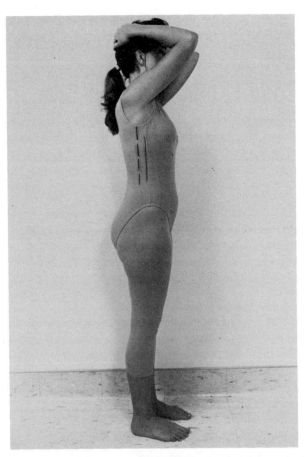

FIGURE 1–2. The midcoronal plane separates the lateralized body into equal anterior and posterior halves (*anterior line*). The midaxillary line extends from the axilla (*posterior, broken line*).

CRANIAL BASELINES AND LANDMARKS

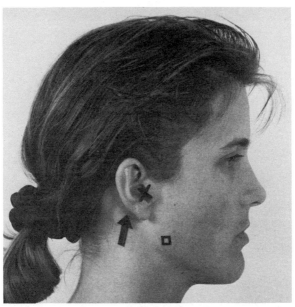

FIGURE 1–3. External acoustic meatus (EAM) (marked by *X*), gonion (*square*), and mastoid tip (*arrow*).

COMMON ERROR: Before palpating for body landmarks, always ask the patient if there is any tenderness or soreness in the area of palpation.

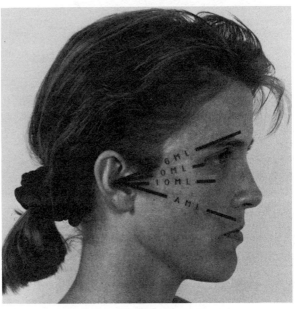

FIGURE 1–4. From the superior, the glabellomeatal line (GML), the orbitomeatal line (OML), the infraorbitomeatal line (IOML), and the acanthomeatal line (AML).

COMMON ERROR: Before palpating for body landmarks, always ask the patient if there is any tenderness or soreness in the area of palpation.

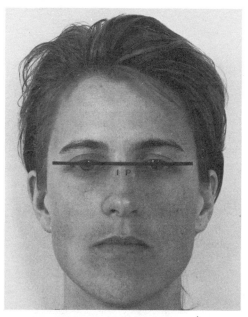

FIGURE 1–5. Interpupillary line (IP).

COMMON ERROR: Before palpating for body landmarks, always ask the patient if there is any tenderness or soreness in the area of palpation.

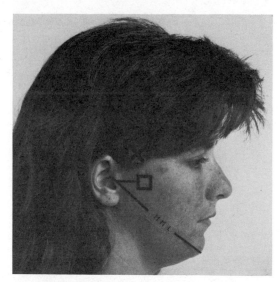

FIGURE 1–6. Temporomandibular joint (*box*) 1 inch (5 cm) anterior to EAM and sella turcica ¾ inch (1.9 cm) anterior from EAM, and then superior from that point (*X*). Mentomeatal line (MML) (*lower line*).

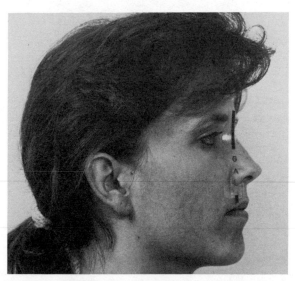

FIGURE 1–7. Glabelloalveolar line (GAL).

COMMON ERROR: Before palpating for body landmarks, always ask the patient if there is any tenderness or soreness in the area of palpation.

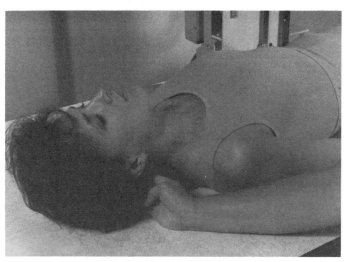

FIGURE 1–8. Palpation for base of skull.

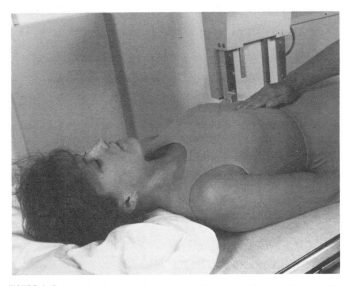

FIGURE 1–9. Palpation for xiphoid process (ensiform process) at T-10 (see also Fig. 1–11).

COMMON ERROR: Before palpating for body landmarks, always ask the patient if there is any tenderness or soreness in the area of palpation.

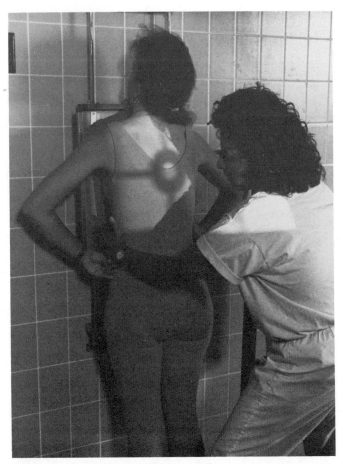

FIGURE 1–10. Assessment of lateral ribs for inclusion on chest or bilateral rib films. Check the inferior, lateral rib margins with the borders of the film by placing your hands on the patient's sides. Now, extend your fingers so that the tips touch the film or film holder. You can ensure that the lateral aspects of the lung fields are included on the film by assessing your fingertip position relative to the film borders. Include a sufficient border of ½ to 1 inch (1.25 to 2.54 cm) of film space on each side of your fingertips in order to allow for rib expansion upon full inspiration of the patient.

COMMON ERROR: Before palpating for body landmarks, always ask the patient if there is any tenderness or soreness in the area of palpation.

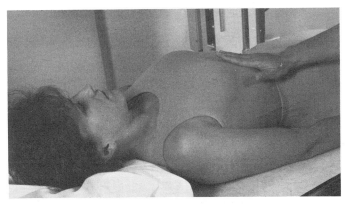

FIGURE 1–11. When palpating for the anterior costal margin, use the *flat* part of the fingers to find the highest point first. Follow the margin laterally to find the end of the ribs (or superiorly to the xiphoid process) in order to locate bony thorax landmarks.

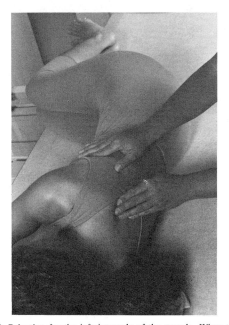

FIGURE 1–12. Palpation for the inferior angle of the scapula. When the scapula of interest is traumatized, use the opposite scapula for palpation in localizing landmarks.

COMMON ERROR: Before palpating for body landmarks, always ask the patient if there is any tenderness or soreness in the area of palpation.

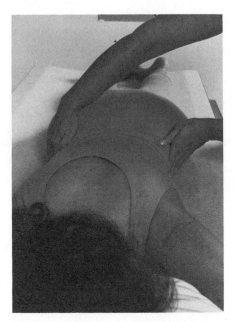

FIGURE 1–13. For difficult-to-palpate, recumbent patients (supine or prone), use both hands to localize the iliac crests. For hypersthenic patients, have them elevate the side closest to you for ease of either iliac crest or anterior superior iliac spine (ASIS) landmark location on that side. Never probe with pointed fingers; use flattened fingers to avoid patient discomfiture.

COMMON ERROR: Before palpating for body landmarks, always ask the patient if there is any tenderness or soreness in the area of palpation.

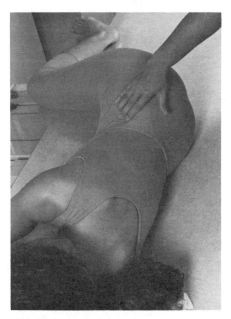

FIGURE 1–14. For lateralized patients, find the iliac crest by using flattened fingers. Start high just below the waist and move from the superior to the inferior. For hypersthenic patients, start at the ASIS (see Fig. 1–15) and then move superiorly and posteriorly to the iliac crest.

COMMON ERROR: Before palpating for body landmarks, always ask the patient if there is any tenderness or soreness in the area of palpation.

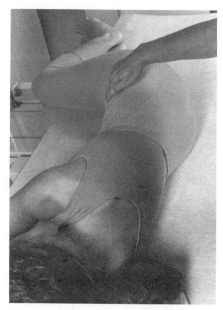

FIGURE 1–15. For lateralized patients, the ASIS is easily located due to the abdominal mass falling away from the side up.

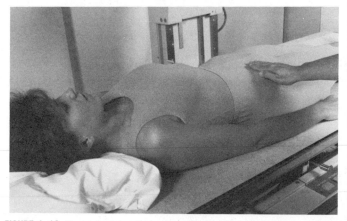

FIGURE 1–16. For supinated patients, the ASIS is easily located with the flattened fingers.

COMMON ERROR: Before palpating for body landmarks, always ask the patient if there is any tenderness or soreness in the area of palpation.

BODY LANDMARKS OF EXTREMITIES

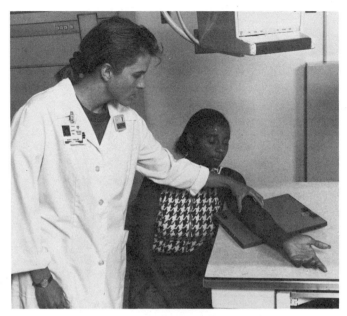

FIGURE 1–17. The epicondyles of the humerus must be level for several AP projections of the arm. The epicondyles of the humerus are easily palpated with your thumb and second finger. Assess for patient tenderness before palpating.

COMMON ERROR: Before palpating for body landmarks, always ask the patient if there is any tenderness or soreness in the area of palpation.

LOCALIZING THE SYMPHYSIS PUBIS VIA THE HIP

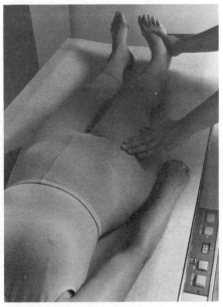

FIGURE 1–18. Many technologists do not use the greater trochanter of the femur to find the level of the symphysis pubis because of the difficulty encountered in localizing the trochanter. For patients with good range of motion and no trauma to the hip, place the flattened fingers of the left hand (or right hand if applicable) on the lateral and *anterior* aspect of the hip. Take the opposite hand and gently rotate the entire lower leg internally. The greater trochanter will be easily palpated by its movement during the lower leg rotation. If it is not localized, gently rock the lower leg back and forth until the trochanter is located. Generally, the error in localizing comes from a too low position on the lateral aspect of the hip. When located, the symphysis pubis lies in the same transverse plane as the greater trochanter. *Do not use this method on the side of any hip or lower leg injuries.* Perform the assessment on the uninjured side.

COMMON ERROR: Before palpating for body landmarks, always ask the patient if there is any tenderness or soreness in the area of palpation.

HOW TO LOCATE THE FEMORAL HEAD AND NECK

Finding the ASIS is the first step in localizing the femoral head and neck. It is relatively easy to find on patients of all classifications of body habitus. With the patient supinated, simply place the flattened fingers over the area of the superior, lateral ilium (see Fig 1–16). The bony prominence of the ASIS should be evident. If not, simply range an inch (2.54 cm) or so up and side to side with the flattened fingers. Because direct probing can cause bruising, try to avoid it.

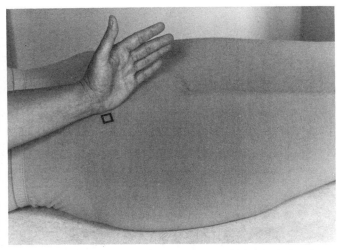

FIGURE 1–19. Place the heel of the hand at the ASIS (see *box* in figure).

COMMON ERROR: Before palpating for body landmarks, always ask the patient if there is any tenderness or soreness in the area of palpation.

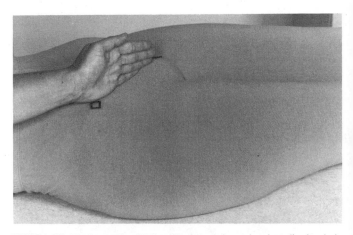

FIGURE 1–20. The femoral head is found by formulating an imaginary line by placing the heel of the left or right hand on the ASIS of the side of interest (see *square* in figure). Swing the hand and extended fingers toward and stop at the midsagittal plane (MSP). This hand alignment forms the baseline for another measurement.

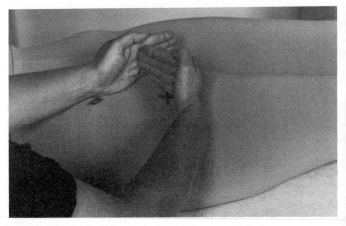

FIGURE 1–21. Find the point that represents the center of the line extending from the ASIS (*square*) to MSP formed by the extended hand. The center will be found along the palmar surface of the hand at the metacarpophalangeal joints. Now form a "T" at this line with your extended opposite hand by measuring a 2- to 3-inch (5- to 8-cm) perpendicular line from the center of the first line. This "leg of the T" measurement is usually found at the proximal, interphalangeal joints of the opposite hand (see *X* in figure).

COMMON ERROR: Before palpating for body landmarks, always ask the patient if there is any tenderness or soreness in the area of palpation.

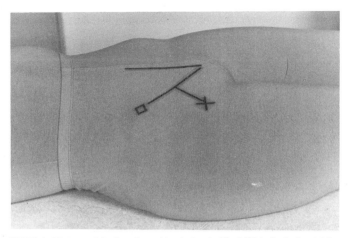

FIGURE 1–22. Map of the lines formed by the hands. The MSP is the horizontal line, the ASIS is the square, and the X is the femoral neck area.

COMMON ERROR: Before palpating for body landmarks, always ask the patient if there is any tenderness or soreness in the area of palpation.

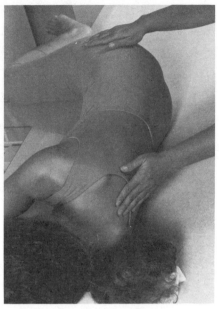

FIGURE 1–23. Checking for true lateralization on a lateral recumbent patient.

COMMON ERROR: Before palpating for body landmarks, always ask the patient if there is any tenderness or soreness in the area of palpation.

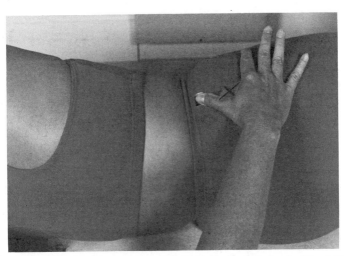

FIGURE 1–24. Palpation method to localize L5-S1 (*X*). Place the thumb of the right hand at the most superior aspect of the iliac crest and align the second finger with the ASIS.

COMMON ERROR: Before palpating for body landmarks, always ask the patient if there is any tenderness or soreness in the area of palpation.

C H A P T E R

Chest and Bony Thorax

CHEST: PA

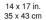

14 x 17 in.
35 x 43 cm

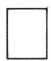

14 x 17 in.
35 x 43 cm

14 x 17 in.
35 x 43 cm

14 x 17 in.
35 x 43 cm

FILM: Use crosswise for hypersthenic patient. Collimate to the area of interest.

CR: Perpendicular to the midsagittal plane at the level of T-6. (Use T2-3 at the level of the suprasternal or jugular notch to locate T-6).

Collimate to the size of the film or smaller.

POSITION: Patient should be upright (orthostatic). The patient may be seated.

A chest stand or chest film holder usually without a grid (72 inches or 183 cm SID*) or with an air gap† (120 inches or 305 cm SID) is used.

The anterior chest is touching the film or film holder.

Weight should be evenly balanced on each foot.

Place the patient's chin on the chin rest.

Have the patient place the hands on the hips.

Roll the shoulders forward and slightly downward to remove the scapulae from superimposing the lung fields. The shoulders should be level.

Make sure that the shoulders are touching the film. If the patient cannot touch the film with his or her shoulders, turn the patient's hands internally so that the dorsal surfaces of the hands lie against

---

*Source-to-image distance (SID), for most radiography procedures, is usually 40 inches or approximately 100 cm. Chest radiographs are usually taken at 72 inches or 183 (rounded to 200) cm SID.

†Air gap is usually performed with a 10-inch or 15-cm space between the patient and the film in order to allow the dissipation of scattered x-rays. This serves much as a grid functions but without the disadvantages of a grid, namely, grid lines on the finished radiograph (see Fig. 2–1).

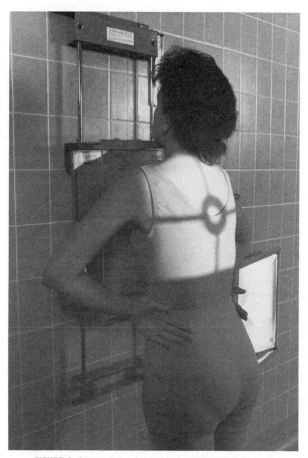

FIGURE 2–1. PA of the chest with shoulders rolled forward.

the hips (Fig. 2–1). Then position each shoulder as close as possible and at the same distance from the film.

The top of the film should be placed 2 inches (5 cm) higher than the shoulders. An exception to this is the hypersthenic patient, for whom the top of the crosswise film should be placed *at* the upper level of the shoulders (the mass of the upper torso is greater and therefore uses the 2 inches of distance routinely allowed).

Check the inferior, lateral rib margins with the borders of the film by placing your hands on the patient's sides. Now, extend your fingers so that the tips touch the film or film holder (see Fig. 1–10). You can ensure that the lateral aspects of the lung fields are included on the film by assessing your fingertip position relative to the film borders. Include a sufficient border of 1/2 to 1 inch

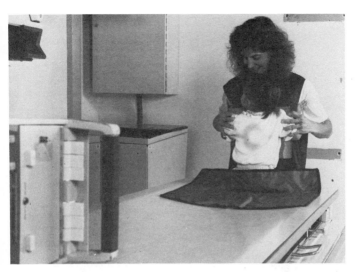

FIGURE 2–2. PA of the chest for a small child when a pediatric restraint device is not available. Use lead gloves if technologist's hands are in primary beam. Have the person holding give instructions to the child to draw the head back into position.

(1.25 to 2.54 cm) of film space on each side of your fingertips in order to allow for rib expansion on full inspiration of the patient.

Have the patient take a deep breath without straining, and make the exposure.

For pediatric patients, when a confinement device is not available, make sure the child's head does not hyperextend and does not superimpose the upper lung fields (Fig. 2–2). If the technologist's hands are in the beam, lead gloves should be worn.

STRUCTURES DEMONSTRATED: The cardiac shadow with both lung fields in their entirety (Fig. 2–3).

The lungs should be aerated up to the ninth or tenth rib.

Exposure taken on full expiration will show more prominent vascular markings. Studies taking two films with first inspiration and then expiration are used to demonstrate travel of diaphragm and/or presence of pneumothorax.

Both right and left hemidiaphragms in their entirety. The right will normally be elevated due to the mass of the liver.

The sternal or proximal aspects of the clavicles should be equidistant from the thoracic spine. When you see one clavicle on the finished radiograph farther away from the thoracic spine than the other, the patient is rotated toward that side.

NOTE: The source-image distance (SID) for chest radiographs usually is 72 inches (183 cm) or 10 feet (305 cm) for air-gap techniques. This increased SID over other table Bucky exams (usually 40 inches or 102 cm SID) decreases magnification of the cardiac shadow and results in a more accurate measurement of the cardiac shadow.

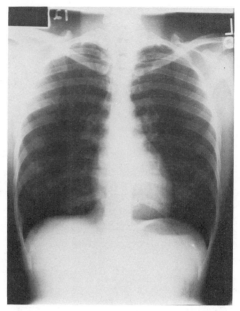

FIGURE 2–3. PA chest x-ray with proximal clavicles equidistant from thoracic spine.

COMMON ERRORS: (1) Insufficient aeration of the lungs. (2) Technique either too light or too dark. A commonly used criterion for technique assessment is to be able to barely see the thoracic spine through the cardiac shadow on the finished radiograph. Use a high kVp, low mAs technique. (3) Rotation.

TECHNIQUE
KV _____ MA _____ SECS _____ MAS _____ CALIPER _____ cm
_____ :1 GRID / B / none SCREEN: RE / High / Par / Detail / None
SID: _____ Rm _____ ADULT / CHILD age: _____ mos. / yrs.
HABITUS: Hyper / s / hypo / a   XS   S   M   L   XL   XXL

CHEST: LATERAL

14 x 17 in.
35 x 43 cm

14 x 17 in.
35 x 43 cm

14 x 17 in.
35 x 43 cm

14 x 17 in.
35 x 43 cm

FILM: Use crosswise for hypersthenic patient. Collimate to the area of interest.

CR: Perpendicularly at midthorax at level of T-6. Use tip of scapula, T-7 (see Fig. 1–12) to locate centering level.

POSITION: The patient is standing (orthostatic) at the chest stand (Fig. 2–4).

Left side is against the film, arms crossed over head. Without bending, have the patient's left shoulder touch the film or film holder to avoid sway.

Patient's posture should be adjusted to place hips in alignment under the shoulders.

Head up, eyes straight ahead.

Place the anterior and posterior surfaces of the thorax equidistant from the right and left edges of film. Place the midaxillary plane (see Fig. 1–2) in the middle of the film. If the upper body then extends beyond the right border of the film, place the posterior surface at the left border of the film and assess the anterior again. If the chest still extends beyond either film border (as it would for a hypersthenic patient), use the film crosswise.

Make sure the body is not rotated. Assess this by placing the right and left shoulders so that they directly superimpose each other. The arms should be in identical positions over the patient's head (Fig. 2–5).

Have the patient take a deep breath without straining, and make the exposure.

STRUCTURES DEMONSTRATED: The unrotated, superimposed lungs in their entirety (Fig. 2–6). An example of rotation is given in Figure 2–7.

A left lateral will demonstrate the heart, aorta, and all left-sided pulmonary lesions, infiltrates, and lobular fissures.

A right lateral will demonstrate right-sided pulmonary lesions, infiltrates, and lobular fissures.

COMMON ERRORS: (1) Rotation. The posterior ribs will not be superimposed over each other. Do not confuse rib magnification of the side farther from the film as rotation. Posterior ribs will never be precisely superimposed due to object-image distance (OID) magnification of the upper ribs. The ribs of the side farther from the film will always be magnified. Knowing this, however,

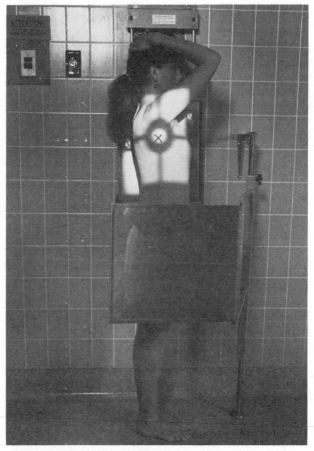

FIGURE 2–4. Left lateral chest with pelvis shield in place.

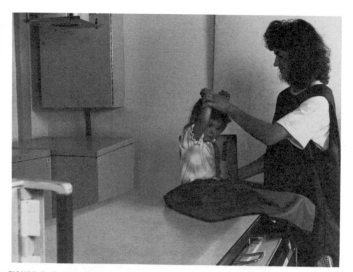

FIGURE 2–5. Left lateral chest of a small child when a pediatric restraint device is not available. Notice apron used as gonadal shield.

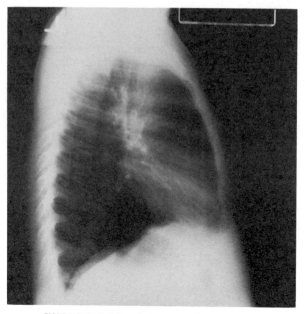

FIGURE 2–6. Left lateral chest x-ray with no rotation.

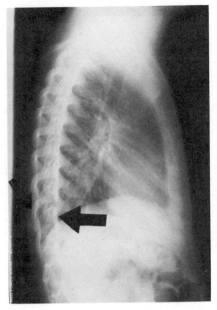

FIGURE 2–7. Left lateral chest x-ray with rotation. The posterior ribs are significantly rotated. The magnified right ribs *(small arrow)* are rotated posteriorly from the left ribs *(large arrow)*. Longitudinal collimation should be better (tighter).

is useful in order to identify which way to correct for a lateral chest that has to be repeated because of rotation (Fig. 2–7). (2) The upper lung area, the apices, are sometimes obliterated by the upper arms when patients are too debilitated to place the arms in the overhead position. Have the patient elevate the arms as much as possible. Have the patient grasp an IV pole to increase arm elevation and to stabilize position.

TECHNIQUE

KV _____ MA _____ SECS _____ MAS _____ CALIPER _____ cm

_____ :1 GRID / B / none SCREEN: RE / High / Par / Detail / None

SID: _____ Rm _____ ADULT / CHILD age: _____ mos. / yrs.

HABITUS: Hyper / s / hypo / a   XS   S   M   L   XL   XXL

CHEST: AP LORDOTIC

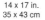
14 x 17 in.
35 x 43 cm

14 x 17 in.
35 x 43 cm

14 x 17 in.
35 x 43 cm

14 x 17 in.
35 x 43 cm

FILM: Collimate to the area of interest.

CR: A cephalic 20-degree angle is used (Fig. 2–8) or the patient's upper body is hyperextended (Fig. 2–9). For bilateral apices, center midsagittally at the level of the sternoclavicular (jugular) notch at T2-3.

POSITION: With the patient's back against the film, center the midsagittal plane to the center of the film.

Make sure that the shoulders are level and both are touching the film or film holder.

The feet are apart and the weight should be evenly balanced.

NOTE: When the patient is ambulatory, another method for a lordotic chest is to lean the patient back against the film. The patient can be positioned about a half step away from the film holder and asked to hyperextend the upper body so that the back

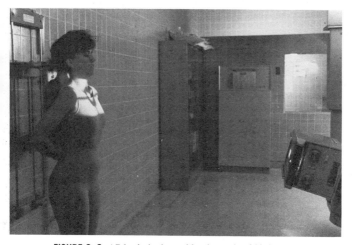

FIGURE 2–8. AP lordotic chest with tube angle of 20 degrees.

is supported by the filmholder or table (Fig. 2–9). No tube angle is required for this method.

STRUCTURES DEMONSTRATED: The apices (the area of the lungs above the clavicles) are free from superimposition of the clavicles.

The clavicles are thrown superiorly, above the apical lung fields (Fig. 2–10).

COMMON ERROR: Not enough angulation. The clavicles are superimposed over the apices. The clavicles must be projected so that they do not obstruct the apices.

TECHNIQUE

KV _____ MA _____ SECS _____ MAS _____ CALIPER _____ cm

_____ :1 GRID / B / none SCREEN: RE / High / Par / Detail / None

SID: _____ Rm _____ ADULT / CHILD age: _____ mos. / yrs.

HABITUS: Hyper / s / hypo / a   XS   S   M   L   XL   XXL

NOTES:

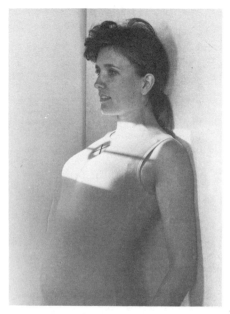

FIGURE 2–9. AP lordotic chest with no tube angle and patient's upper body hyperextended.

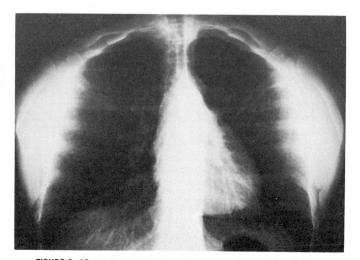

FIGURE 2–10. AP lordotic chest x-ray (Courtesy of Becky Moe, R.T.).

CHEST: AP

   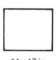

| 14 x 17 in. | 14 x 17 in. | 14 x 17 in. | 14 x 17 in. |
| 35 x 43 cm | 35 x 43 cm | 35 x 43 cm | 35 x 43 cm |

FILM: Use the film crosswise for a hypersthenic patient. Collimate to the area of interest.

CR: Perpendicular to film at level of T-6. For gurney, tabletop, or portable chests, use as close as possible to 72 inches SID or at least 1 to 2 meters.[1] For portable chest radiography, traction bars can limit the SID (see Fig. 8–2). In that case, try to have a minimum of 60 inches (152 cm) SID.

POSITION: The patient can be upright, sitting, or fully recumbent (Fig. 2–11). An upright study is preferable owing to the lower intrathoracic pressure from gravitational lowering of the abdominal viscera. The AP is generally utilized for portable studies or for patients who are unable to stand (see Fig. 8–1).

The film is placed behind the back of the patient while the patient is in the recumbent position or in the Fowler's position (a semi-erect position in which the patient's head is elevated at least 18 inches or 46 cm).

Make sure the upper edge of the film extends 2 inches above the shoulders (or at a level with the shoulders if the patient is hypersthenic).

Center the midsagittal plane to the center of the film. If the lateral margins of the ribs extend out of the film area, use the film crosswise.

Have the patient take a deep breath without straining. If the patient is comatose or on a respirator, make the exposure when the patient is at the fullest stage of inspiration and use a very short exposure time.

STRUCTURES DEMONSTRATED: The cardiac shadow with both lung fields in their entirety (Fig. 2–12). The cardiac shadow will be slightly enlarged as compared with the PA projection of the chest.

The lungs should be aerated up to the ninth or tenth rib.

An exposure taken on full expiration will show more prominent vascular markings. Studies taking two films with first inspiration and then expiration demonstrate travel of diaphragm and/or presence of pneumothorax.

Both right and left hemidiaphragms in their entirety. The right will normally be elevated due to the liver mass.

The medial aspects of the clavicles should be equidistant from the thoracic spine. The unequal position of the proximal clavicles from midline indicates patient rotation.

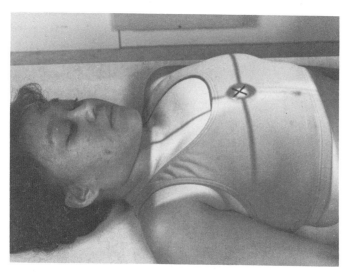

FIGURE 2–11. Recumbent AP chest.

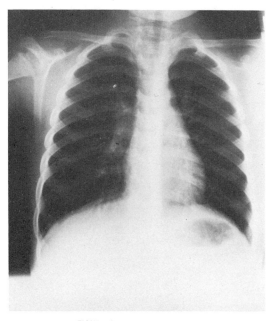

FIGURE 2–12. AP chest x-ray.

COMMON ERROR: The tube is not perpendicular to the film. Since this is usually a bedside or recumbent study, the SID is often not at the appropriate or optimal distance. Make sure the central ray is perpendicular to the film while using the correct SID, or try to adjust the plane of the collimator face so that it is parallel to the plane of the film while maintaining the correct SID. Taking this precaution will avoid the "flying clavicles" or lordotic-like chest film that is caused by poor tube-to-film longitudinal, angled alignment.

TECHNIQUE

KV _____ MA _____ SECS _____ MAS _____ CALIPER _____ cm

_____ :1 GRID / B / none SCREEN: RE / High / Par / Detail / None

SID: _____ Rm _____ ADULT / CHILD age: _____ mos. / yrs.

HABITUS: Hyper / s / hypo / a   XS   S   M   L   XL   XXL

NOTES:

STERNUM: RAO

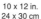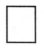

| 10 x 12 in. | 10 x 12 in. | 11 x 14 in. | 11 x 14 in. |
| 24 x 30 cm | 24 x 30 cm | 30 x 35 cm | 30 x 35 cm |

FILM: Use table Bucky or grid. Collimate to the area of interest.
CR: Perpendicular to the center of the film when the top of the film is placed 2 inches, or 5 cm, above the level of the sternoclavicular or jugular notch.
POSITION: The recumbent patient is semipronated on the right side. Place the patient's right arm down by that side, and the left arm up by the pillow. Flex the patient's left knee (Fig. 2–13).

The patient is obliqued 15 to 30 degrees depending on the anterior-to-posterior measurement of the thorax. An asthenic patient (shallow thorax) will require a greater obliquity than a hypersthenic (deep thorax) patient. The amount of obliquity must be enough to avoid superimposition of the thoracic spine and sternum, yet not so much as to move the sternum out of the shadow of the heart. The cardiac shadow will act as a natural filter in this obliquity.

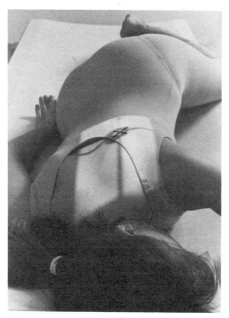

FIGURE 2–13. Right anterior oblique (RAO) position for the sternum.

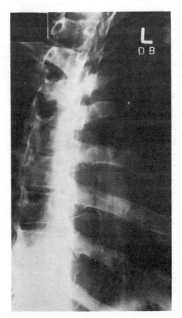

FIGURE 2–14. RAO sternum x-ray with breathing technique. (Courtesy of David Buckley, R.T.).

NOTE: The use of a short SID is not advised. The increased radiation dose to the patient is prohibitive to using short SIDs.
STRUCTURES DEMONSTRATED: The slightly, obliqued sternum in its entirety.

The sternum will be demonstrated within the cardiac shadow (Fig. 2–14).

If a breathing technique is used, the bronchial markings will be blurred.
COMMON ERROR: *(1) The sternum is barely visible due to over-penetration. Make sure you use a breathing technique or full expiration to make the lung density as uniform as possible. (2) The sternum is overobliqued out of the cardiac shadow. Use only as much obliquity as is needed to avoid superimposition of the sternum over the thoracic spine.*

TECHNIQUE
KV _____ MA _____ SECS _____ MAS _____ CALIPER _____ cm
_____ :1 GRID / B / none SCREEN: RE / High / Par / Detail / None
SID: _____ Rm _____ ADULT / CHILD age: _____ mos. / yrs.
HABITUS: Hyper / s / hypo / a   XS   S   M   L   XL   XXL

STERNUM: LATERAL

| 10 x 12 in. | 10 x 12 in. | 11 x 14 in. | 11 x 14 in. |
| 24 x 30 cm | 24 x 30 cm | 30 x 35 cm | 30 x 35 cm |

FILM: Use table Bucky or grid. Collimate to the area of interest.
CR: Perpendicular to the body of the sternum in its lateral aspect.
Place the top of the film 2 inches or 5 cm above the sternoclavicular
or jugular notch.
POSITION: Patients may be recumbent for an upright study (Fig.
2–15), dorsal decubitus study (Fig. 2–16), lateralized at the chest

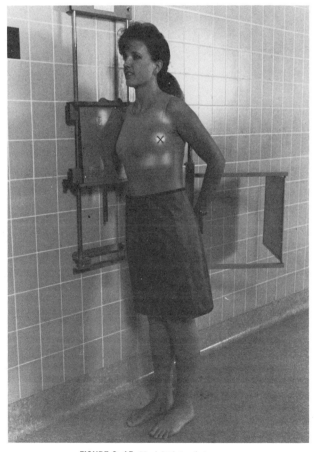

FIGURE 2–15. Upright lateral sternum.

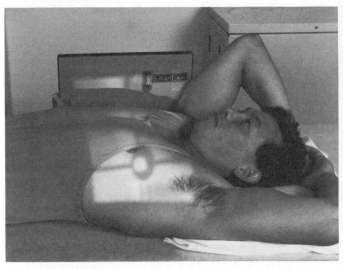

FIGURE 2–16. Recumbent, crosstable lateral sternum (dorsal decubitus).

board, or lateralized on the x-ray table, depending on their condition. Use 72 inches or 183 cm SID.

When the patient is *upright*, rotate the shoulders posteriorly with the arms behind the back (see Fig. 2–15).

When the patient is *recumbent and lateralized*, both arms should be over the head if tolerated.

When a *dorsal decubitus position* with a horizontal beam is used for the multiple trauma patient, use close collimation to reduce scattered radiation (Fig. 2–16). One may not elect to use a grid due to the increased OID. The increased OID will allow falloff of the scattered radiation before it reaches the film.

You may use an SID greater than 40 inches or 100 cm to minimize the increased OID magnification effects.

Use full inspiration. This moves the sternum out while increasing the contrast between lung and bone.

STRUCTURES DEMONSTRATED: The lateralized sternum in its entirety (Fig. 2–17).

The sternoclavicular articulations.

The xiphoid (ensiform) process is seen when of sufficient density or calcification.

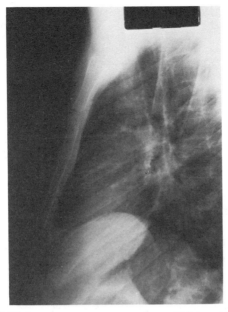

FIGURE 2–17. Lateral sternum x-ray centered toward left to avoid blocker.

COMMON ERRORS: (1) Overpenetration. The sternum is relatively free from superimposition in the lateral aspect. (2) Underpenetration. When the patient is large-breasted or is hypersthenic, the technique must be increased accordingly. (3) Superimposition of the soft tissue of the upper arm in an upright study. The arms must be elevated together or placed behind the back together so that they are out of the area of interest.

TECHNIQUE

KV _____ MA _____ SECS _____ MAS _____ CALIPER _____ cm

_____ :1 GRID / B / none SCREEN: RE / High / Par / Detail / None

SID: _____ Rm _____ ADULT / CHILD age: _____ mos. / yrs.

HABITUS: Hyper / s / hypo / a   XS   S   M   L   XL   XXL

RIBS: AP

FILM
Bilateral Ribs: Collimate to the area of interest.

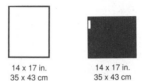

14 x 17 in.   14 x 17 in.
35 x 43 cm   35 x 43 cm

Unilateral Ribs: Collimate to the area of interest.

14 x 17 in.   14 x 17 in.   11 x 14 in.   11 x 14 in.
35 x 43 cm   35 x 43 cm   30 x 35 cm   30 x 35 cm

Bilateral Lower Ribs

11 x 14 in.   11 x 14 in.   14 x 17 in.   14 x 17 in.
30 x 35 cm   30 x 35 cm   35 x 43 cm   35 x 43 cm

Unilateral Lower Ribs

10 x 12 in.   10 x 12 in.   10 x 12 in.   10 x 12 in.
24 x 30 cm   24 x 30 cm   24 x 30 cm   24 x 30 cm

CR
Bilateral Ribs: Place the top of the film just above the base of the neck (3 to 4 inches or 8 to 10 cm superior to the sternal notch), and center to the midpoint of the film.
Unilateral Ribs: Place the top of the film just above the base of the neck (3 to 4 inches or 8 to 10 cm superior to the sternal notch), and center longitudinally to the midpoint of the film while centering transversely to the midpoint of the injured side (Fig. 2–18).
POSITION: If the patient is ambulatory, perform upright. However, because ribs are most likely to be requested on patients with multiple trauma, the procedure would likely be performed with the patient recumbent.

The patient is supinated with a pad under the knees, if the patient's injuries permit.
Bilateral Study: Center the midsagittal plane to the table (Fig. 2–19).

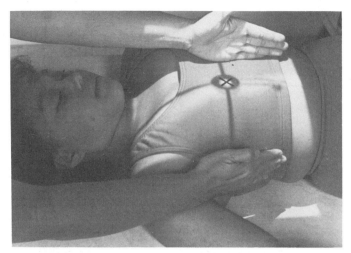

FIGURE 2–18. AP unilateral right ribs showing centering assessment.

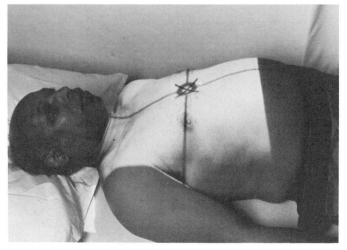

FIGURE 2–19. AP bilateral ribs. Make sure you move pillow away from area of interest.

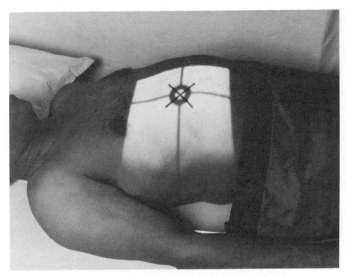

FIGURE 2–20. AP unilateral lower ribs.

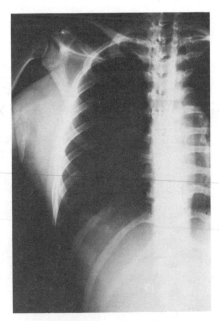

FIGURE 2–21. AP unilateral ribs x-ray.

Bilateral Lower Rib Study: While having the patient remain in the same position as stated above (Fig. 2–20), place the bottom edge of a transverse 11 × 14 inch (30 × 35 cm) or 14 × 17 inch (35 × 43 cm) film cassette at the level of the iliac crest. Center the CR to the film. Use a gallbladder scout technique on full expiration.

Unilateral Study: Center the transverse midpoint of the side of interest to the table (that is, the middle of the right side or the middle of the left side of the patient's thorax). To find the transverse midpoint, measure from the patient's midsagittal plane to the injured side's lateral border (see Fig. 2–18).

Make sure the patient is not rotated. Check that the shoulders and hips are in the same transverse planes.

From the anatomical position, place the arm of the side of interest away from the body. If the patient tolerates, internally (medially) rotate the entire arm in order to move the scapula away from the area of interest. An alternate arm position is to raise the flexed arm over the head.

Unilateral Lower Rib Study: While having the patient remain in the same position as stated above, place the bottom edge of the 10 × 12 inch (24 × 30 cm) film cassette 2 inches above the iliac crest. Palpate the uninjured side to make sure you include all of the lower ribs. Center the CR to the film. Use a gallbladder scout technique on full expiration.

STRUCTURES DEMONSTRATED: The ribs above (Fig. 2–21) and below the diaphragm (Fig. 2–22).

The posterior aspect of the middle and upper ribs.

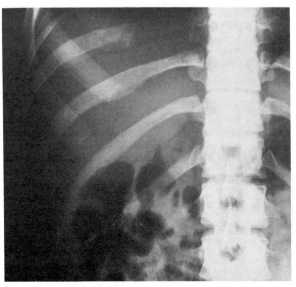

FIGURE 2–22. AP unilateral lower ribs x-ray.

COMMON ERRORS: (1) Underpenetration. Make sure when you are formulating your technique (or borrowing one from another technologist) that the respiratory instructions are clear. Some technologists use suspended respiration, some use quiet breathing with a longer exposure time, and others use full inspiration with a reduced technique. The reduced technique is necessary due to the blackening effect of the increased volume of air. (2) The upper ribs are clipped off of the film. Make sure you place the top of the film sufficiently above the level of the first rib. If you place the film at the level of the first rib, the divergence of the x-ray beam will cause the first rib to be cast out of the filming area.

TECHNIQUE

KV _____ MA _____ SECS _____ MAS _____ CALIPER _____ cm

_____ :1 GRID / B / none SCREEN: RE / High / Par / Detail / None

SID: _____ Rm _____ ADULT / CHILD age: _____ mos. / yrs.

HABITUS: Hyper / s / hypo / a   XS   S   M   L   XL   XXL

NOTES:

RIBS: AP OBLIQUES

FILM
Bilateral Ribs: Collimate to the area of interest.

| 14 x 17 in. | 14 x 17 in. | 14 x 17 in. | 14 x 17 in. |
| 35 x 43 cm | 35 x 43 cm | 35 x 43 cm | 35 x 43 cm |

Unilateral Ribs: Collimate to the area of interest.

| 14 x 17 in. | 14 x 17 in. | 11 x 14 in. | 11 x 14 in. |
| 35 x 43 cm | 35 x 43 cm | 30 x 35 cm | 30 x 35 cm |

Bilateral Lower Ribs

| 11 x 14 in. | 11 x 14 in. | 14 x 17 in. | 14 x 17 in. |
| 30 x 35 cm | 30 x 35 cm | 35 x 43 cm | 35 x 43 cm |

Unilateral Lower Ribs

| 10 x 12 in. | 10 x 12 in. | 10 x 12 in. | 10 x 12 in. |
| 24 x 30 cm | 24 x 30 cm | 24 x 30 cm | 24 x 30 cm |

CR
Bilateral Ribs: Place the top of the film just above the base of the neck (3 to 4 inches or 8 to 10 cm superior to the sternal notch), and center to the midpoint of the film.
Unilateral Ribs: Place the top of the film just above the base of the neck (3 to 4 inches or 8 to 10 cm superior to the sternal notch). Center longitudinally to the midpoint of the film, while centering transversely to the midpoint of the side of interest. Find the transverse midpoint by measuring from the midsternum to the lateral border (see Fig. 2–18).
POSITION: If the patient is ambulatory, perform upright standing or seated. This will not only avoid excessive movement but also produce less discomfort to the patient when performed upright. When the patient is recumbent, the side down is demonstrated; therefore, the patient will be placing weight on the injured side.

However, because ribs are likely to be requested on patients with multiple trauma, the procedure would likely be performed with the patient recumbent.

The patient is obliqued 45 degrees from supine toward the side of injury (Fig. 2–23).

Bilateral Study: Palpate the thoracic spinous processes. Center the point 3 inches (7 to 8 cm) anterior to the thoracic spinous processes to the center of the table.

Bilateral Lower Rib Study: While having the patient remain in the same position as stated above, place the bottom edge of a transverse 11 × 14 inch (30 × 35 cm) or 14 × 17 inch (35 × 43 cm) film cassette at the level of the iliac crest. Center the CR to the film. Use a gallbladder scout technique on full expiration.

Unilateral Study: Center the transverse midpoint of the side of interest to the table—that is, the middle of the right side or the middle of the left side of the patient's obliqued thorax. Find this midpoint by measuring from the spinous process of a middle thoracic vertebra to the lateral border of the side of interest. Center this midpoint to the center of the x-ray table (Fig. 2–23).

Make sure the patient is obliqued 45 degrees. Check that the shoulders and hips are in the same planes.

Place the arm of the side of interest away from the body.

Unilateral Lower Rib Study: While having the patient remain in the same position as stated above, place the bottom edge of the 10 × 12 inch (24 × 30 cm) film cassette 2 inches above the iliac crest. Palpate the uninjured side to make sure you include all of the lower ribs. Center the CR to the film. Use a gallbladder scout technique on full expiration.

STRUCTURES DEMONSTRATED: Obliqued axillary ribs of side down (Fig. 2–24).

For a bilateral study, perform both obliques (right and left posterior oblique [RPO and LPO]).

The ribs of the side up will be severely foreshortened; however, the proximal articulations of the ribs of the side up will be well demonstrated.

The thoracic spine will be superimposed over the ribs of the side up.

The fullest extent of the lung of the side down.

COMMON ERROR: (1) Underpenetration. Make sure when you are formulating your technique (or borrowing one from another technologist) that the respiratory instructions are consistent. Some technologists use suspended respiration, some use quiet breathing with a longer exposure time, and others use full inspiration with a reduced technique. The technique reduction is necessary due to the blackening effect of the increased volume of air. (2) The upper ribs are clipped off of the film. Make sure you place the top of the film sufficiently above the level of the first rib or base of the neck. If you place the film at the level of the first rib, the divergence of the x-ray beam will cause the first rib to be cast out of the filming area.

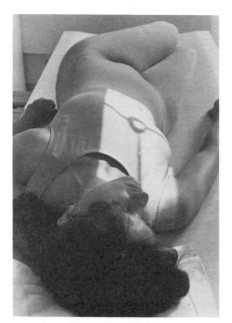

FIGURE 2–23. Unilateral study of the right ribs in the right AP oblique projection (RPO position).

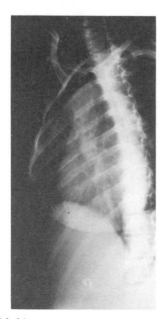

FIGURE 2–24. Posterior oblique x-ray of unilateral ribs.

47

TECHNIQUE

KV _____ MA _____ SECS _____ MAS _____ CALIPER _____ cm
_____ :1 GRID / B / none SCREEN: RE / High / Par / Detail / None
SID: _____ Rm _____ ADULT / CHILD age: _____ mos. / yrs.
HABITUS: Hyper / s / hypo / a   XS   S   M   L   XL   XXL

NOTES:

RIBS: PA

FILM
Bilateral Ribs: Collimate to the area of interest.

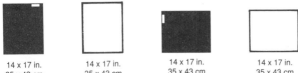

| 14 x 17 in. | 14 x 17 in. | 14 x 17 in. | 14 x 17 in. |
| 35 x 43 cm | 35 x 43 cm | 35 x 43 cm | 35 x 43 cm |

Unilateral Ribs: Collimate to the area of interest.

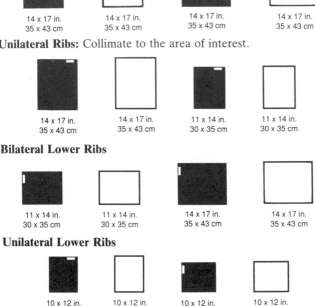

| 14 x 17 in. | 14 x 17 in. | 11 x 14 in. | 11 x 14 in. |
| 35 x 43 cm | 35 x 43 cm | 30 x 35 cm | 30 x 35 cm |

Bilateral Lower Ribs

| 11 x 14 in. | 11 x 14 in. | 14 x 17 in. | 14 x 17 in. |
| 30 x 35 cm | 30 x 35 cm | 35 x 43 cm | 35 x 43 cm |

Unilateral Lower Ribs

| 10 x 12 in. | 10 x 12 in. | 10 x 12 in. | 10 x 12 in. |
| 24 x 30 cm | 24 x 30 cm | 24 x 30 cm | 24 x 30 cm |

CR
Bilateral Ribs: Place the top of the film just above the base of the neck (3 to 4 inches or 8 to 10 cm superior to the sternal notch), and center to the midpoint of the film.
Unilateral Ribs: Place the top of the film just above the base of the neck (3 to 4 inches or 8 to 10 cm superior to the sternal notch), and center longitudinally to the midpoint of the film while centering transversely to the midpoint of the injured side (measure from the spinous processes to the lateral aspect of the ribs).
POSITION: If the patient is ambulatory, perform upright. However, because ribs are most likely to be requested on patients with multiple trauma, the procedure would likely be performed with the patient recumbent.
Bilateral Study: Center the midsagittal plane to the table. Assess the rib borders. Make sure they are included within the borders of the film (Fig. 2–25).

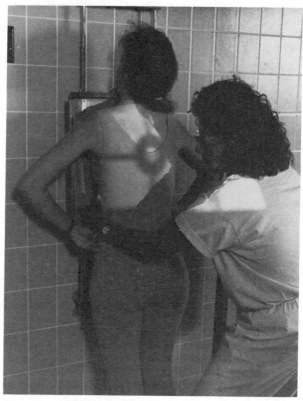

FIGURE 2–25. PA projection of bilateral ribs.

Bilateral Lower Rib Study: While having the patient remain in the same position as stated above, place the bottom edge of a transverse 11 × 14 inch (30 × 35 cm) or 14 × 17 inch (35 × 43 cm) film cassette at the level of the iliac crest. Center the CR to the film. Use a gallbladder scout technique on full expiration.

Unilateral Study: Center the transverse midpoint of the side of interest to the table (that is, the middle of the right side or the middle of the left side of the patient's thorax). To find the transverse midpoint, measure from the patient's midsagittal plane to the injured side's lateral border.

Place the arm of the side of interest away from the body.

Make sure the patient is not rotated. Check that the shoulders and hips are in the same transverse planes.

Unilateral Lower Rib Study: While having the patient remain in the same position as stated above, place the bottom edge of the 10 × 12 inch (24 × 30 cm) film cassette 2 inches above the iliac crest. Palpate the uninjured side to make sure you include all of

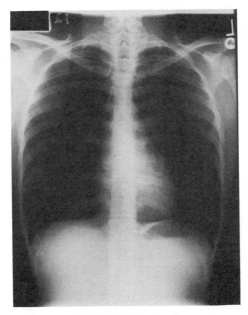

FIGURE 2–26. PA ribs x-ray.

the lower ribs. Center the CR to the film. Use a gallbladder scout technique on full expiration.

STRUCTURES DEMONSTRATED: The ribs above the diaphragm and below the diaphragm (Fig. 2–26).

The anterior aspect of the middle and upper ribs.

COMMON ERRORS: (1) Underpenetration. Make sure when you are formulating your technique (or borrowing one from another technologist) that the respiratory instructions are clear. Some technologists use suspended respiration, some use quiet breathing with a longer exposure time, and others use full inspiration with a reduced technique. The reduced technique is necessary due to the blackening effect of the increased volume of air. (2) The upper ribs are clipped off of the film. Make sure you place the top of the film sufficiently above the level of the first rib. If you place the film at the level of the first rib, the divergence of the x-ray beam will cause the first rib to be cast out of the filming area.

TECHNIQUE

KV _____ MA _____ SECS _____ MAS _____ CALIPER _____ cm

_____ :1 GRID / B / none SCREEN: RE / High / Par / Detail / None

SID: _____ Rm _____ ADULT / CHILD age: _____ mos. / yrs.

HABITUS: Hyper / s / hypo / a   XS   S   M   L   XL   XXL

RIBS: PA OBLIQUES

FILM

Bilateral Ribs: Collimate to the area of interest.

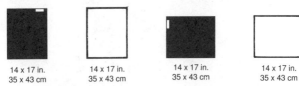

14 x 17 in.   14 x 17 in.   14 x 17 in.   14 x 17 in.
35 x 43 cm   35 x 43 cm   35 x 43 cm   35 x 43 cm

Unilateral Ribs: Collimate to the area of interest.

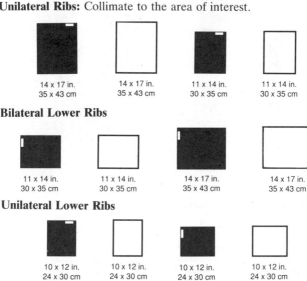

14 x 17 in.   14 x 17 in.   11 x 14 in.   11 x 14 in.
35 x 43 cm   35 x 43 cm   30 x 35 cm   30 x 35 cm

Bilateral Lower Ribs

11 x 14 in.   11 x 14 in.   14 x 17 in.   14 x 17 in.
30 x 35 cm   30 x 35 cm   35 x 43 cm   35 x 43 cm

Unilateral Lower Ribs

10 x 12 in.   10 x 12 in.   10 x 12 in.   10 x 12 in.
24 x 30 cm   24 x 30 cm   24 x 30 cm   24 x 30 cm

NOTE: Position the patient first and then adjust the level of the film and central ray. Then only one readjustment is necessary. This recommendation would be invalid if the patient could not tolerate maintaining the position.

CR

Bilateral Ribs: Place the top of the film just above the base of the neck (3 to 4 inches or 8 to 10 cm superior to the sternal notch). Center to the midpoint of the film.

Unilateral Ribs: Place the top of the film just above the base of the neck (3 to 4 inches or 8 to 10 cm superior to the sternal notch). Center the patient longitudinally to the midpoint of the film, while centering the patient transversely to the midpoint of the side of interest. (To find the transverse midpoint, measure from a middle thoracic spinous process to the lateral border and find the center point. Place that point at the center of the x-ray table.)

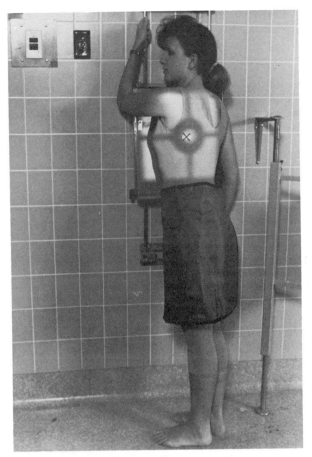

FIGURE 2–27. RAO position of bilateral ribs.

POSITION: If the patient is ambulatory, perform upright standing or seated. This may avoid excessive pressure on the thorax. The RAO (Fig. 2–27) and LAO (Fig. 2–28) positions produce less discomfort to the patient if performed upright. The side up is demonstrated; therefore, patients do not have to place their weight on the injured side. However, because ribs are likely to be requested on patients with multiple trauma, the procedure would likely be performed with the patient recumbent. Depending on injuries, rather than turn the recumbent patient over for the PA oblique, an AP oblique projection might be more appropriate.

The patient's injured side is obliqued 45 degrees away from the film.

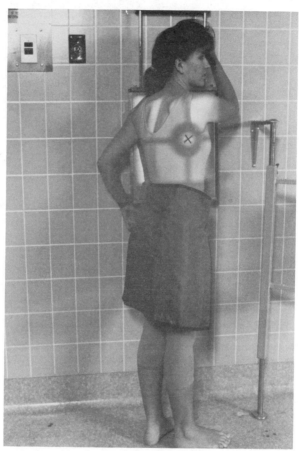

FIGURE 2–28. Left anterior oblique (LAO) position of bilateral ribs.

Bilateral Study: Center the point 3 inches (7 to 8 cm) from the midthoracic spinous process at the inferior border of the scapula to the table, or simply find the center point of the left to right width of the ribs. Center that point to the center of the x-ray table. Make sure that the lateral aspects of the ribs are included on the film.

Bilateral Lower Rib Study: While having the patient remain in the same position as stated above, place the bottom edge of a transverse 11 × 14 inch (30 × 35 cm) or 14 × 17 inch (35 × 43 cm) film cassette at the level of the iliac crest. Center the CR to the film. Use a gallbladder scout technique on full expiration.

Unilateral Study: Center the transverse midpoint of the side of interest to the table (that is, the middle of the right side or the middle of the left side of the patient's thorax). To find the transverse midpoint, measure the side starting at a middle thoracic spine process and ending at the lateral border.

Make sure the patient is obliqued 45 degrees. Check that the shoulders and hips are in the same planes.

Place the arm of the side of interest away from the body.

Unilateral Lower Rib Study: While having the patient remain in the same position as stated above, place the bottom edge of the 10 × 12 inch (24 × 30 cm) film cassette 2 inches above the iliac crest. Palpate the uninjured side to make sure you include all of the lower ribs. Center the CR to the film. Use a gallbladder scout technique on full expiration.

STRUCTURES DEMONSTRATED: Axillary ribs of side up (Fig. 2–29).

The fullest extent of the lung of the side up.

For bilateral study, perform both obliques (RAO and LAO).

The ribs of the side down will be severely foreshortened; however, the proximal articulations of the ribs of the side down will be well demonstrated.

The thoracic spine will be superimposed over the ribs of the side down.

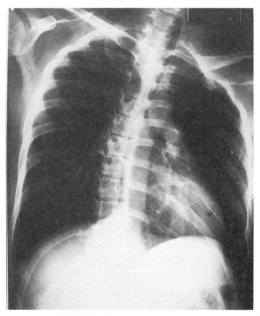

FIGURE 2–29. Bilateral RAO of ribs.

COMMON ERRORS: (1) Underpenetration. Make sure when you are formulating your technique (or borrowing one from another technologist) that the respiratory instructions are clear. Some technologists use suspended respiration, some use quiet breathing with a longer exposure time, and others use full inspiration with a reduced technique due to the blackening effect of the increased volume of air. (2) The upper ribs are clipped off of the film. Make sure you place the top of the film sufficiently above the level of the first rib. If you place the film at the level of the first rib, the divergence of the x-ray beam will cause the first rib to be cast out of the filming area.

TECHNIQUE

KV _____ MA _____ SECS _____ MAS _____ CALIPER _____ cm

_____ :1 GRID / B / none SCREEN: RE / High / Par / Detail / None

SID: _____ Rm _____ ADULT / CHILD age: _____ mos. / yrs.

HABITUS: Hyper / s / hypo / a   XS   S   M   L   XL   XXL

NOTES:

3

Upper Extremities

FIRST DIGIT: AP

| 8 x 10 in. | 8 x 10 in. | 8 x 10 in. |
| 20 x 24 cm | 20 x 24 cm | 20 x 24 cm |

FILM: No grid or table Bucky. Use tabletop only. Collimate to the area of interest.

CR: Perpendicular to first metacarpophalangeal joint (Fig. 3–1).

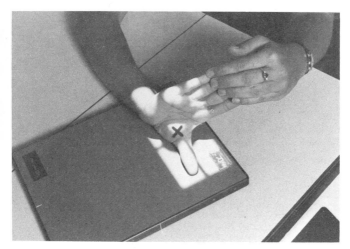

FIGURE 3–1. AP first digit (thumb).

POSITION: Rotate the forearm, wrist, and hand of the injured side by extreme inversion.

Place the dorsal side of the thumb on the film.

The patient may hold the rest of the fingers away from the thumb with the uninjured hand (Fig. 3–1).

Turn the film to center the thumb within one third of the film area provided.

STRUCTURES DEMONSTRATED: The entire first digit in the dorsal aspect (Fig. 3–2).

This part-film contact allows increased detail over the PA projection.

There is a loss of detail proximal to the first metacarpophalangeal articulation due to musculature of the thenar eminence and the presence of a fat pad.

COMMON ERROR: Underpenetration of the proximal thumb. If within the area injured, the thenar pad at the base of the thumb must be considered in formulation of your technique. Be careful not to overcorrect and end up overpenetrating the distal thumb.

TECHNIQUE

KV _____ MA _____ SECS _____ MAS _____ CALIPER _____ cm

_____ :1 GRID / B / none SCREEN: RE / High / Par / Detail / None

SID: _____ Rm _____ ADULT / CHILD age: _____ mos. / yrs.

HABITUS: Hyper / s / hypo / a   XS   S   M   L   XL   XXL

NOTES:

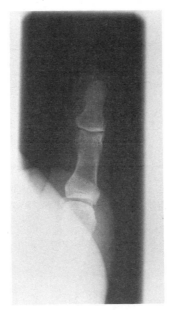

FIGURE 3–2. AP first digit (thumb) x-ray.

FIRST DIGIT: PA

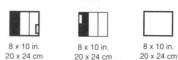

8 x 10 in. 8 x 10 in. 8 x 10 in.
20 x 24 cm 20 x 24 cm 20 x 24 cm

FILM: No grid or table Bucky. Use tabletop only. Collimate to the area of interest.

CR: Perpendicular to first metacarpophalangeal joint.

POSITION: Place hand in extension with ulnar side down on film.

Thumb should be placed parallel to surface of film and abducted slightly (Fig. 3–3).

Immobilize and support thumb with radiolucent sponge.

STRUCTURES DEMONSTRATED: A magnified first digit is seen.

The first carpometacarpal joint is included (Fig. 3–4).

COMMON ERROR: The carpometacarpal joint is not included on the film.

TECHNIQUE

KV _____ MA _____ SECS _____ MAS _____ CALIPER _____ cm

_____ :1 GRID / B / none SCREEN: RE / High / Par / Detail / None

SID: _____ Rm _____ ADULT / CHILD age: _____ mos. / yrs.

HABITUS: Hyper / s / hypo / a XS S M L XL XXL

NOTES:

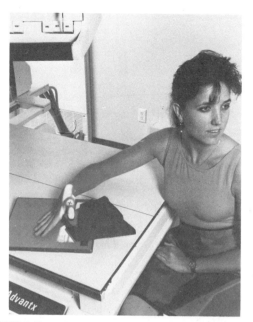

FIGURE 3–3. PA first digit (thumb) with use of radiolucent sponge.

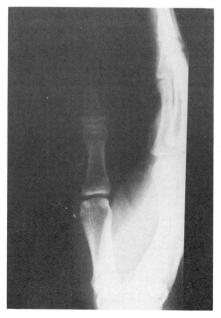

FIGURE 3–4. PA first digit (thumb) x-ray. Collimation was larger than usual due to search for foreign bodies (see fb at MCP joint).

FIRST DIGIT: PA OBLIQUE

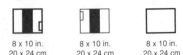

8 x 10 in.
20 x 24 cm

8 x 10 in.
20 x 24 cm

8 x 10 in.
20 x 24 cm

FILM: No grid or table Bucky. Use tabletop only. Collimate to the area of interest.

CR: Perpendicularly at the first metacarpophalangeal joint.

POSITION: Begin with hand flat (pronated) as if for PA hand. Abduct the thumb slightly.

Align the longitudinal axis of the thumb to the film space provided, or simply turn the film cassette in order to center the thumb to the film (Fig. 3–5). Adjust the CR and collimation again.

STRUCTURES DEMONSTRATED: Obliquity of the first digit with the carpometacarpal joint included (Fig. 3–6).

COMMON ERROR: Not including the first carpometacarpal joint on the film.

TECHNIQUE

KV _____ MA _____ SECS _____ MAS _____ CALIPER _____ cm

_____ :1 GRID / B / none SCREEN: RE / High / Par / Detail / None

SID: _____ Rm _____ ADULT / CHILD age: _____ mos. / yrs.

HABITUS: Hyper / s / hypo / a   XS   S   M   L   XL   XXL

NOTES:

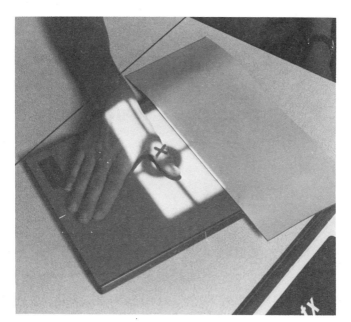

FIGURE 3–5. PA oblique first digit (thumb). Second exposure of three-exposures-on-one film.

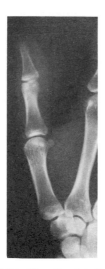

FIGURE 3–6. PA oblique first digit (thumb) x-ray.

FIRST DIGIT: LATERAL

8 x 10 in.
20 x 24 cm

8 x 10 in.
20 x 24 cm

8 x 10 in.
20 x 24 cm

FILM: No grid or table Bucky. Use tabletop only. Collimate to the area of interest.

CR: Perpendicularly to first metacarpophalangeal joint.

POSITION: Pronate hand with digits curled. This will arch the palmar surface of hand (Fig. 3–7).

Slightly elevate ulnar side of wrist to complete lateralization of thumb. Align the longitudinal axis of the thumb to the film or simply turn the film in order to center the thumb to the film. Adjust the CR and collimation again.

STRUCTURES DEMONSTRATED: Both the anterior and posterior aspects of the first digit are seen in profile.

The first carpometacarpal joint is seen.

The joint spaces are open (Fig. 3–8).

COMMON ERROR: Underpenetration of the proximal thumb.

COMMENT: If in the area of injury, the thenar muscle pad at the base of the thumb must be considered in formulation of your technique. Be careful not to overcorrect and end up overpenetrating the distal thumb.

TECHNIQUE

KV _____ MA _____ SECS _____ MAS _____ CALIPER _____ cm

_____ :1 GRID / B / none SCREEN: RE / High / Par / Detail / None

SID: _____ Rm _____ ADULT / CHILD age: _____ mos. / yrs.

HABITUS: Hyper / s / hypo / a   XS   S   M   L   XL   XXL

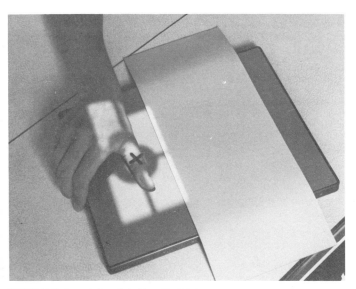

FIGURE 3–7. Lateral first digit (thumb). Third exposure of three-exposures-on-one film.

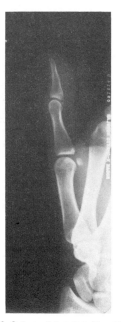

FIGURE 3–8. Lateral first digit (thumb) x-ray.

DIGITS #2–5: PA

| 8 x 10 in. | 8 x 10 in. | 8 x 10 in. | 10 x 12 in. |
| 20 x 24 cm | 20 x 24 cm | 20 x 24 cm | 24 x 30 cm |

FILM: No grid or table Bucky. Use tabletop only. Collimate to the area of interest.

CR: Perpendicularly at the proximal interphalangeal joint.

POSITION: Patient is seated with arm resting on table (Fig. 3–9).

Palmar surface of hand flat against film.

Isolate digit of interest by separating fingers slightly.

Center the digit of interest within one third of film area (Fig. 3–10).

STRUCTURES DEMONSTRATED: PA projection of any one of the second through fifth digits.

All joint spaces are open with no rotation of the digit.

The metacarpophalangeal joint is included (Fig. 3–11).

COMMON ERROR: The digit is not flat against the film. When collimating to the digit of interest, it is advised to numerically mark the digit of interest with a lead number: 2, 3, 4, or 5. The severity of the collimation sometimes makes it difficult to distinguish one digit from another.

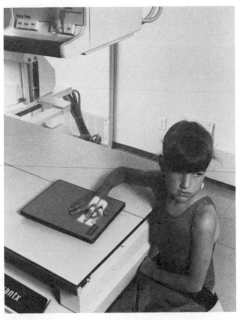

FIGURE 3–9. PA #2 digit. First exposure of three-exposures-on-one film.

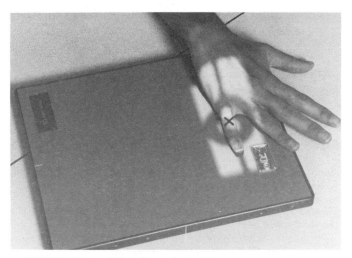

FIGURE 3–10. PA #5 digit. First exposure of three-exposures-on-one film.

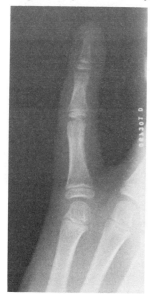

FIGURE 3–11. PA #3 digit x-ray.

TECHNIQUE

KV _____ MA _____ SECS _____ MAS _____ CALIPER _____ cm

_____ :1 GRID / B / none SCREEN: RE / High / Par / Detail / None

SID: _____ Rm _____ ADULT / CHILD   age: _____ mos. / yrs.

HABITUS: Hyper / s / hypo / a   XS   S   M   L   XL   XXL

DIGITS #2–5: PA OBLIQUE

8 x 10 in. 20 x 24 cm	8 x 10 in. 20 x 24 cm	8 x 10 in. 20 x 24 cm	10 x 12 in. 24 x 30 cm

FILM: No grid or table Bucky. Use tabletop only. Collimate to the area of interest.

CR: Perpendicularly at the proximal interphalangeal joint.

POSITION: Rest forearm on table. Hand resting on ulnar side.

Elevate radial side of hand 45 degrees.

The digit of interest slightly flexed and touching film, or use step-wedge radiolucent sponge to elevate distal digit to same level as proximal digit (Fig. 3–12).

STRUCTURES DEMONSTRATED: Obliquity of digit of interest. The distal joint spaces will be closed when the digit is flexed. When a sponge is used to elevate the digit, the medial aspects of the joint spaces will be opened.

All soft tissue and bony anatomy distal to the metacarpophalangeal joint (Fig. 3–13).

COMMON ERROR: Do not allow the digit to curl too much—use extended digit while maintaining the proper degree of obliquity.

TECHNIQUE

KV _____ MA _____ SECS _____ MAS _____ CALIPER _____ cm

_____ :1 GRID / B / none SCREEN: RE / High / Par / Detail / None

SID: _____ Rm _____ ADULT / CHILD age: _____ mos. / yrs.

HABITUS: Hyper / s / hypo / a   XS   S   M   L   XL   XXL

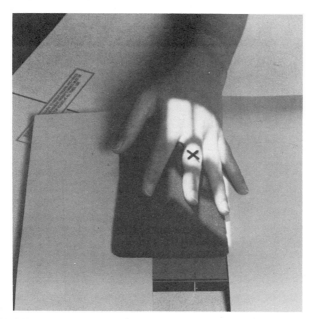

FIGURE 3–12. PA oblique #3 digit. Second exposure of three-exposures-on-one film.

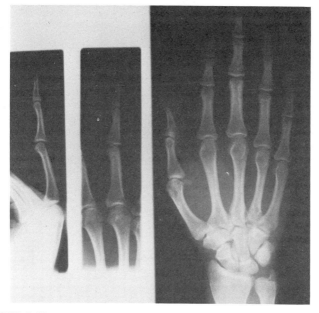

FIGURE 3–13. An example of a 3-on-1 finger routine x-ray. Full PA hand (right), finger of interest PA oblique (center), and lateral (left).

DIGITS #2–5: LATERAL

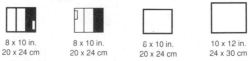

| 8 x 10 in. | 8 x 10 in. | 8 x 10 in. | 10 x 12 in. |
| 20 x 24 cm | 20 x 24 cm | 20 x 24 cm | 24 x 30 cm |

FILM: No grid or table Bucky. Use tabletop only. Collimate to the area of interest.

CR: Perpendicularly at the proximal interphalangeal joint.

#2 DIGIT POSITION: Rotate hand in extreme internal rotation (see AP thumb position).

The hand is inverted completely with the radial aspect of the digit on the film (Fig. 3–14).

All digits are flexed except the second digit.

Extend the second digit.

Lateralize the second digit by controlling the rotation of the wrist.

#3 THROUGH #5 DIGIT POSITION: The hand rests on its ulnar aspect.

All digits are flexed except the digit of interest.

Extend the digit of interest. If the patient can tolerate it, use a small radiolucent sponge for extension (Fig. 3–15).

Lateralize the digit of interest by controlling the rotation of the wrist.

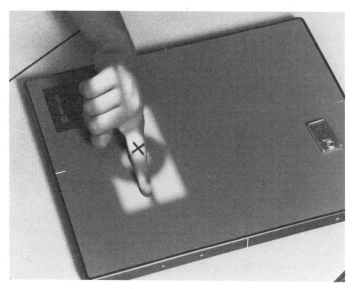

FIGURE 3–14. Lateral #2 digit. Third exposure of three-exposures-on-one film.

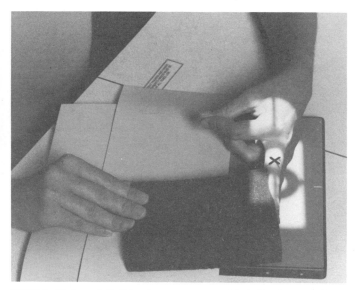

FIGURE 3–15. Lateral #3 digit using sponge to extend (only if patient can tolerate it). Third exposure of three-exposures-on-one film.

Elevate the distal digit to level of proximal digit.

A radiolucent, fanned sponge is recommended.

STRUCTURES DEMONSTRATED: The lateral aspect of the digit of interest with no rotation from the lateral (Fig. 3–16).

All joint spaces are open (unless closed due to condition or trauma).

The metacarpophalangeal joint of the digit of interest is included on the film.

COMMON ERROR: Superimposition of the bases of other than the digit of interest. Be sure the digit of interest is extended as much as practicable. The closure of the hand in a tighter grip will remove the bases of the other digits. Instruct the patient to use the thumb to tighten the grip.

TECHNIQUE

KV _____ MA _____ SECS _____ MAS _____ CALIPER _____ cm

_____ :1 GRID / B / none SCREEN: RE / High / Par / Detail / None

SID: _____ Rm _____ ADULT / CHILD age: _____ mos. / yrs.

HABITUS: Hyper / s / hypo / a   XS   S   M   L   XL   XXL

NOTES:

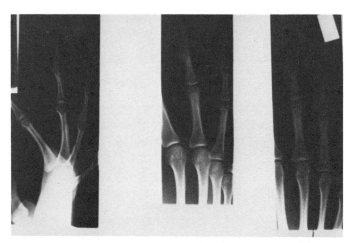

FIGURE 3–16. Lateral #3 digit x-ray (left). An example of a 3-on-1 finger routine—PA (right), PA oblique (center), and lateral (left). (In this film, notice that using the same technique for all three positions does not result in optimal contrast.)

HAND: PA

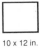

| 8 x 10 in. | 8 x 10 in. | 10 x 12 in. | 10 x 12 in. |
| 20 x 24 cm | 20 x 24 cm | 24 x 30 cm | 24 x 30 cm |

FILM: No grid or table Bucky. Use tabletop only. Collimate to the area of interest.

CR: Perpendicular to third metacarpophalangeal joint.

POSITION: Remove all jewelry.

Rest forearm on table for support.

Spread fingers slightly.

Palmar surface of hand flat against film (Fig. 3–17).

Include carpals (at the very minimum, include the distal row).

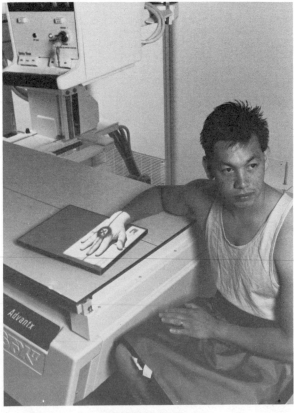

FIGURE 3–17. PA hand.

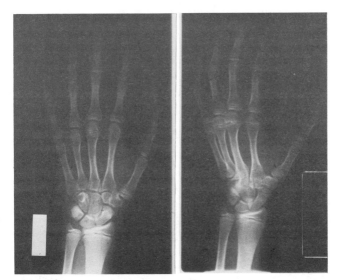

FIGURE 3–18. X-ray of PA hand (left) and PA oblique hand (right).

STRUCTURES DEMONSTRATED: PA projection of #2, 3, 4, 5 digits.

PA oblique projection of #1 digit.

PA projection of metacarpals and carpals (Fig. 3–18).

COMMON ERROR: Hand and digits not flattened completely. Use AP projection if patient unable to flatten hand or digits to demonstrate open joint spaces. Use a technique that demonstrates soft tissue as well as bony trabeculation.

TECHNIQUE

KV _____ MA _____ SECS _____ MAS _____ CALIPER _____ cm

_____ :1 GRID / B / none SCREEN: RE / High / Par / Detail / None

SID: _____ Rm _____ ADULT / CHILD age: _____ mos. / yrs.

HABITUS: Hyper / s / hypo / a   XS   S   M   L   XL   XXL

HAND: PA OBLIQUE

| 8 x 10 in. | 8 x 10 in. | 10 x 12 in. | 10 x 12 in. |
| 20 x 24 cm | 20 x 24 cm | 24 x 30 cm | 24 x 30 cm |

FILM: No grid or table Bucky. Use tabletop only. Collimate to the area of interest.

CR: Perpendicular to third metacarpophalangeal joint.

POSITION: Rest forearm on table.

Hand resting on ulnar side.

Elevate radial side of hand 45 degrees. This results in an anterior oblique position with a lateral rotation (Fig. 3–19).

Digits slightly flexed and touching film, or use step-wedge radiolucent sponge.

STRUCTURES DEMONSTRATED: Obliquity of phalanges, metacarpals, and carpals (Fig. 3–20).

Soft tissue of hand.

Minimal overlap of #3, 4, and 5 metacarpals at their bases.

COMMON ERROR: Incorrect degree of obliquity. The use of a 45-degree radiolucent angle or step-wedge for support of the hand is recommended to minimize patient motion, maximize patient comfort, and allow for exact replication of obliquities. Many technologists use the "OK" position of the hand for this routine (first and second phalanges—fingertips touching).

TECHNIQUE

KV _____ MA _____ SECS _____ MAS _____ CALIPER _____ cm

_____ :1 GRID / B / none SCREEN: RE / High / Par / Detail / None

SID: _____ Rm _____ ADULT / CHILD age: _____ mos. / yrs.

HABITUS: Hyper / s / hypo / a XS S M L XL XXL

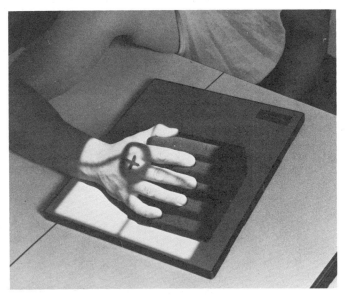

FIGURE 3–19. PA oblique hand.

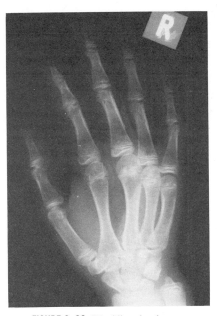

FIGURE 3–20. PA oblique hand x-ray.

HAND: LATERAL

8 x 10 in.
20 x 24 cm

8 x 10 in.
20 x 24 cm

FILM: No grid or table Bucky. Use tabletop only. Collimate to the area of interest.

CR: Perpendicular to second metacarpophalangeal joint.

POSITION: Place hand in extension with ulnar side down on film.

Thumb should be in PA projection while supported and immobilized with radiolucent sponge (Fig. 3–21).

Digits may be fanned to include study of digits (Fig. 3–21).

A lateral in flexion may be taken to demonstrate a carpal boss, that is, a bony growth usually at the base of the third metacarpal.

STRUCTURES DEMONSTRATED: Phalanges, metacarpals, and carpals superimposed in lateral aspect. When digits are fanned with the hand lateralized, the lateral aspect of the phalanges is also demonstrated (Fig. 3–22).

Demonstration of anterior or posterior displacement of fractures or foreign bodies.

COMMON ERROR: Underpenetration. A significant increase in kilovoltage over the PA hand technique is necessary for this projection.

TECHNIQUE

KV _____ MA _____ SECS _____ MAS _____ CALIPER _____ cm

_____ :1 GRID / B / none SCREEN: RE / High / Par / Detail / None

SID: _____ Rm _____ ADULT / CHILD age: _____ mos. / yrs.

HABITUS: Hyper / s / hypo / a   XS   S   M   L   XL   XXL

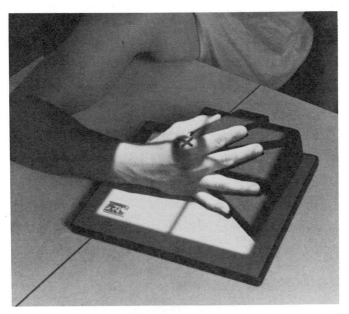

FIGURE 3–21. Lateral hand.

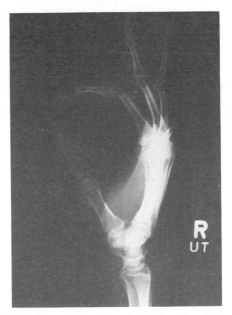

FIGURE 3–22. Lateral hand x-ray in "OK" position of fingers.

BALLCATCHER'S POSITION—NORGAARD METHOD[2]
(AP OBLIQUE HANDS)

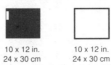

| 10 x 12 in. | 10 x 12 in. |
| 24 x 30 cm | 24 x 30 cm |

FILM: No grid or table Bucky. Use tabletop only. Collimate to the area of interest.

CR: Perpendicular to center of film. A particular anatomical part will not be centered to the central ray due to the large area surveyed (Fig. 3–23).

POSITION: Place both hands palmar surface up on film.

COMMENT: The hands in a "cupped" position will usually accommodate arthritic patients as it is sometimes difficult for them to extend the hands and digits for a PA oblique projection.

Ulnar surfaces of hands are touching film, with radial aspect elevated to 45-degree obliquities. Use radiolucent 45-degree angle sponges to stabilize the dorsal surfaces of the hands.

Digits cupped in relaxed flexion.

Hands should be placed on film so that all parts of phalanges, metacarpals, and carpals are seen.

STRUCTURES DEMONSTRATED: Demonstrates joint spaces of the hand with the distal, metacarpal heads free from superimposition (Fig. 3–24).

This position demonstrates the diagnosis of rheumatoid arthritis, a loss of the outline of the bone with accompanying demineralization.

COMMON ERROR: Overpenetration. A lighter technique is necessary. As arthritis is a bony degenerative disease, less kilovoltage is needed.

TECHNIQUE

KV _____ MA _____ SECS _____ MAS _____ CALIPER _____ cm

_____ :1 GRID / B / none SCREEN: RE / High / Par / Detail / None

SID: _____ Rm _____ ADULT / CHILD age: _____ mos. / yrs.

HABITUS: Hyper / s / hypo / a   XS   S   M   L   XL   XXL

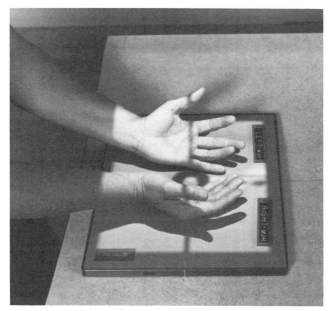

FIGURE 3–23. AP oblique (ballcatcher's) hands. (Notice the isolation of the pisiform in the wrist with medial rotation.)

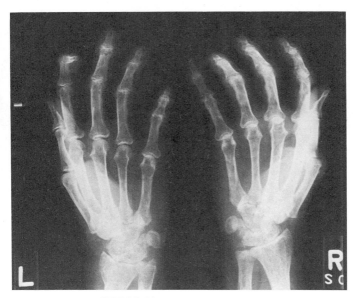

FIGURE 3–24. AP oblique hands x-ray.

WRIST: PA

10 x 12 in.
24 x 30 cm

8 x 10 in.
20 x 24 cm

8 x 10 in.
20 x 24 cm

FILM: No grid or table Bucky. Use tabletop only. Collimate to the area of interest.

CR: Perpendicularly to the midcarpal area just medial to ulnar prominence.

POSITION: Rest entire forearm on table with patient seated (Fig. 3–25). Pronate the hand and wrist (palmar surface on film).

Center wrist to film area.

Curl digits to bring the anterior surface of the wrist in closer contact with film.

Align the hand, wrist, and forearm longitudinally on the film.

NOTE: When moving a fracture, support the entire hand, wrist, and forearm. Minimize movement of the extremity by first taking the x-ray position already approximated by the patient's position, and then move the limb for the remaining positions. On post reductions, only the AP and lateral projections are usually taken. A wet plaster cast needs more kVp than a dry one. A fiberglass cast generally requires less technique than a plaster cast. Be careful, however, of abnormally thick casts, which may throw your techniques off.

STRUCTURES DEMONSTRATED: Carpals in relationship to each other. Proximal row from radial (lateral) side: scaphoid (navicular), lunate (semilunar), triquetrum (cuneiform, or triangular), and pisiform. Distal row from radial (lateral) side: trapezium (greater multangular), trapezoid (lesser multangular), capitate (os magnum or capitatum) and hamate (unciform).

The carpometacarpal joints are included.

The distal radius and ulna are included. The distal ulna is slightly obliqued in the PA projection (Fig. 3–26).

COMMON ERROR: The wrist is not flat against the film's surface. To correct, slightly curl the digits. Do not extend the digits.

TECHNIQUE

KV _____ MA _____ SECS _____ MAS _____ CALIPER _____ cm

_____ :1 GRID / B / none SCREEN: RE / High / Par / Detail / None

SID: _____ Rm _____ ADULT / CHILD age: _____ mos. / yrs.

HABITUS: Hyper / s / hypo / a   XS   S   M   L   XL   XXL

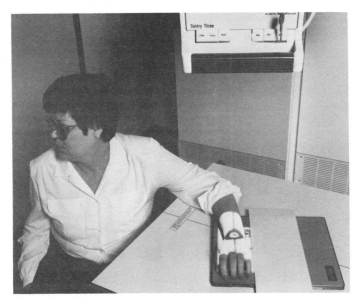

FIGURE 3–25. Right PA wrist with fingers curled. First exposure of three-exposures-on-one film.

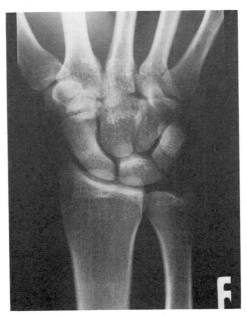

FIGURE 3–26. PA wrist x-ray. Increasing object-to-image distance produces magnification, a desired result to study the small bones of the wrist.

WRIST: PA OBLIQUE

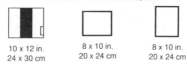

10 x 12 in.
24 x 30 cm

8 x 10 in.
20 x 24 cm

8 x 10 in.
20 x 24 cm

FILM: No grid or table Bucky. Use tabletop only. Collimate to the area of interest.

CR: Perpendicularly at the navicular or highest point of wrist on the radial aspect.

POSITION: Rest entire forearm on table with patient seated.

Place the hand and wrist in 45-degree semipronation with the ulnar side down (Fig. 3–27). This results in an anterior oblique position with a lateral rotation.

Center the wrist to the area provided.

Use radiolucent sponge to support the radial side of the hand and wrist.

NOTE: When moving a fracture, support the entire hand, wrist, and forearm. Minimize movement of the extremity by first taking the x-ray position already approximated by the patient's position, and then move the limb for the remaining positions. On post reductions, only the AP and lateral projections are usually taken. A wet plaster cast needs more kVp than a dry one. A fiberglass cast generally requires less technique than a plaster cast. Be careful, however, of abnormally thick casts, which may throw your techniques off.

STRUCTURES DEMONSTRATED: The carpals on the lateral or radial side of the wrist are best demonstrated (Fig. 3–28).

The scaphoid (navicular) is free from superimposition.

NOTE: The AP oblique projection of the wrist will isolate the pisiform with good demonstration of the triangular and hamate. The carpals on the medial or ulnar side of the wrist will be best demonstrated by this projection, the AP oblique wrist.

COMMON ERROR: Underpenetration due to not increasing the technique from the PA projection. Each projection of the wrist routine requires a slight adjustment in technique because of the variation in structure density. Usually a 2 kilovoltage increase is customary from the PA to the PA oblique and another 2 kilovoltage increase from the PA oblique to the lateral wrist projection. (However, this incremental change is approximate and may not be exact because of variations such as screens, single-phase versus three-phase equipment, SID, tube age, etc.).

TECHNIQUE

KV _____ MA _____ SECS _____ MAS _____ CALIPER _____ cm

_____ :1 GRID / B / none SCREEN: RE / High / Par / Detail / None

SID: _____ Rm _____ ADULT / CHILD age: _____ mos. / yrs.

HABITUS: Hyper / s / hypo / a   XS   S   M   L   XL   XXL

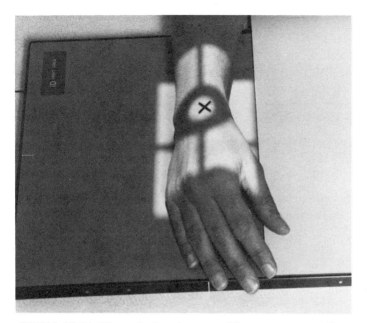

FIGURE 3–27. PA oblique wrist. Second exposure of three-exposures-on-one film.

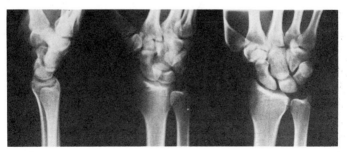

FIGURE 3–28. PA oblique wrist x-ray (center), PA (right), and lateral (left) wrist routine.

WRIST: LATERAL

10 x 12 in.
24 x 30 cm

6 x 10 in.
20 x 24 cm

8 x 10 in.
20 x 24 cm

FILM: No grid or table Bucky. Use tabletop only. Collimate to the area of interest.

CR: At the midcarpal area on radial side. Perpendicularly between the trapezium (greater multangular) and the scaphoid (navicular).

POSITION: Support the forearm by resting it on the table.

Patient is seated.

The wrist is resting on its ulnar surface.

The wrist's anterior and posterior (dorsal) surfaces are perpendicular to the film (Fig. 3–29).

Lateralize the wrist by adjusting its rotation (see Common Errors).

NOTE: When moving a fracture, support the entire hand, wrist, and forearm. Minimize movement of the extremity by first taking the x-ray position already approximated by the patient's position, and then move the limb for the remaining positions. On post reductions, only the AP and lateral projections are usually taken. A wet plaster cast needs more kVp than a dry one. A fiberglass cast generally requires less technique than a plaster cast. Be careful, however, of abnormally thick casts, which may throw off your techniques.

STRUCTURES DEMONSTRATED: The carpals are superimposed laterally to demonstrate any anterior or posterior displacement of fractures (Fig. 3–30).

The first carpometacarpal joint is well demonstrated.

COMMON ERRORS: (1) Underpenetration due to significant density increase over PA. (2) The distal radius and ulna will not be directly superimposed. If this habitually occurs in your positioning, after lateralizing the wrist use a very slight lateral or external rotation of the hand and wrist to ensure placement of the ulna over the middle of the distal radius.

When the radius is found to be posterior to the ulna on the resultant film, the motion to correct if the film is repeated is to slightly invert (internally rotate) the hand and wrist from the original position. Conversely, when the ulna is found to be anterior to the radius, the motion to correct should be to slightly evert (externally rotate) the hand and wrist from the original position.

TECHNIQUE

KV _____ MA _____ SECS _____ MAS _____ CALIPER _____ cm

_____ :1 GRID / B / none SCREEN: RE / High / Par / Detail / None

SID: _____ Rm _____ ADULT / CHILD age: _____ mos. / yrs.

HABITUS: Hyper / s / hypo / a   XS   S   M   L   XL   XXL

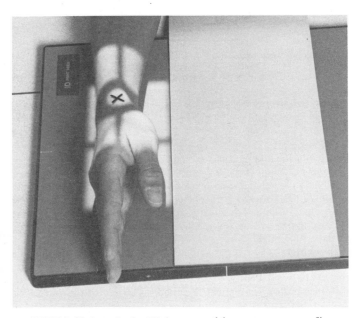

FIGURE 3–29. Lateral wrist. Third exposure of three-exposures-on-one film.

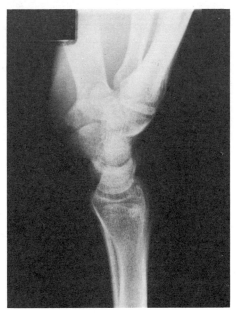

FIGURE 3–30. Lateral wrist x-ray.

WRIST: CARPAL TUNNEL

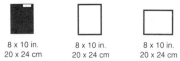

8 x 10 in.   8 x 10 in.   8 x 10 in.
20 x 24 cm   20 x 24 cm   20 x 24 cm

FILM: No grid or table Bucky. Use tabletop only. Collimate to the area of interest.

CR

Inferosuperior: Use a 25- to 35-degree, proximal angle directed along the longitudinal axis of the forearm. Center to the heel or base of the hand. If the forearm is flat on the film, use 35 degrees; if slightly elevated, use 25 degrees.

NOTE: Do not use the overhead distance indicators to measure the source-to-image distance (SID). Always use the tape measure along the path of the central ray to measure to the tabletop when using a tube angle.

Superoinferior: Use a perpendicular CR aligned distally along the longitudinal axis of the forearm and wrist.

POSITION

Inferosuperior: The patient is seated on a chair at the end of the x-ray table.

Pronate the forearm, wrist, and hand on the film.

With the opposite hand, have the patient hyperextend the digits of the side of interest. Keep the anterior surface of the forearm on the film. Sometimes, due to discomfort, injury, or limited range of motion, the anterior surface of the forearm will be elevated (Fig. 3–31).

Superoinferior: The patient is standing with the back to the film, reaching back to place the palm of the side of interest on the film (Fig. 3–32). The heel or base of the hand will be elevated.

STRUCTURES DEMONSTRATED: The carpal canal (tunnel or sulcus) (Fig. 3–33).

Demonstration of the palmar aspect of the scaphoid (navicular), the capitate (os magnum), the hook or hamulus of the hamate (unciform), and the pisiform.

***COMMON ERRORS:** (1) Distortion due to excessive angulation. In the inferosuperior projection with the forearm elevated from the film, you do not need as much angle. (2) Superimposition of the forearm over the carpal canal. In the superoinferior projection, the elbow must be flexed enough so that it is not in direct alignment over the wrist. To correct, have the patient move his or her body slightly away from the film.*

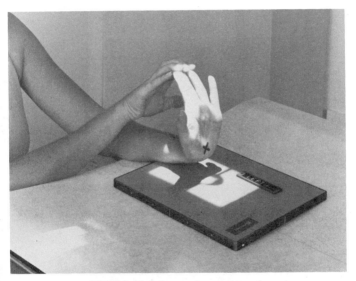

FIGURE 3–31. Inferosuperior carpal tunnel.

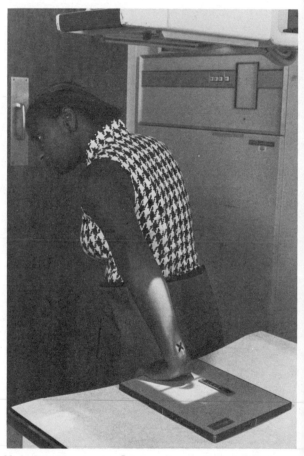

FIGURE 3–32. Superoinferior carpal tunnel. Remember to turn the lead half apron around to place it between patient and x-ray beam.

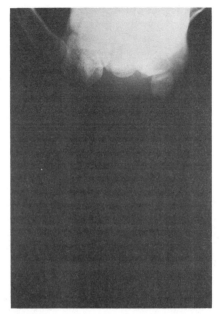

FIGURE 3–33. Carpal tunnel or carpal sulcus x-ray.

TECHNIQUE

KV _____ MA _____ SECS _____ MAS _____ CALIPER _____ cm

_____ :1 GRID / B / none SCREEN: RE / High / Par / Detail / None

SID: _____ Rm _____ ADULT / CHILD age: _____ mos. / yrs.

HABITUS: Hyper / s / hypo / a   XS   S   M   L   XL   XXL

NOTES:

WRIST: SCAPHOID (NAVICULAR)—
STECHER'S METHOD[3]

8 x 10 in.
20 x 24 cm

8 x 10 in.
20 x 24 cm

8 x 10 in.
20 x 24 cm

FILM: Use tabletop only. Collimate to the area of interest.

CR: Use a 20-degree angle proximally along the longitudinal axis of the hand, wrist, and forearm. Enter the scaphoid (proximal row, lateral aspect).

NOTE: Do not use the overhead distance indicators to measure the SID. Always use the tape measure along the path of the central ray to measure to the tabletop when using a tube angle.

If an angle sponge is used to elevate the distal end of the film (Fig. 3–34), place the CR perpendicularly to the scaphoid bone (proximal row, lateral aspect).

POSITION: Rest entire forearm on table with patient seated. Pronate the hand and wrist (palmar surface on film).

Extend the digits.

Center wrist to film area.

Align the hand, wrist, and forearm longitudinally on the film.

If no CR angulation is used, elevate the distal aspect of the film with a 20-degree angle sponge (Fig. 3–34).

STRUCTURES DEMONSTRATED: The scaphoid (navicular) free from superimposition (Fig. 3–35).

COMMON ERROR: Not enough angulation to free the scaphoid from superimposition.

TECHNIQUE

KV _____ MA _____ SECS _____ MAS _____ CALIPER _____ cm

_____ :1 GRID / B / none SCREEN: RE / High / Par / Detail / None

SID: _____ Rm _____ ADULT / CHILD age: _____ mos. / yrs.

HABITUS: Hyper / s / hypo / a   XS   S   M   L   XL   XXL

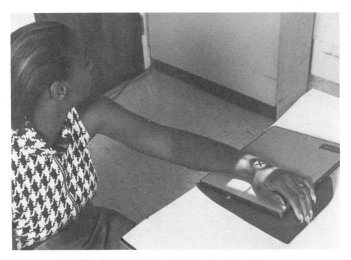

FIGURE 3–34. Scaphoid (navicular) wrist with angle sponge.

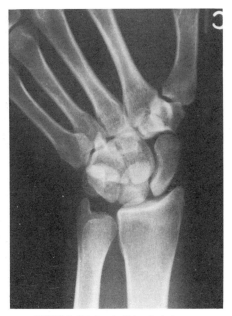

FIGURE 3–35. Scaphoid (navicular) x-ray.

WRIST: ULNAR AND RADIAL FLEXION

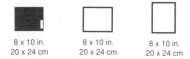

8 x 10 in.   8 x 10 in.   8 x 10 in.
20 x 24 cm   20 x 24 cm   20 x 24 cm

FILM: No grid or table Bucky. Use tabletop only. Collimate to the area of interest.

CR: Perpendicularly to the midcarpal area just medial to ulnar prominence.

POSITION: Rest entire forearm on table with patient seated.
  Pronate the hand and wrist (palmar surface on film).
  Center wrist to film area.

Radial Flexion: While the palm is flat against the film, move the fingers and palm toward the thumb side (radial) of the hand as far as possible (Fig. 3–36).

Ulnar Flexion: While the palm is flat against the film, move the fingers and palm away from the thumb side of the hand, toward the ulnar side as far as possible (Fig. 3–37).

STRUCTURES DEMONSTRATED: For ulnar flexion (radial deviation), the scaphoid (navicular) with its surrounding joint spaces open (Fig. 3–38).

  For radial flexion (ulnar deviation), the medial carpal bones with their surrounding joint spaces open.

COMMON ERROR: Central ray is not centered. The movement of the hand causes the CR to be corrected.

NOTES:

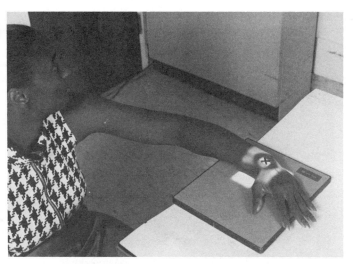

FIGURE 3–36. Radial flexion (ulnar deviation) PA wrist.

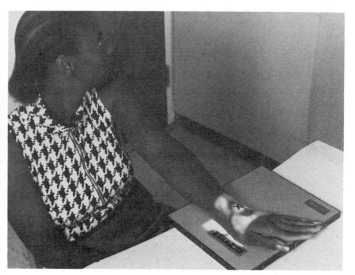

FIGURE 3–37. Ulnar flexion (radial deviation) PA wrist.

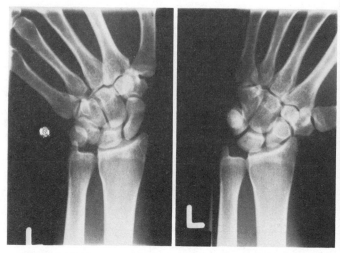

FIGURE 3–38. Ulnar flexion (left) and radial flexion (right) left wrist x-ray.

TECHNIQUE

KV _____ MA _____ SECS _____ MAS _____ CALIPER _____ cm
_____ :1 GRID / B / none SCREEN: RE / High / Par / Detail / None
SID: _____ Rm _____ ADULT / CHILD age: _____ mos. / yrs.
HABITUS: Hyper / s / hypo / a   XS   S   M   L   XL   XXL

FOREARM: AP

11 x 14 in.
30 x 35 cm

11 x 14 in.
30 x 35 cm

11 x 14 in.
30 x 35 cm

10 x 12 in.
24 x 30 cm.

10 x 12 in.
24 x 30 cm

7 x 17 in.
18 x 43 cm

FILM: No grid or table Bucky. Use tabletop only. Collimate to the area of interest.

CR: Perpendicularly to midshaft (midforearm) equidistant from the wrist and elbow.

POSITION: Patient is seated with arm extended on tabletop (Fig. 3–39).

Supinate the hand with elbow in full extension.

Humerus should be flat against the tabletop. Have patient lean forward to lower level of humerus.

Include both articulations; if not possible, then include the joint closest to injury.

If mothers help position their child, always ask if there is a possibility of their being pregnant. If not, make sure you use shielding for them as well as for the patient (Fig. 3–40).

NOTE: When moving a fracture, support the entire hand, wrist, and forearm. Minimize movement of the extremity by first taking the x-ray position already approximated by the patient's position, and then move the limb for the remaining positions. On post reductions, only the AP and lateral projections are usually taken. A wet plaster cast needs more kVp than a dry one. A fiberglass cast generally requires less technique than a plaster cast. Be careful, however, of abnormally thick casts, which may throw your techniques off.

STRUCTURES DEMONSTRATED: The AP projection of the forearm demonstrates the radius and ulna free from most superimposition.

The entire shafts of the radius and ulna are seen (Fig. 3–41).

COMMON ERROR: The hand and wrist are not fully supinated. The elbow is underpenetrated. The humerus is not on the same level or plane as the forearm.

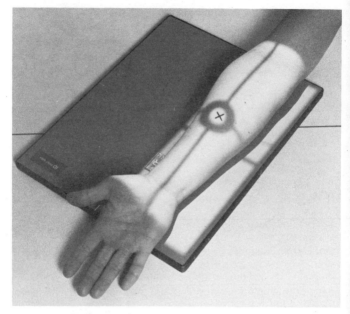

FIGURE 3–39. AP forearm. First exposure of two-exposures-on-one film.

TECHNIQUE

KV _____ MA _____ SECS _____ MAS _____ CALIPER _____ cm

_____ :1 GRID / B / none SCREEN: RE / High / Par / Detail / None

SID: _____ Rm _____ ADULT / CHILD age: _____ mos. / yrs.

HABITUS: Hyper / s / hypo / a   XS   S   M   L   XL   XXL

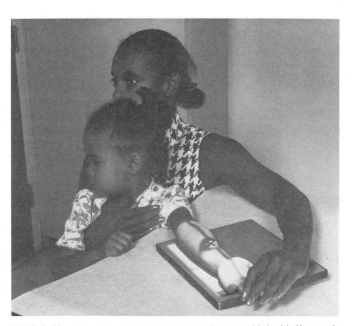

FIGURE 3–40. AP forearm of pediatric patient and parent with lead half apron for radiation protection.

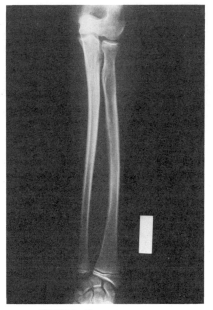

FIGURE 3–41. AP forearm x-ray.

FOREARM: LATERAL

11 x 14 in.	11 x 14 in.	**10 x 12 in.**	11 x 14 in.	7 x 17 in.
30 x 35 cm	30 x 35 cm	**24 x 30 cm.**	30 x 35 cm	18 x 43 cm

FILM: No grid or table Bucky. Use tabletop only. Collimate to the area of interest.

CR: Perpendicularly to midshaft (midforearm), equidistant from both articulations.

POSITION: Patient is seated with arm resting on table (Fig. 3–42).

The elbow is flexed 90 degrees.

Lateralize the hand and wrist (resting on ulnar side).

Humerus must be on same level as forearm. Have patient lean forward in order to place humerus flat against table.

Turn the film to accommodate the length of the forearm.

Have the patient turn the face away from the beam (Fig. 3–43).

NOTE: When moving a fracture, support the entire hand, wrist, and forearm. Minimize movement of the extremity by first taking the x-ray position already approximated by the patient's position, and then move the limb for the remaining positions. On post reductions, only the AP and lateral projections are usually taken. A wet plaster cast needs more kVp than a dry one. A fiberglass cast generally requires less technique than a plaster cast. Be careful, however, of abnormally thick casts, which may throw your techniques off.

STRUCTURES DEMONSTRATED: Both joints, wrist and elbow, are included.

The distal radius and ulna are directly superimposed.

The shafts are fully demonstrated (Fig. 3–44).

COMMON ERRORS: The distal radius and ulna are not directly superimposed. If this habitually occurs in your positioning, and assuming there has been internal rotation error, after lateralizing the wrist, use a very slight lateral or external rotation of the hand and wrist to ensure placement of the ulna over the middle of the distal radius.

When the radius is found to be posterior to the ulna on the resultant film, the motion to correct if repeated is to slightly internally rotate the hand and wrist from the original position. Conversely, when the ulna is found to be posterior to the radius, the motion to correct should be to slightly externally rotate the hand and wrist from the original position.

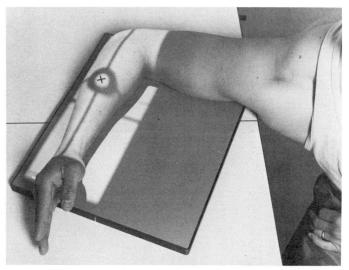

FIGURE 3–42. Lateral forearm. Second exposure of two-exposures-on-one film. Notice that the upper arm is placed on the same level as the forearm.

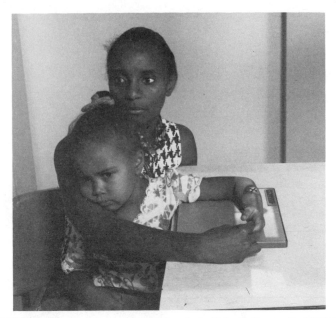

FIGURE 3–43. Lateral forearm of pediatric patient with lead half apron for radiation protection.

TECHNIQUE

KV _____ MA _____ SECS _____ MAS _____ CALIPER _____ cm

_____ :1 GRID / B / none SCREEN: RE / High / Par / Detail / None

SID: _____ Rm _____ ADULT / CHILD age: _____ mos. / yrs.

HABITUS: Hyper / s / hypo / a   XS   S   M   L   XL   XXL

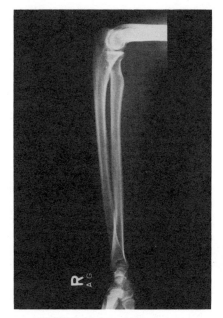

FIGURE 3–44. Lateral forearm x-ray.

NOTES:

ELBOW: AP

10 x 12 in.
24 x 30 cm

10 x 12 in.
24 x 30 cm

10 x 12 in.
24 x 30 cm

10 x 12 in.
24 x 30 cm

8 x 10 in.
20 x 24 cm

FILM: No grid or table Bucky. Use tabletop only. Collimate to the area of interest.

CR: Perpendicularly at midjoint (antecubital fossa).

POSITION: Patient seated with extended arm resting on table.

Supinate the hand with elbow in full extension.

Humerus should be flat against the tabletop. Have patient lean forward to lower level of humerus (Fig. 3–45).

Center the extended elbow to the film.

NOTE: When moving a fracture, support the entire hand, wrist, forearm, and elbow. Minimize movement of the extremity by first taking the x-ray position already approximated by the patient's position, and then move the limb for the remaining positions. On post reductions, only the AP and lateral projections are usually taken. A wet plaster cast requires more kVp than a dry one. A fiberglass cast generally requires less technique than a plaster cast. Be careful, however, of abnormally thick casts, which may throw your techniques off.

STRUCTURES DEMONSTRATED: The distal humerus is seen along with slight radial and ulnar superimposition.

The proximal ulna is superimposed over the elbow joint space (Fig. 3–46).

COMMON ERROR: The hand is not fully supinated. The AP elbow is often underpenetrated. It requires as much kilovoltage and milliamperage as the lateral projection due to the superimposition of radius, ulna, and humerus.

TECHNIQUE

KV _____ MA _____ SECS _____ MAS _____ CALIPER _____ cm

_____ :1 GRID / B / none SCREEN: RE / High / Par / Detail / None

SID: _____ Rm _____ ADULT / CHILD age: _____ mos. / yrs.

HABITUS: Hyper / s / hypo / a   XS   S   M   L   XL   XXL

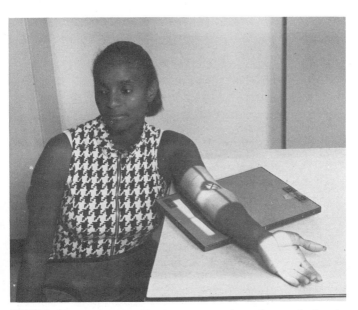

FIGURE 3–45. Left AP elbow. The upper arm must be on the same level as the elbow. First exposure of two-exposures-on-one film.

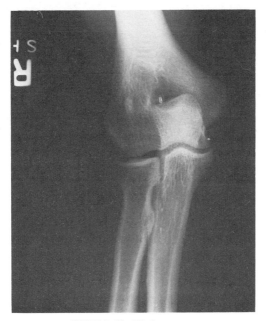

FIGURE 3–46. AP elbow x-ray.

ELBOW: AP EXTERNAL (LATERAL) OBLIQUE

10 x 12 in.	10 x 12 in.	10 x 12 in.	8 x 10 in.	8 x 10 in.
24 x 30 cm	24 x 30 cm	24 x 30 cm	20 x 24 cm	20 x 24 cm

FILM: No grid or table Bucky. Use tabletop only. Collimate to the area of interest.

CR: Perpendicularly at midjoint at highest point elevated from table.

POSITION: Patient is seated with elbow fully extended on film.

The hand is supinated to separate the radius and ulna.

From the anterior, rotate the elbow laterally (externally) 45 degrees. Make sure this motion originates at the shoulder. The entire arm is obliqued (Fig. 3–47).

Center the elbow to the film area.

NOTE: This position is not recommended for a suspected fracture of the humerus. On post reductions, only the AP and lateral projections are usually taken.

STRUCTURES DEMONSTRATED: This obliquity best demonstrates the relationship of the radial head with the capitellum (capitulum) of the humerus (Fig. 3–48).

COMMON ERROR: Underrotation or overrotation. The radial head must be free from superimposition.

TECHNIQUE

KV _____ MA _____ SECS _____ MAS _____ CALIPER _____ cm

_____ :1 GRID / B / none SCREEN: RE / High / Par / Detail / None

SID: _____ Rm _____ ADULT / CHILD age: _____ mos. / yrs.

HABITUS: Hyper / s / hypo / a   XS   S   M   L   XL   XXL

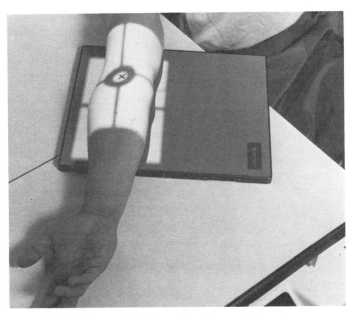

FIGURE 3–47. Right AP external oblique. Second exposure of two-exposures-on-one film.

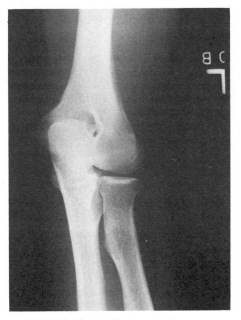

FIGURE 3–48. Left AP external oblique x-ray.

ELBOW: LATERAL

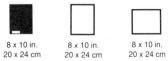

| 8 x 10 in. | 8 x 10 in. | 8 x 10 in. |
| 20 x 24 cm | 20 x 24 cm | 20 x 24 cm |

FILM: No grid or table Bucky. Use tabletop only. Collimate to the area of interest.

CR: Perpendicularly, midjoint on lateral surface at flexed joint intersection.

POSITION: Patient is seated with arm resting on table.

The elbow is flexed 90 degrees.

Lateralize the hand and wrist (resting on ulnar side).

Humerus must be on same level as forearm. Have patient lean forward in order to place humerus flat against table (Fig. 3–49).

Turn the film to accommodate centering of the elbow in flexion.

NOTE: When moving a fracture, support the entire hand, wrist, forearm, and elbow. Minimize movement of the extremity by first taking the x-ray position already approximated by the patient's position, and then move the limb for the remaining positions. On post reductions, only the AP and lateral projections are usually taken. A wet plaster cast needs more kVp than a dry one. A fiberglass cast generally requires less technique than a plaster cast. Be careful, however, of abnormally thick casts, which may throw your techniques off.

STRUCTURES DEMONSTRATED: The olecranon process is seen in profile.

The lateral aspects of the distal humerus and proximal radius and ulna are seen (Fig. 3–50).

COMMON ERROR: The humeral condyles are not directly super-imposed due to the elevation of the humerus. The humerus must be placed on the same level as the forearm and elbow.

TECHNIQUE

KV _____ MA _____ SECS _____ MAS _____ CALIPER _____ cm
_____ :1 GRID / B / none SCREEN: RE / High / Par / Detail / None
SID: _____ Rm _____ ADULT / CHILD age: _____ mos. / yrs.
HABITUS: Hyper / s / hypo / a   XS   S   M   L   XL   XXL

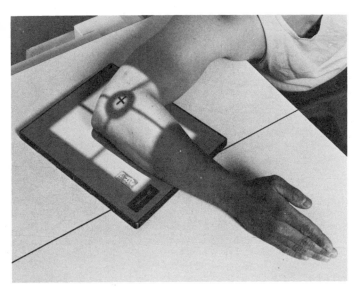

FIGURE 3–49. Lateral right elbow. The upper arm must be on the same level as the elbow.

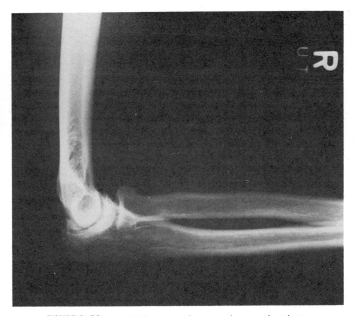

FIGURE 3–50. Lateral elbow x-ray demonstrating more long bone.

ELBOW: AP INTERNAL (MEDIAL) OBLIQUE

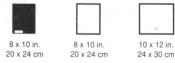

| 8 x 10 in. | 8 x 10 in. | 10 x 12 in. |
| 20 x 24 cm | 20 x 24 cm | 24 x 30 cm |

FILM: No grid or table Bucky. Use tabletop only. Collimate to the area of interest.

CR: Midjoint at highest point elevated from table.

POSITION: Patient is seated with elbow fully extended on film.

The hand is pronated to visualize the coronoid process of the ulna. This action should also rotate the elbow medially or internally 45 degrees. Make sure the hand motion rotates the elbow and shoulder position as well. The entire arm is obliqued medially (Fig. 3–51).

Center the elbow to the film area.

NOTE: This position is not recommended for suspected fracture. On post reductions, only the AP and lateral projections are usually taken.

STRUCTURES DEMONSTRATED: This obliquity best demonstrates the relationship of the coronoid process of the ulna with the trochlea of the humerus (Fig. 3–52).

The proper obliquity will free the radial head from superimposition over the coronoid process.

The medial condyle of the humerus is isolated.

COMMON ERROR: Underrotation. If the coronoid process is not free from superimposition, the obliquity is less than 45 degrees.

TECHNIQUE

KV _____ MA _____ SECS _____ MAS _____ CALIPER _____ cm

_____ :1 GRID / B / none SCREEN: RE / High / Par / Detail / None

SID: _____ Rm _____ ADULT / CHILD age: _____ mos. / yrs.

HABITUS: Hyper / s / hypo / a   XS   S   M   L   XL   XXL

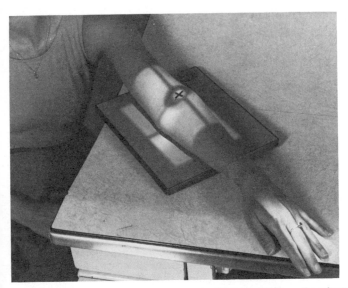

FIGURE 3–51. AP internal oblique elbow. The hand is rotated to lie on the palmar surface.

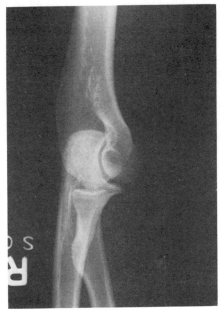

FIGURE 3–52. AP internal oblique elbow x-ray.

HUMERUS: AP

7 x 17 in.
18 x 43 cm

7 x 17 in.
18 x 43 cm

11 x 14 in.
30 x 35 cm

**10 x 12 in.
24 x 30 cm.**

11 x 14 in.
30 x 35 cm

FILM: Tabletop use. However, if the thickness of the humerus is greater than 10 cm to 12 cm (4 to 5 inches),[4, 5] use a grid. Collimate to the area of interest.

CR: Perpendicularly at anterior surface midshaft, equidistant from each articulation.

POSITION: *If a fracture is suspected, take an "as is" scout for initial assessment (see Comment, below).*

Patient may be standing at chest board or be recumbent on the x-ray table (Fig. 3–53).

If the patient can tolerate it, an upright study is generally more comfortable due to the ease of manipulation of the body with less movement of the injured arm.

Include both articulations.

The body along with the upper extremity is placed in the anatomical position.

An imaginary coronal plane through the epicondyles of the distal humerus should be parallel with the plane of the film. This verifies the anatomical position (see Fig. 1–16). Slightly abduct the arm.

COMMENT: Whenever the arm is fractured or when the range of motion is severely impaired, instead of moving the arm, oblique the patient's entire body (usually 40 degrees toward injured side when patient is cradling arm to side) to achieve the proper AP projection. This is ideally done when patient is sitting or standing.

STRUCTURES DEMONSTRATED: The entire humerus is seen.

The greater tubercle (tuberosity) is seen in profile on the lateral aspect of the humeral head. This denotes true anatomical position (Fig. 3–54).

COMMON ERROR: Lead blocker over area of interest. The film must be placed in order to avoid positioning the lead blocker over any anatomy of interest.

TECHNIQUE

KV _____ MA _____ SECS _____ MAS _____ CALIPER _____ cm

_____ :1 GRID / B / none SCREEN: RE / High / Par / Detail / None

SID: _____ Rm _____ ADULT / CHILD age: _____ mos. / yrs.

HABITUS: Hyper / s / hypo / a   XS   S   M   L   XL   XXL

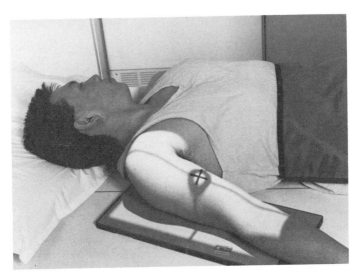

FIGURE 3–53. AP humerus.

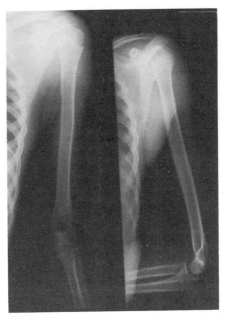

FIGURE 3–54. AP humerus (left) and lateral humerus (right) x-ray.

HUMERUS: LATERAL

| 7 x 17 in. | 7 x 17 in. | 11 x 14 in. | 11 x 14 in. | 10 x 12 in. |
| 18 x 43 cm | 18 x 43 cm | 30 x 35 cm | 30 x 35 cm | 24 x 30 cm. |

FILM: Match the long axis of the film to the length of the humerus. Commonly tabletop use. However, if the thickness of the humerus is greater than 3 to 4 inches (8 to 10 cm), use a grid. Collimate to the area of interest.

CR: Perpendicularly to midshaft, equidistant from each end.

POSITION: Patient may be recumbent supine (Fig. 3–55), sitting, or standing upright.

When placing the patient recumbent, have the patient support the upper arm and shoulder and/or place a radiolucent sponge under the upper arm. Do not elevate the arm, but simply support

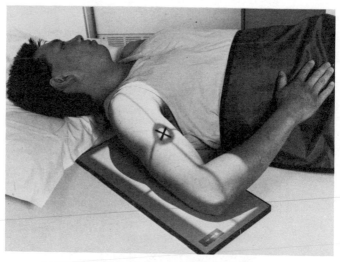

FIGURE 3–55. Lateral humerus recumbent.

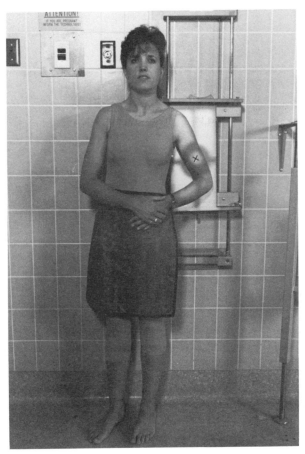

FIGURE 3–56. Lateral humerus upright.

it so the use of the sponge does not stress the shoulder or upper arm.

With a suspected fracture, do not attempt to move or adjust the humerus—take it "as is" or see method B.

Fair–Good Mobility

Method A. If the patient has a relatively good range of motion and slight or no discomfort from the anatomical position, the palmar surface of the hand is placed against the hip (internally rotating the wrist and forearm) while moving the elbow away from the body (see Fig. 3–55). This places the coronal plane through the epicondyles perpendicular to the film and results in a 90-degree flexion at the elbow. The ulnar aspect is closest to the film.

If the recumbent patient has only fair movement, ease the humerus away from the body. Have the patient lay the hand on the abdomen if tolerated. Notice that this will elevate the shoulder slightly (Fig. 3–56). *However, if a fracture is suspected, take an "as is" scout for initial assessment.*

Poor Mobility

Method B. For severe trauma, a transthoracic projection[6] (with the use of a grid) is useful when the arm has limited or no range of motion. The unaffected arm is elevated above the head. The injured shoulder is dropped below the level of the unaffected shoulder (this avoids superimposition). The proximal shoulder is positioned midthorax to the midcoronal plane, just anteriorly to the lateral thoracic spine and posteriorly to the sternum (Fig. 3–57). Full inspiration improves the penetrability of this exposure, and a breathing technique will allow more detail of the humerus within the lung fields. A breathing technique requires the use of a long exposure time (3 to 4 seconds) to allow blurring of the lung markings. The patient is instructed to breathe softly and shallowly while the exposure is made. *With a suspected fracture, do not attempt to move or adjust the humerus—take it as is!*

NOTES:

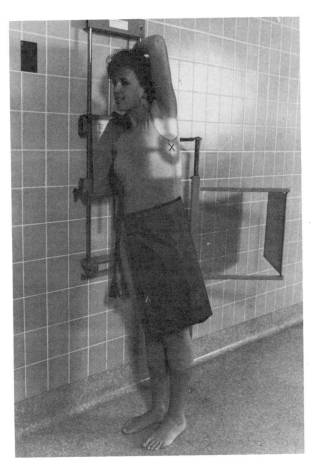

FIGURE 3–57. Lateral humerus transthoracic.

STRUCTURES DEMONSTRATED: Both joints are included. The lateral aspect of the humerus is seen with the greater tubercle (tuberosity) on the lateral aspect (external rotation). The epicondyles of the humerus should be directly superimposed, but due to the elevation of the forearm and hand (see Fig. 3–56), they are not always superimposed.

The transthoracic method will demonstrate possible fracture or dislocation of the proximal humerus with either anterior or posterior displacement of the proximal humerus (see Fig. 3–58).

COMMON ERRORS: Method A: *The humerus is not in a true lateral position. The epicondyles must be directly superimposed at the elbow. The technique is either too dark at the distal humerus or too light at the shoulder.* Method B: *A grid must be used. The humeral head should not be superimposed over the thoracic spine. Placement of the humeral head must be anterior to the thoracic spine, yet posterior to the sternum within the lung fields (10 degrees right or left posterior oblique [RPO or LPO]).*

COMMENT: The use of a grid is optional in Method A. The recommended thickness of part for the use of a grid is 10 cm to 12 cm (4 to 5 inches)[7, 8] and over.

TECHNIQUE

KV _____ MA _____ SECS _____ MAS _____ CALIPER _____ cm

_____ :1 GRID / B / none SCREEN: RE / High / Par / Detail / None

SID: _____ Rm _____ ADULT / CHILD age: _____ mos. / yrs.

HABITUS: Hyper / s / hypo / a XS S M L XL XXL

NOTES:

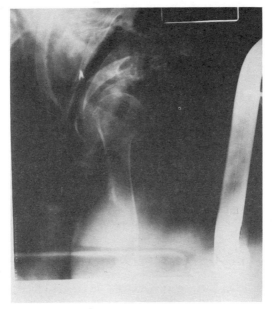

FIGURE 3–58. Lateral transthoracic humerus x-ray (patient in wheelchair).

SHOULDER: AP EXTERNAL ROTATION

10 x 12 in.
24 x 30 cm

10 x 12 in.
24 x 30 cm

10 x 12 in.
24 x 30 cm

10 x 12 in.
24 x 30 cm

FILM: Use table Bucky or grid. Collimate to the area of interest.
CR: Coracoid process, medial to the humeral head (in actual practice, some technologists center at midscapula 2 to 3 inches below the coracoid process in order to include more of the humerus on the film).
POSITION: The patient can be upright (orthostatic), sitting, or supine.
   Center the shoulder to the center of the grid or table Bucky.
   Abduct the arm slightly in the anatomical position.
   Then rotate the entire arm externally, that is, toward the lateral aspect (Fig. 3–59).
STRUCTURES DEMONSTRATED: The clavicle and scapula are seen in their entirety.
   The proximal humerus is seen with the greater tubercle (tuberosity) in profile on the lateral aspect of the humeral head (Fig. 3–60).
   Range-of-motion studies such as the shoulder routine assess joint competency while demonstrating possible calcium deposits.
COMMON ERROR: The humerus is not rotated sufficiently to see the greater tubercle (tuberosity) on the lateral aspect of the humeral head. Do not ask the patient to rotate the arm any more than what is comfortable. A shoulder rotation study should not be performed when a fracture or dislocation is suspected.

TECHNIQUE

KV _____ MA _____ SECS _____ MAS _____ CALIPER _____ cm
_____ :1 GRID / B / none SCREEN: RE / High / Par / Detail / None
SID: _____ Rm _____ ADULT / CHILD age: _____ mos. / yrs.
HABITUS: Hyper / s / hypo / a   XS   S   M   L   XL   XXL

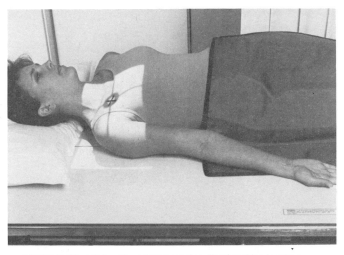

FIGURE 3–59. AP shoulder external rotation. Hand position is palm up.

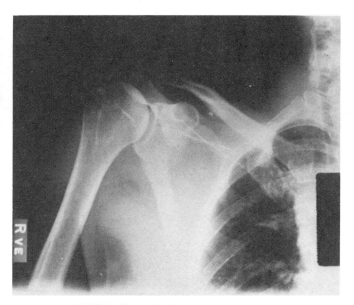

FIGURE 3–60. AP shoulder external rotation x-ray.

SHOULDER: AP NEUTRAL POSITION

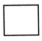

10 x 12 in.
24 x 30 cm

10 x 12 in.
24 x 30 cm

10 x 12 in.
24 x 30 cm

10 x 12 in.
24 x 30 cm

FILM: Use table Bucky or grid. Collimate to the area of interest.
CR: Coracoid process, medial to the humeral head (in actual practice, some technologists center at midscapula 2 to 3 inches below the coracoid process in order to include more of the humerus on the film).
POSITION: The patient can be upright (orthostatic), sitting, or supine.

Center the shoulder to the center of the grid or table Bucky.

Rotate the hand, forearm, and elbow slightly internally from the anatomical position so that the cupped hand is lateralized and the elbow is medially obliqued (Fig. 3–61).
STRUCTURES DEMONSTRATED: The clavicle and scapula are seen in their entirety.

The proximal humerus is seen with the posterior aspect of the greater tubercle (tuberosity) slightly in profile. The majority of the greater tubercle should be found on the anterior aspect of the humeral head (Fig. 3–62).

When this projection is included in the shoulder routine, complete range of motion is assessed.

This projection when taken alone serves as a survey film of the shoulder while demonstrating possible calcium deposits.

***COMMON ERROR: Do not ask the patient to rotate the arm any more than what is comfortable.* A shoulder rotation study should not be performed when a fracture or dislocation is suspected.**

TECHNIQUE

KV _____ MA _____ SECS _____ MAS _____ CALIPER _____ cm
_____ :1 GRID / B / none SCREEN: RE / High / Par / Detail / None
SID: _____ Rm _____ ADULT / CHILD age: _____ mos. / yrs.
HABITUS: Hyper / s / hypo / a   XS   S   M   L   XL   XXL

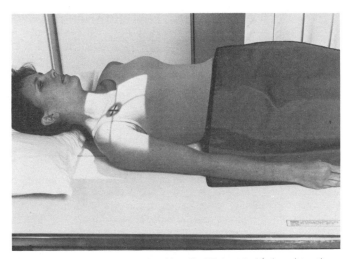

FIGURE 3–61. AP shoulder neutral position. Hand is lateral with the wrist resting on its ulnar aspect.

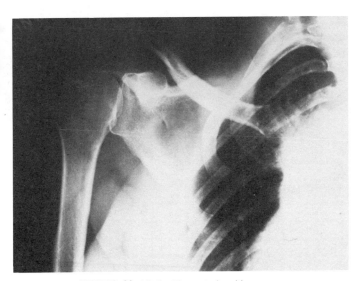

FIGURE 3–62. AP shoulder neutral position x-ray.

SHOULDER: AP INTERNAL ROTATION

10 x 12 in.
24 x 30 cm

10 x 12 in.
24 x 30 cm

10 x 12 in.
24 x 30 cm

10 x 12 in.
24 x 30 cm

FILM: Use table Bucky or grid. Collimate to the area of interest.
CR: Coracoid process, medial to the humeral head (in actual practice, most technologists center at midscapula 2 to 3 inches below the coracoid in order to include more of the humerus on the film).
POSITION: The patient can be upright (orthostatic), sitting, or supine.

Center the shoulder to the center of the grid or table Bucky.

Abduct the arm slightly in the anatomical position.

Rotate the entire arm internally (toward the medial). The hand should rest on its radial surface (Fig. 3–63).

If the shoulder-to-film or -table distance increases by more than 1 or 2 inches, roll the patient up 20 degrees toward the injured side to reduce the increased object-image distance (OID).

NOTE: A shoulder rotation study should not be performed when a fracture or dislocation is suspected.

STRUCTURES DEMONSTRATED: The clavicle and scapula are seen in their entirety.

The proximal humerus is seen with the lesser tubercle (tuberosity) in profile on the medial aspect of the humeral head (Fig. 3–64).

Because this routine demonstrates range of motion (from external rotation to internal rotation), obtain a patient history.

This routine assesses directional joint competency while demonstrating possible calcium deposits.

COMMON ERRORS: (1) The humerus is not rotated sufficiently to see the lesser tubercle (tuberosity) on the medial aspect of the humeral head. Do not force the patient to rotate the arm any more than what is comfortable. A shoulder rotation study should not be performed when a fracture or dislocation is suspected. (2) Overpenetration. Calcium deposits may be missed radiographically if the film is overexposed.

TECHNIQUE

KV _____ MA _____ SECS _____ MAS _____ CALIPER _____ cm

_____ :1 GRID / B / none SCREEN: RE / High / Par / Detail / None

SID: _____ Rm _____ ADULT / CHILD age: _____ mos. / yrs.

HABITUS: Hyper / s / hypo / a   XS   S   M   L   XL   XXL

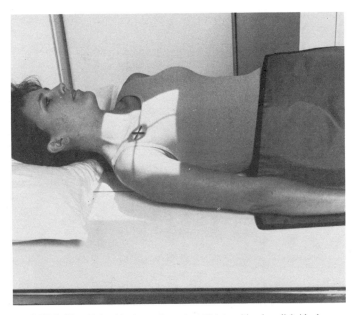

FIGURE 3–63. AP shoulder internal rotation. Wrist position is radial side down.

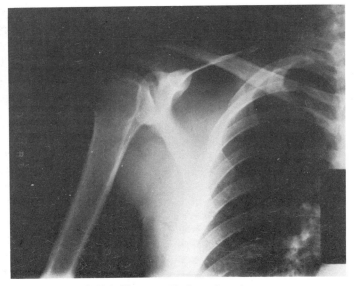

FIGURE 3–64. AP shoulder internal rotation x-ray.

AP OBLIQUE SHOULDER FOR GLENOID FOSSA

8 x 10 in.
20 x 24 cm

8 x 10 in.
20 x 24 cm

8 x 10 in.
20 x 24 cm

8 x 10 in.
20 x 24 cm

FILM: Use table Bucky or grid. Collimate to the area of interest.
CR: Perpendicular and immediately adjacent to the humeral head at its medial side.
POSITION: The patient can be upright (orthostatic), sitting, or supinated.

Center the head of the humerus to the center of the grid or table Bucky.

Abduct the upper arm slightly while placing the hand on the abdomen. The humeral head will be internally rotated.

Oblique the patient toward the side of interest 35 to 45 degrees (Fig. 3–65).

An alternate hand position is palm up for an external rotation of the humeral head.

STRUCTURES DEMONSTRATED: A detailed view of the glenoid fossa in profile (on edge) and the humeral head (Fig. 3–66).

COMMON ERROR: The kilovoltage needs to be increased when close collimation is used. Smaller, closely collimated fields produce less scattered radiation. Because there is less blackening effect with less scatter, technique must be increased to compensate for this event.[9]

TECHNIQUE

KV _____ MA _____ SECS _____ MAS _____ CALIPER _____ cm

_____ :1 GRID / B / none SCREEN: RE / High / Par / Detail / None

SID: _____ Rm _____ ADULT / CHILD age: _____ mos. / yrs.

HABITUS: Hyper / s / hypo / a   XS   S   M   L   XL   XXL

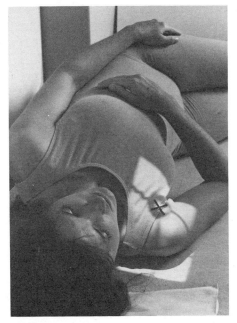

FIGURE 3–65. AP oblique shoulder for glenoid fossa.

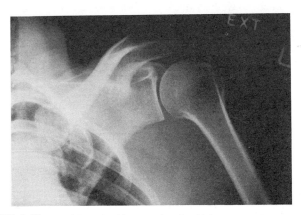

FIGURE 3–66. AP oblique shoulder x-ray for glenoid fossa external rotation with hand palm up.

CLAVICLE: AP

10 x 12 in.   10 x 12 in.   11 x 14 in.
24 x 30 cm   24 x 30 cm   30 x 35 cm

FILM: Use a grid or table Bucky if part thickness is over 3 to 4 inches (8 to 10 cm). Collimate to the area of interest.

CR: Midshaft of the clavicle equidistant from the articular ends.

POSITION: Patient may be supine (Fig. 3–67) or upright (Fig. 3–68).

If the patient can tolerate them, the upright and seated positions generally are less painful.

Shoulders should be even and level.

Center the middle of the clavicle to the center of the film.

If the patient is upright, brace him or her against the film or film holder to avoid body sway.

STRUCTURES DEMONSTRATED: The clavicle is projected over the upper ribs. Both articulations should be seen in their entirety (Fig. 3–69).

COMMON ERROR: Film too dark. Shoulder technique is often used incorrectly since the clavicle requires less technique. The clavicle is often clipped at the medial end; it must be seen in its entirety. The midshaft of the clavicle should be centered to the film. Place the blocker out of the area of interest.

TECHNIQUE

KV _____ MA _____ SECS _____ MAS _____ CALIPER _____ cm

_____ :1 GRID / B / none SCREEN: RE / High / Par / Detail / None

SID: _____ Rm _____ ADULT / CHILD age: _____ mos. / yrs.

HABITUS: Hyper / s / hypo / a XS S M L XL XXL

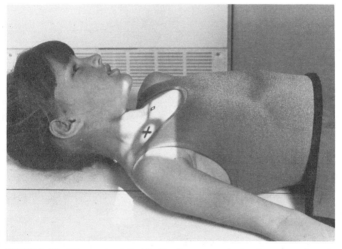

FIGURE 3–67. AP recumbent clavicle. Small square marks jugular or sternal notch.

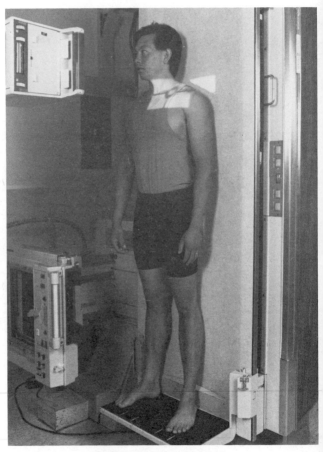

FIGURE 3–68. AP clavicle upright.

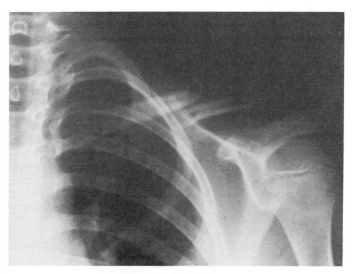

FIGURE 3–69. AP clavicle x-ray.

CLAVICLE: AP SEMI-AXIAL (ANGLED)

10 x 12 in.   10 x 12 in.   11 x 14 in.
24 x 30 cm   24 x 30 cm   30 x 35 cm

FILM: Use a grid or table Bucky if part thickness is over 3 to 4 inches (8 to 10 cm). Collimate to the area of interest.

CR: Midshaft of the clavicle with a 10- to 15-degree cephalic angle.

For an asthenic patient, use a 15-degree cephalic angle; for a hypersthenic patient, use a 10-degree cephalic angle. The reason for the difference is that the recumbent, hypersthenic patient's clavicle is already elevated superiorly from the table and thus needs less of an angle to decrease superimposition over the ribs.

NOTE: Do not use the overhead distance indicators to measure the SID. Always use the tape measure along the path of the central ray to measure to the tabletop when using a tube angle.

POSITION: Patient may be upright or supine (Fig. 3–70).

If the patient can tolerate them, the upright and seated positions generally are less painful.

Shoulders should be even and level.

Center the middle of the clavicle to 1 inch below the center of the film (the angle will throw the clavicle back up to the center of the film).

If the patient is upright, brace him or her against film or film holder to avoid body sway.

STRUCTURES DEMONSTRATED: The clavicle is projected above the upper margin of the scapula to increase visualization of fracture (Fig. 3–71).

If the clavicle needs to be demonstrated above the rib margin, increase the angle to 25 to 30 degrees. This, however, will increase distortion.

COMMON ERROR: Film too dark. Shoulder technique is often used incorrectly since the clavicle requires less technique. The clavicle is often clipped at the medial end; it must be seen in its entirety. The midshaft of the clavicle should be centered to the film. Place the blocker out of the area of interest.

TECHNIQUE

KV _____ MA _____ SECS _____ MAS _____ CALIPER _____ cm

_____ :1 GRID / B / none SCREEN: RE / High / Par / Detail / None

SID: _____ Rm _____ ADULT / CHILD age: _____ mos. / yrs.

HABITUS: Hyper / s / hypo / a   XS   S   M   L   XL   XXL

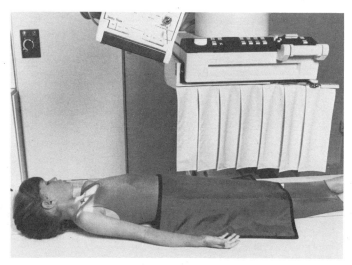

FIGURE 3–70. AP semi-axial clavicle.

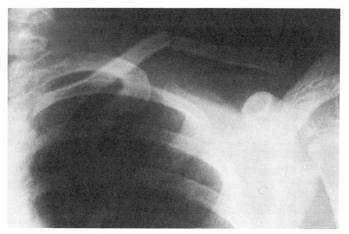

FIGURE 3–71. AP semi-axial clavicle x-ray.

SHOULDER: ACROMIOCLAVICULAR JOINTS

FILM

Bilateral Study: The use of a grid is not necessary.

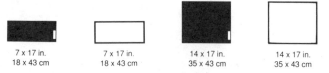

| 7 x 17 in. | 7 x 17 in. | 14 x 17 in. | 14 x 17 in. |
| 18 x 43 cm | 18 x 43 cm | 35 x 43 cm | 35 x 43 cm |

Hypersthenic Patients: Use two films for separate exposures, right side and left side, respectively.

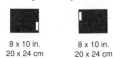

| 8 x 10 in. | 8 x 10 in. |
| 20 x 24 cm | 20 x 24 cm |

CR: Perpendicular and centered to the sternal notch for a bilateral study. Center to the distal end of the clavicle for a separate exposure of each side.

POSITION: The patient can be upright (orthostatic),* sitting, or supine.

Center the midsagittal plane at the level of the sternal notch to the center of the film for a single-exposure bilateral study (Fig. 3–72).

Center the distal clavicle to the center of the film for two separate exposures of a bilateral study.

Rotate the hand, forearm, and elbow slightly externally in the anatomical position so that the hands are palm out (see Fig. 1–1). Have the patient suspend respiration for the first exposure or set of exposures. Change the film cassette(s).

Have the patient hold equal weights (3 to 5 pounds) in each hand (Fig. 3–73). Mark the film(s) "with weight." Suspend respiration and make the second exposure or set of exposures.

STRUCTURES DEMONSTRATED: The bilateral acromioclavicular joints (AC joints) without weights and with weights for comparison (Fig. 3–74).

These studies demonstrate the integrity or degree of separation of the AC joints due to a tear in the acromioclavicular joint capsule.

COMMON ERROR: Do not ask the patient to rotate the arm any more than what is comfortable. **A shoulder rotation study should not be performed when a fracture or dislocation is suspected.**

---

*The SID is usually 72 inches or 183 cm (rounded to 200 cm) to reduce magnification distortion.

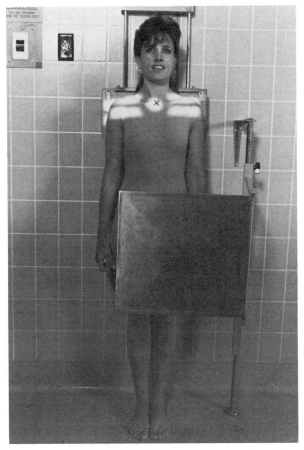

FIGURE 3–72 AP acromioclavicular (AC) joints without weights with pelvis shield in place.

TECHNIQUE

KV _____ MA _____ SECS _____ MAS _____ CALIPER _____ cm

_____ :1 GRID / B / none SCREEN: RE / High / Par / Detail / None

SID: _____ Rm _____ ADULT / CHILD age: _____ mos. / yrs.

HABITUS: Hyper / s / hypo / a   XS   S   M   L   XL   XXL

NOTES:

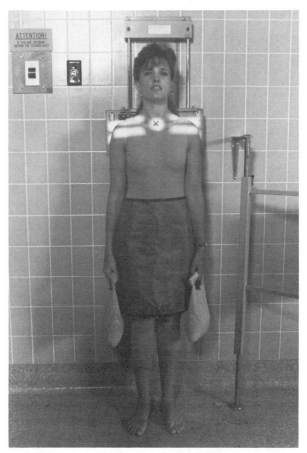

FIGURE 3–73. AP AC joints with weights with patient wearing lead half apron.

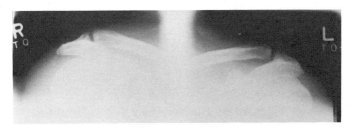

FIGURE 3–74. Bilateral, two exposures on one film, AP AC joints x-ray. One set of films *must* be marked as to with weights or without weights.

SCAPULA: AP

10 x 12 in.   10 x 12 in.
24 x 30 cm   24 x 30 cm

FILM: Use the table Bucky or a grid. Make sure the bottom of the film includes level of T-7 (bottom of scapula). Collimate to the area of interest.

CR: Midscapula, 2 to 3 inches below level of coracoid process.

POSITION: The patient is supine and, if tolerated, can be slightly rolled up on side of interest (5- to 10-degree obliquity) to place the scapula in a true anterior-to-posterior aspect.

Excellent to Good Mobility: With patient supine (Fig. 3–75) or upright (Fig. 3–76), abduct the hand and forearm by raising the hand and flexing the elbow to place the dorsum of the hand against the table. This flattens the scapula to allow a relatively undistorted assessment of the bone.

Poor Mobility: Take film with patient "as is" for initial assessment. If the patient can tolerate, the upright and seated positions generally are less painful. Shoulders should be even and level. Center the middle of the scapula to the center of the film. If the patient is upright, brace him or her against film or film holder to avoid body sway.

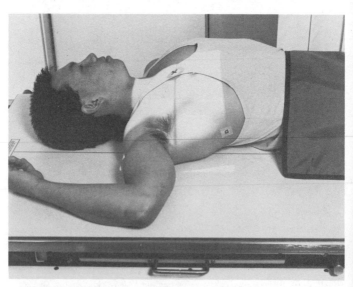

FIGURE 3–75. AP scapula recumbent. Square marks inferior border of scapula.

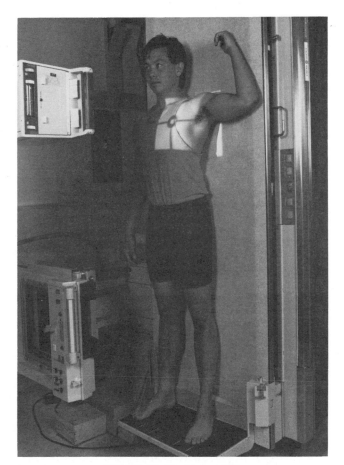

FIGURE 3–76. AP scapula upright.

STRUCTURES DEMONSTRATED: The entire posterior aspect of scapula with the lateral border free from superimposition (Fig. 3–77).

COMMON ERROR: Film underpenetrated. The detail of the thicker part of the scapula (the lateral or axillary border) is seen as "white-out" as compared with the medial border, which is thinner. To aid visualization, use either cessation of respiration to evenly distribute densities of the lung or use a "breathing" technique. A breathing technique means to use a long exposure time (3 to 4 seconds) in order to allow blurring of the lung markings. The patient is instructed to breathe softly and shallowly while the exposure is made.

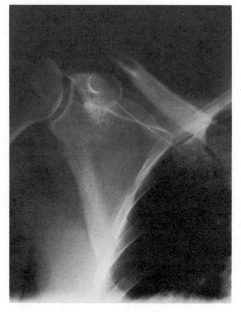

FIGURE 3–77. AP scapula x-ray.

TECHNIQUE

KV _____ MA _____ SECS _____ MAS _____ CALIPER _____ cm
_____ :1 GRID / B / none SCREEN: RE / High / Par / Detail / None
SID: _____ Rm _____ ADULT / CHILD age: _____ mos. / yrs.
HABITUS: Hyper / s / hypo / a   XS   S   M   L   XL   XXL

NOTES:

SCAPULA: LATERAL

  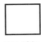

10 x 12 in.
24 x 30 cm

10 x 12 in.
24 x 30 cm

10 x 12 in.
24 x 30 cm

FILM: Use the table Bucky or a grid.

CR: Midscapula on medial (vertebral) border if RAO or LAO, or on lateral (axillary) border if RPO or LPO position (Fig. 3–78).

POSITION: If the patient can tolerate them, the upright and seated positions generally are less painful (either AP or PA). Center the middle of the scapula to the center of the film.

If the patient is upright, brace him or her against film or film holder to avoid body sway.

Excellent Mobility: An upright or supine position used is the arm "wrap" method. Take the arm of the side of interest and have the patient grasp the posterior aspect of the opposite shoulder or back of the neck and elevate the elbow while facing the film. This rolls the shoulder of the injured side and lateralizes the scapula of the side of interest. Oblique the patient only enough to place the body of the scapula end-on-end (medial border superimposed on lateral border). The less mobile the patient in "wrapping," the more you must increase the obliquity of the body of the patient to compensate (Fig. 3–78).

Poor Mobility: An upright method for either the single-trauma (Fig. 3–79) or recumbent, multiple-injury patient is to slightly oblique the patient away from the side of interest 15 to 30 degrees. If the patient can tolerate, move the arm of the side of interest so that the hand is touching the opposite hip. The better the arm motion, the less obliquity needed.

Glenohumeral Joint: To visualize the glenohumeral joint for fracture or dislocation, position the patient's arm of the side of interest down by the side or on the hip, if tolerated by the patient (also known as the "Y" position, Fig. 3–80).

Acromion and Coracoid Process: Place the hand and forearm of the side of interest on top of the patient's head, if tolerated by the patient (Fig. 3–81).

STRUCTURES DEMONSTRATED: The lateral and medial borders of the scapula should be superimposed. The entire scapula should be seen (Fig. 3–82). AP obliques show side up.

COMMON ERRORS: (1) Patient's scapula obliqued instead of lateralized. If the x-ray is taken in an AP oblique projection (RPO or LPO positions) and if only the lateral border is superimposed over the ribs, then the patient is not obliqued enough. If only the medial border is superimposed over the ribs, then the patient is obliqued too much. Reverse the positions (RAO or LAO) and use the same respective corrective measures. (2) Technique too light to visualize the superior aspect of the scapula.

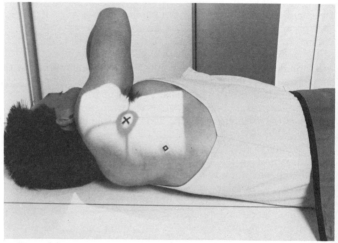

FIGURE 3–78. Lateral scapula recumbent with arm wrap. Diamond marks inferior border of scapula.

NOTES:

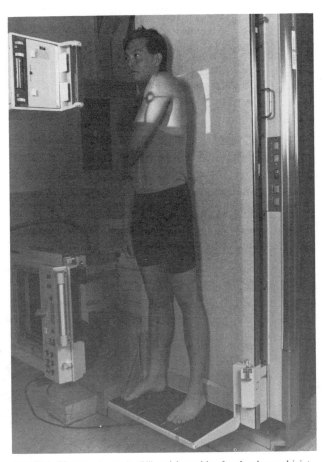

FIGURE 3–79. Lateral scapula "Y" upright position for glenohumeral joint.

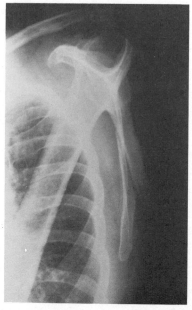

FIGURE 3–80. Fractured, lateral scapular "Y" x-ray with arm crossed over to opposite hip. Make sure the upper as well as the lower portion of the scapula is included on the film. (Courtesy of Maureen Wade, S.R.T.)

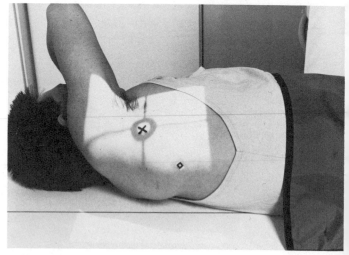

FIGURE 3–81. Lateral scapula with elevated arm position for the acromion and coracoid process.

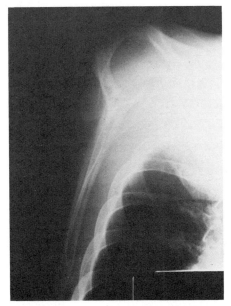

FIGURE 3–82. Lateral scapula x-ray with arm wrap.

TECHNIQUE

KV _____ MA _____ SECS _____ MAS _____ CALIPER _____ cm

_____ :1 GRID / B / none SCREEN: RE / High / Par / Detail / None

SID: _____ Rm _____ ADULT / CHILD age: _____ mos. / yrs.

HABITUS: Hyper / s / hypo / a XS S M L XL XXL

Lower Extremities

TOES: DORSOPLANTAR (AP)

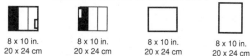

| 8 x 10 in. | 8 x 10 in. | 8 x 10 in. | 8 x 10 in. |
| 20 x 24 cm | 20 x 24 cm | 20 x 24 cm | 20 x 24 cm |

FILM: No grid or table Bucky. Use tabletop only. Collimate to the area of interest.

CR: For entire distal foot, at the 2nd metatarsophalangeal joint.

For isolation of 1st (great) toe, at 1st metatarsophalangeal joint.

For isolation of 2nd through 5th toes, at the proximal interphalangeal joint of each (Fig. 4–1).

Perpendicular or with a 10-degree cephalic (proximal) angle in order to flatten the curled toes.

POSITION: The patient is supinated recumbent on the table or is sitting up on the table.

Help the patient flex his or her knee while placing the patient's distal toes flat against the surface of the film.

The plantar surface is flat against the film, and the toes are centered to the film. If the film slides on the tabletop away from the patient, have the patient slightly increase the flexion of the knee or simply place a sandbag against the distal edge of the film.

Place the hip, knee, and foot in the same longitudinal plane.

NOTE: Use a plantodorsal projection or PA projection of the toes when toes are excessively curled (i.e., hammertoes).

STRUCTURES DEMONSTRATED: Demonstration of the entire foot (Fig. 4–2, on left) or only the distal metatarsals, metatarsophalangeal joints, and complete phalanx (or phalanges) of interest (Fig. 4–8, on left).

COMMON ERROR: Overpenetration of the distal phalanges. Do not use a foot technique for toes. Toes require less technique than the foot.

TECHNIQUE

KV _____ MA _____ SECS _____ MAS _____ CALIPER _____ cm

_____ :1 GRID / B / none SCREEN: RE / High / Par / Detail / None

SID: _____ Rm _____ ADULT / CHILD age: _____ mos. / yrs.

HABITUS: Hyper / s / hypo / a   XS   S   M   L   XL   XXL

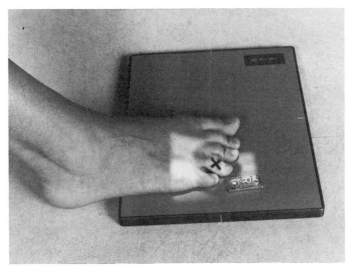

FIGURE 4–1. AP projection 4th toe.

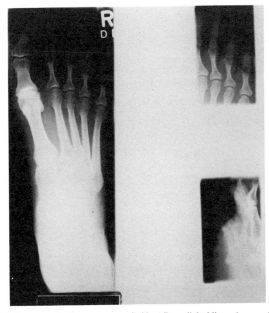

FIGURE 4–2. AP projection toes x-ray (left), AP medial oblique (upper right), and lateral toes (lower right).

TOES: AP MEDIAL (INTERNAL) OBLIQUE

| 8 x 10 in. | 8 x 10 in. | 8 x 10 in. | 8 x 10 in. |
| 20 x 24 cm | 20 x 24 cm | 20 x 24 cm | 20 x 24 cm |

FILM: No grid or table Bucky. Use tabletop only. Collimate to the area of interest.

CR: Perpendicular.

For entire distal foot, at the 2nd metatarsophalangeal joint.

For isolation of 1st (great) toe, at 1st metatarsophalangeal joint.

For isolation of 2nd through 5th toes, at the proximal interphalangeal joint of each (Fig. 4–3).

POSITION: Place the toes flat on the unexposed side of film cassette.

Internally rotate the foot 45 degrees medially. The lateral toes (#3, 4, and 5) will be elevated slightly from the surface of the film. Use a radiolucent sponge for support if necessary for patient comfort and stabilization.

STRUCTURES DEMONSTRATED: The entire phalanges (Fig. 4–4), 1 through 5, or the toe of interest in the oblique aspect (Fig. 4–2, upper right, and Fig. 4–8, middle).

COMMON ERROR: Not enough obliquity. If this projection is used in lieu of a lateral projection, the degree of obliquity must be severe in order to view the posterior aspect of the phalanges.

TECHNIQUE

KV _____ MA _____ SECS _____ MAS _____ CALIPER _____ cm

_____ :1 GRID / B / none SCREEN: RE / High / Par / Detail / None

SID: _____ Rm _____ ADULT / CHILD age: _____ mos. / yrs.

HABITUS: Hyper / s / hypo / a   XS   S   M   L   XL   XXL

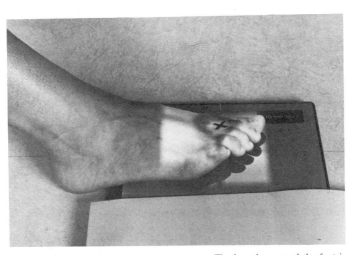

FIGURE 4–3. AP medial oblique projection toes. The lateral aspect of the foot is elevated off of the film.

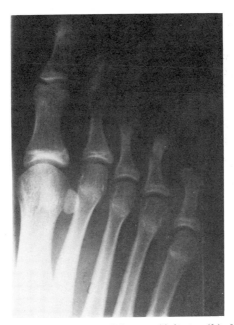

FIGURE 4–4. AP medial oblique x-ray of the toes with fracture (fx) of 4th proximal phalanx (also see Fig. 4–2, upper right).

TOES: LATERAL

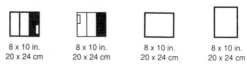

8 x 10 in.   8 x 10 in.   8 x 10 in.   8 x 10 in.
20 x 24 cm   20 x 24 cm   20 x 24 cm   20 x 24 cm

FILM: No grid or table Bucky. Use tabletop only. Collimate to the area of interest.

CR: For isolation of 1st (great) toe, perpendicular at 1st metatarsophalangeal joint (Fig. 4–5).

For isolation of 2nd through 5th toes, at the proximal interphalangeal joint of each (Fig. 4–6).

POSITION: Place the foot on the medial aspect if the toe of interest is #1 or #2 (see Fig. 4–5).

Place the foot on its lateral surface if the toe of interest is #3, #4, or #5.

Test the range of motion by asking the patient to fan, or extend the toes if comfortably able to do so. (This should not be attempted if a severe fracture is suspected.) Depending upon this ability, isolate the remaining toes out of the area of interest by using a small wedge of radiolucent sponge between the uninjured toe and the injured toe, or simply lateralize the toe of interest when a good range of motion is exhibited upon fanning the toes. Taping can be used if it doesn't place stress upon the injury (Fig. 4–6).

NOTES:

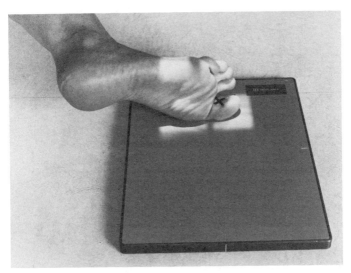

FIGURE 4–5. Lateral #1 toe. Use a lateral-to-medial projection.

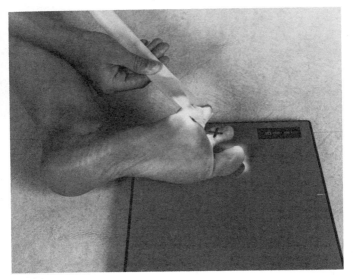

FIGURE 4–6. Lateral #2 toe (use tape only if patient can tolerate it; take care not to manipulate injured toe).

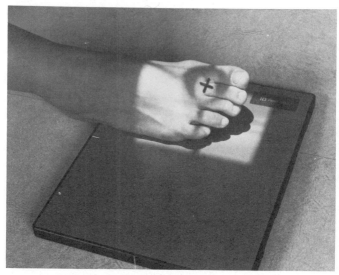

FIGURE 4–7. AP lateral oblique projection of the toes.

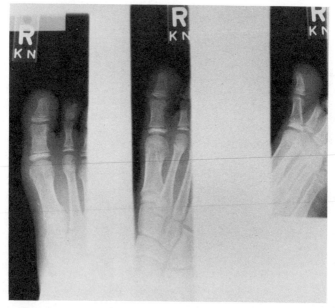

FIGURE 4–8. Example of three-view routine of individual toe. PA (left), PA oblique (center), lateral (left) of right 1st toe x-ray.

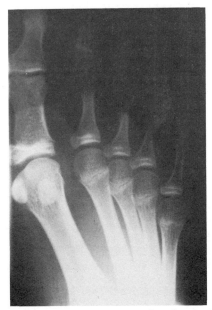

FIGURE 4–9. AP lateral oblique x-ray of the toes. Sometimes used when individual lateral toe positioning is unsuccessful.

NOTE: Should all else fail in the attempt to lateralize individual toes, both an AP lateral (external) oblique and AP medial (internal) oblique of the toes may be helpful in the absence of a lateral projection (Fig. 4–7).

STRUCTURES DEMONSTRATED: The toe of interest in a lateral aspect free from superimposition of the noninjured toes (Fig. 4–2, lower right, and Fig. 4–8, right).

The metatarsophalangeal articulation should be included. If the individual toe cannot be isolated, a lateral oblique is performed (Fig. 4–9).

COMMON ERROR: Superimposition. Use an increased technique from the AP or AP medial oblique. If there is some unavoidable superimposition, the toe of interest can still be visualized with a slightly increased technique.

TECHNIQUE

KV _____ MA _____ SECS _____ MAS _____ CALIPER _____ cm

_____ :1 GRID / B / none SCREEN: RE / High / Par / Detail / None

SID: _____ Rm _____ ADULT / CHILD age: _____ mos. / yrs.

HABITUS: Hyper / s / hypo / a   XS   S   M   L   XL   XXL

SESAMOIDS: TANGENTIAL

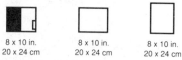

| 8 x 10 in. | 8 x 10 in. | 8 x 10 in. |
| 20 x 24 cm | 20 x 24 cm | 20 x 24 cm |

FILM: No grid or table Bucky. Use tabletop only. Collimate to the area of interest.

CR: Perpendicularly, on the plantar surface at the 1st metatarso-phalangeal articulation.

POSITION

Method A: The patient is supine on the table with legs extended.

The foot is comfortably dorsiflexed; the toes are pulled back (hyperextended). If the patient is unable to maintain this position, a length of gauze, a Penrose surgical drain, or other type of elastic tourniquet with the patient applying gentle pressure may be used in order to hyperextend the toes (Fig. 4–10). Place the plantar aspect of the 1st metatarsophalangeal joint just beyond the plane of the plantar surface of the calcaneus and distal phalanx.

Method B: The patient is pronated on the table with legs extended.

The weight of the lower leg is placed upon the fully extended toes. The foot is not dorsiflexed. The calcaneus must be positioned so as not to superimpose the sesamoids of the 1st metatarsopha-langeal articulation. This can be controlled by increasing or decreasing the flexion of the foot at the metatarsophalangeal joints (Fig. 4–11).

NOTES:

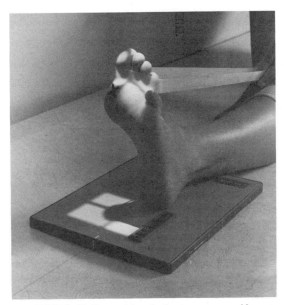

FIGURE 4–10. Tangential projection toes-up sesamoids.

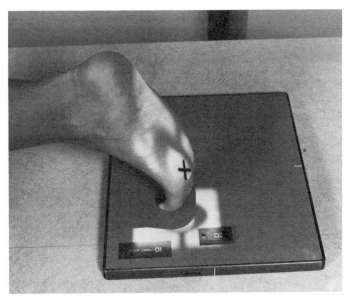

FIGURE 4–11. Tangential projection toes-down sesamoids.

STRUCTURES DEMONSTRATED: A magnified tangential projection of the first metatarsal head with the sesamoids isolated from superimposition (Fig. 4–12).
COMMON ERROR: Method A—superimposition of the sesamoids by overpositioning! Simply think of this as an AP ankle position with the centering over the sesamoids (Fig. 4–13). Method B— lack of sufficient extension at the metatarsophalangeal articulations, causing superimposition of the calcaneus and sesamoids.

TECHNIQUE

KV _____ MA _____ SECS _____ MAS _____ CALIPER _____ cm
_____ :1 GRID / B / none SCREEN: RE / High / Par / Detail / None
SID: _____ Rm _____ ADULT / CHILD age: _____ mos. / yrs.
HABITUS: Hyper / s / hypo / a   XS   S   M   L   XL   XXL

NOTES:

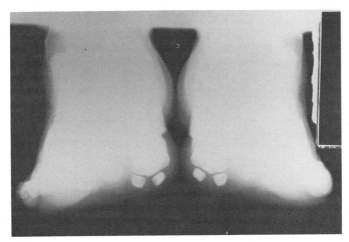

FIGURE 4–12. Bilateral, tangential projection sesamoids x-ray (use tighter collimation and marker).

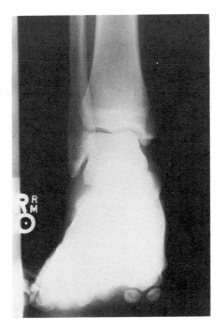

FIGURE 4–13. An AP x-ray of the dorsiflexed ankle with wider than usual collimation demonstrating a tangential view of the sesamoids.

FOOT: DORSOPLANTAR (AP)

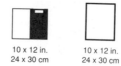

10 x 12 in.   10 x 12 in.
24 x 30 cm   24 x 30 cm

FILM: No grid or table Bucky. Use tabletop only. Collimate to the area of interest.

CR: Either: (1) perpendicular centered midfoot at the level of the 3rd metatarsal's base, or (2) use a 10-degree cephalic (proximal) angle centered at the midfoot level of the base of the 3rd metatarsal (Fig. 4–14). This opens the tarsal articulations.

NOTE: Whenever an angle is used that is directed toward the lower axial skeleton, lead shielding should be provided to the patient. Do not use the overhead distance indicators to measure the source-to-image distance (SID) for any tube angle. Always use the tape measure along the path of the central ray to measure to the tabletop or film when using a tube angle.

POSITION: The patient is supinated recumbent on the table or is sitting up on the table.

Help the patient bend the knee while placing the patient's foot flat against the surface of one side of the film (Fig. 4–15).

The plantar surface is flat against the film and is centered to the space allotted on the film. To avoid film slippage, have the patient increase the flexion of the knee while using gonadal shielding, or simply place a sandbag against the distal edge of the film.

NOTES:

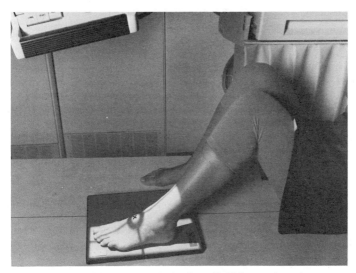

FIGURE 4–14. Left AP projection foot with 10-degree tube angle.

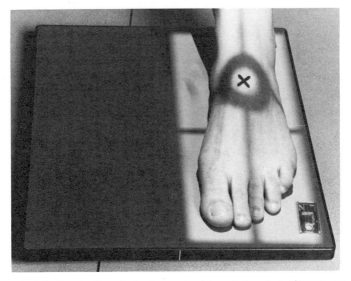

FIGURE 4–15. Left AP projection foot centered for a first exposure of two-on-one film.

Place the hip, knee, and foot in the same longitudinal axis.

Occasionally, a wedge filter attached to the collimator housing is used with the thicker side over the thinnest anatomical area (the toes) in order to mediate the exposure over the greatly differing thicknesses of the foot.

STRUCTURES DEMONSTRATED: All tarsals distal to the talus, all metatarsals, phalanges with sesamoids usually found at the 1st metatarsophalangeal articulation on the plantar surface of the foot (Fig. 4–16). The use of an angle (see CR, above) demonstrates the open tarsal articulations.

NOTE: When taking x-rays for congenital deformities of the feet (i.e., talipes equinovarus), do not attempt to correct the position of the foot. Take the routine projections "as is."

COMMON ERROR: Underpenetration of the tarsals. Adjust your technique for the area of injury. Lower the technique for injury to the distal foot and increase from this technique when the area of interest is the midfoot, or proximal foot. The use of a step-wedge filter attached to the collimator is also recommended.

TECHNIQUE

KV _____MA _____SECS _____MAS _____CALIPER _____cm

_____ :1 GRID / B / none SCREEN: RE / High / Par / Detail / None

SID: _____ Rm _____ ADULT / CHILD   age: _____ mos. / yrs.

HABITUS: Hyper / s / hypo / a   XS   S   M   L   XL   XXL

NOTES:

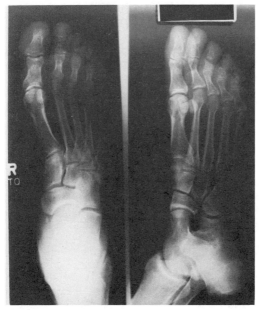

FIGURE 4–16. AP projection (left) and AP internal (medial) oblique projection (right) of the right foot x-ray.

FOOT: AP MEDIAL (INTERNAL) OBLIQUE

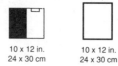

10 x 12 in.   10 x 12 in.
24 x 30 cm   24 x 30 cm

FILM: No grid or table Bucky. Use tabletop only. Collimate to the area of interest.

CR: Perpendicular to the midfoot, dorsal surface, at the level of the base of the 3rd metatarsal.

POSITION: Place foot flat on unexposed side of film cassette.

Internally rotate the foot 30 to 45 degrees medially. The lateral aspect of the foot should be elevated no more than 1 inch (2.5 cm) from the film's surface (Fig. 4–17).

NOTE: When taking x-rays for congenital deformities of the feet (i.e., talipes equinovarus), do not attempt to correct the position of the foot. Take the routine projections "as is."

STRUCTURES DEMONSTRATED: This obliquity allows the best demonstration of the articulations located on the lateral aspect of the foot (Fig. 4–18, on right). The opposite oblique, the lateral (external) oblique, will best demonstrate the articulations on the medial side of the foot.

The tarsal articulations on the lateral aspect will be opened.

COMMON ERROR: Underpenetration of the tarsals. Adjust your technique for the area of injury. Lower the technique for injury to the distal foot and increase from this technique when the area of interest is the midfoot, or proximal foot. The use of a step-wedge filter attached to the collimator is also recommended.

TECHNIQUE

KV _____ MA _____ SECS _____ MAS _____ CALIPER _____ cm

_____ :1 GRID / B / none SCREEN: RE / High / Par / Detail / None

SID: _____ Rm _____ ADULT / CHILD age: _____ mos. / yrs.

HABITUS: Hyper / s / hypo / a   XS   S   M   L   XL   XXL

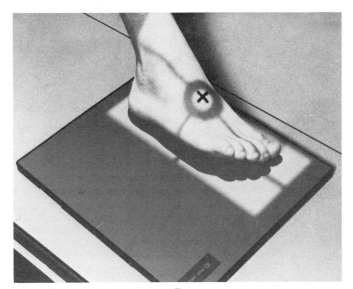

FIGURE 4–17. Right AP internal (medial) oblique projection of foot.

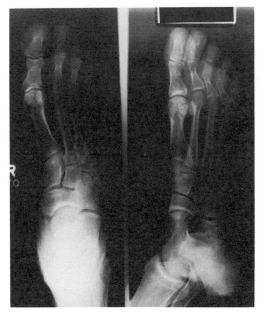

FIGURE 4–18. AP projection (left) and AP internal (medial) oblique projection (right) of the right foot x-ray.

FOOT: LATERAL

10 x 12 in.
24 x 30 cm

10 x 12 in.
24 x 30 cm

FILM: Use tabletop only. Collimate to the area of interest.

CR: Perpendicular to midtarsals, on the medial surface of the foot, near the highest point of the arch (Fig. 4–19).

POSITION: Patient should be recumbent or sitting up on the table.

Turn the patient toward the side of interest.

Sponge the knee in order to correctly lateralize the ankle.

Method A: The leg of the side of interest is rotated so that the foot lies on the lateral (external) surface. This is a medial-to-lateral projection of the foot (Fig. 4–19).

The knee is flexed. Place a support (sponge) under the knee to elevate it slightly. This will prevent the foot from being overrotated.

The foot will be slightly inverted. The plantar surface of the foot will *not* be perpendicular to the film for this position, a "lazy" lateral.

Method B: Take a lateral-to-medial projection of the foot for the position to result in a true lateral.

The foot is lying on its medial (internal) surface (Fig. 4–20).

The plantar surface of the foot must be perpendicular to the film surface in order to be a true lateral.

Center the foot to the film placed lengthwise, or if a large foot, use the film diagonally.

NOTE: When taking x-rays for congenital deformities of the feet (i.e., talipes equinovarus), do not attempt to correct the position of the foot. Take the routine projections "as is."

NOTES:

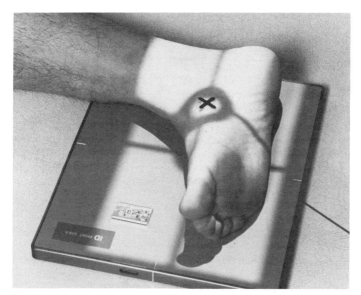

FIGURE 4–19. Lateral foot (mediolateral projection of right foot). A "lazy" lateral that will demonstrate the base of the fifth metatarsal. You can make sure the entire foot (toes and heel) is included on the film and within collimation by simply observing the shadow cast by the collimator light.

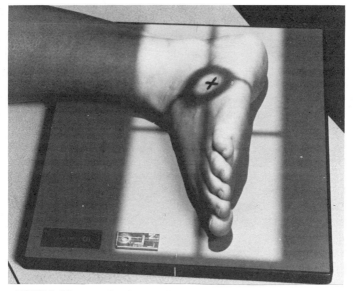

FIGURE 4–20. Lateral foot (lateromedial projection of left foot). A true lateral.

STRUCTURES DEMONSTRATED: The lateral aspect of the foot is demonstrated. This position best demonstrates anterior or posterior displacements of fractures, or foreign bodies.

The tibiotalar articulation is seen.

The base of the 5th metatarsal is isolated in the medial-to-lateral projection (lazy lateral) of the foot (Fig. 4–21). This is a common fracture site of the foot.

COMMON ERROR: Underpenetration of the tarsal area. The technique must be increased over the dorsoplantar and medial oblique projections. Use an ankle technique.

TECHNIQUE

KV _____ MA _____ SECS _____ MAS _____ CALIPER _____ cm

_____ :1 GRID / B / none SCREEN: RE / High / Par / Detail / None

SID: _____ Rm _____ ADULT / CHILD age: _____ mos. / yrs.

HABITUS: Hyper / s / hypo / a XS S M L XL XXL

NOTES:

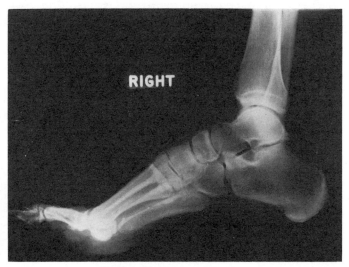

FIGURE 4–21. Mediolateral foot x-ray.

NOTES:

CALCANEUS: PLANTODORSAL

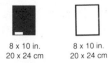

8 x 10 in.   8 x 10 in.
20 x 24 cm   20 x 24 cm

FILM: No grid or table Bucky. Use tabletop only. Collimate to the area of interest.

CR: Enters the plantar surface of the midfoot at a 40-degree cephalic (proximal) angle. Place the central ray midfoot at the base of the 3rd metatarsal joint (Fig. 4–22).

POSITION: The patient is supine on the table. Have him or her sit up if able to assist with the exam.

Place the plantar surface of the foot perpendicularly to the film's surface, toes up. The foot is dorsiflexed, and the toes are pulled back (hyperextended) by using a length of gauze around the foot at the level of the metatarsophalangeal articulations. Have the patient hold the end of the gauze firmly and pull back. This removes the distal metatarsals and phalanges from superimposing the calcaneus.

Do not delay; this position is uncomfortable for the patient to maintain.

NOTE: Whenever you use an angle toward the body or the tube is centered near the abdominal area, use gonadal shielding.

STRUCTURES DEMONSTRATED: The distal calcaneus and tuberosity. The subtalar articulations of the calcaneus if sufficiently penetrated.

The medial aspect should demonstrate the sustentaculum tali and medial tuberosity (Fig. 4–23).

The lateral aspect should demonstrate the lateral process and trochlear process. The lateral aspect can be identified by locating the 5th metatarsal.

COMMON ERROR: Underpenetration. The calcaneus should be penetrated sufficiently that the subtalar joint is demonstrated on the film.

TECHNIQUE

KV _____ MA _____ SECS _____ MAS _____ CALIPER _____ cm

_____ :1 GRID / B / none SCREEN: RE / High / Par / Detail / None

SID: _____ Rm _____ ADULT / CHILD age: _____ mos. / yrs.

HABITUS: Hyper / s / hypo / a   XS   S   M   L   XL   XXL

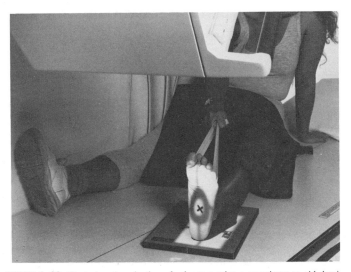

FIGURE 4–22. Plantodorsal projection of calcaneus using a tourniquet to aid dorsiflexion of the foot.

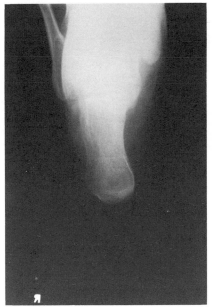

FIGURE 4–23. X-ray of plantodorsal projection of right calcaneus taken for distal aspect (underpenetrated for proximal area).

CALCANEUS: DORSOPLANTAR

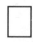

8 x 10 in.   8 x 10 in.   10 x 12 in.   10 x 12 in.
20 x 24 cm   20 x 24 cm   24 x 30 cm   24 x 30 cm

FILM: No grid or table Bucky. Use tabletop only. Collimate to the area of interest.

CR: Enters the Achilles area to penetrate the dorsal surface of the midfoot at a 40-degree caudal (distal) angle (Fig. 4–24).

Place the central ray so that it exits midfoot at the level of the base of the 3rd metatarsal articulation.

POSITION: The patient is pronated on the table. Elevate the ankle with radiolucent sponges until the toes just touch the surface of the table.

Place the plantar surface of the foot perpendicularly to the x-ray table's surface, toes down. Use a film holder or footboard in order for the film to rest against the plantar surface of the foot. The knee may be padded for the plantar surface to be in contact with the film's surface.

Do not delay; this position is sometimes uncomfortable for the patient to maintain for a length of time.

NOTE: Whenever you use an angle toward the body or the tube is centered near the abdominal area, use gonadal shielding.

STRUCTURES DEMONSTRATED: The distal calcaneus and tuberosity. The subtalar articulations of the calcaneus if sufficiently penetrated.

The medial aspect should demonstrate the sustentaculum tali and medial tuberosity (similar to Fig. 4–23).

The lateral aspect should demonstrate the lateral process and trochlear process. The lateral aspect can be identified by locating the 5th metatarsal.

COMMON ERROR: Underpenetration. The calcaneus should be penetrated sufficiently that the subtalar joint is demonstrated on the film.

TECHNIQUE

KV _____ MA _____ SECS _____ MAS _____ CALIPER _____ cm

_____ :1 GRID / B / none SCREEN: RE / High / Par / Detail / None

SID: _____ Rm _____ ADULT / CHILD age: _____ mos. / yrs.

HABITUS: Hyper / s / hypo / a   XS   S   M   L   XL   XXL

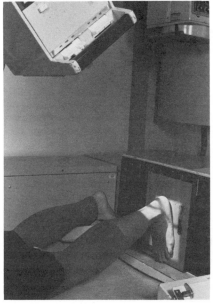

FIGURE 4–24. Dorsoplantar projection of calcaneus using the footboard as a film holder.

CALCANEUS: LATERAL

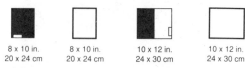

| 8 x 10 in. | 8 x 10 in. | 10 x 12 in. | 10 x 12 in. |
| 20 x 24 cm | 20 x 24 cm | 24 x 30 cm | 24 x 30 cm |

FILM: No grid or table Bucky. Use tabletop only. Collimate to the area of interest.

CR: Perpendicularly to the medial surface of the midcalcaneus (1 inch or 2.54 cm below the medial malleolus).

POSITION: The patient is recumbent and rolled up toward the side of interest for the mediolateral projection (Fig. 4–25).

Slightly dorsiflex the foot if the patient tolerates it; otherwise, take as is if the range of motion is impaired.

Place a sponge under the knee to prevent overrotation.

NOTE: A crosstable lateral of the calcaneus can be taken when fractures are obvious or when the patient is severely debilitated.

STRUCTURES DEMONSTRATED: The entire tibiotalar articulation in profile (Fig. 4–26).

The lateral malleolus will be seen superimposed over the talus.

The sinus tarsi partially open.

The subtalar articulations.

COMMON ERROR: Overrotation, demonstrated by the fibula's extreme posterior position. Pad the knee to avoid overrotation of the calcaneus.

TECHNIQUE

KV _____ MA _____ SECS _____ MAS _____ CALIPER _____ cm

_____ :1 GRID / B / none SCREEN: RE / High / Par / Detail / None

SID: _____ Rm _____ ADULT / CHILD age: _____ mos. / yrs.

HABITUS: Hyper / s / hypo / a   XS   S   M   L   XL   XXL

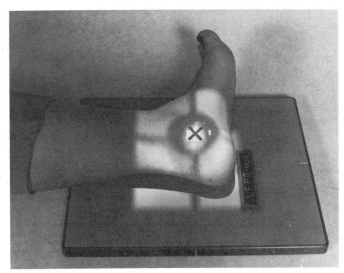

FIGURE 4–25. A mediolateral position of the calcaneus.

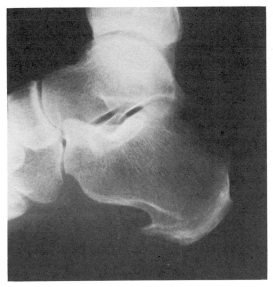

FIGURE 4–26. Lateral calcaneus x-ray.

ANKLE: AP

| 10 x 12 in. | 10 x 12 in. | 8 x 10 in. | 8 x 10 in. |
| 24 x 30 cm | 24 x 30 cm | 20 x 24 cm | 20 x 24 cm |

FILM: No grid or table Bucky. Use tabletop only. Collimate to the area of interest.

CR: Perpendicularly, at the anterior surface, midankle between the medial and lateral malleoli.

POSITION: The patient is supine on the table. The leg of interest is extended, with the knee in alignment with the ankle (Fig. 4–27).

NOTE: When moving a fractured ankle, support the entire lower leg and foot. Minimize movement of the extremity by sliding the film under the gurney (or bed) sheet. On postreductions of the ankle, only the AP and lateral projections are usually taken. A wet plaster cast needs more kVp than a dry one. A fiberglass cast generally requires less technique than a plaster cast. Be careful, however, of abnormally thick casts or abnormally thin partial casts or splints, which may throw your techniques off.

Method A: The plantar surface of the foot is perpendicular to the film's surface, toes up. The foot is dorsiflexed without pulling the toes back (extended) (Fig. 4–28). This moves the calcaneus inferiorly to avoid superimposition of the calcaneus over the distal lateral malleolus. The 3rd metatarsal and phalanx are perpendicular to the film (Fig. 4–27).

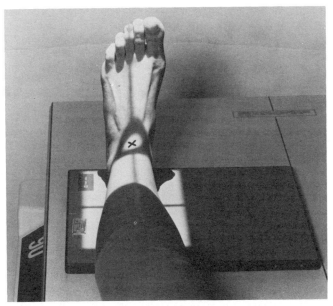

FIGURE 4–27. AP projection of ankle with no obliquity.

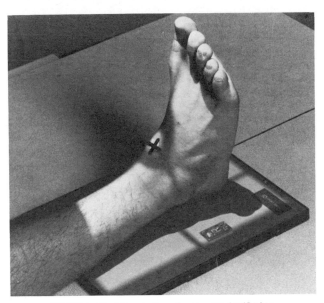

FIGURE 4–28. AP projection of ankle with dorsiflexion.

Method B: The AP is taken with the ankle slightly internally rotated, 5 to 10 degrees. A plane between the internal and external malleoli (the intermalleolar line) will be parallel to the film.[10, 11, 12] Align the 4th metatarsal and phalanx perpendicularly to the film (Fig. 4–29). Make sure the entire foot is dorsiflexed without just simply pulling the toes back.

STRUCTURES DEMONSTRATED

Method A: The ankle mortise is slightly obstructed with slight overlap of the talofibular joint space (Fig. 4–30).

The tibotalar joint space will be open at its medial and superior aspects.

Method B: The ankle mortise is seen in its entirety (Fig. 4–31). The talofibular space is open, isolating the lateral malleolus. The tibiofibular space may be partially obscured.

The surfaces of the talus are relatively free from superimposition on its medial, superior, and lateral aspects.

COMMON ERROR: (1) Insufficient penetration. Trabecular patterns must be demonstrated on the talus. (2) Superimposition of the calcaneus over the lateral malleolus. Not enough dorsiflexion.

TECHNIQUE

KV _____ MA _____ SECS _____ MAS _____ CALIPER _____ cm

_____ :1 GRID / B / none SCREEN: RE / High / Par / Detail / None

SID: _____ Rm _____ ADULT / CHILD age: _____ mos. / yrs.

HABITUS: Hyper / s / hypo / a   XS   S   M   L   XL   XXL

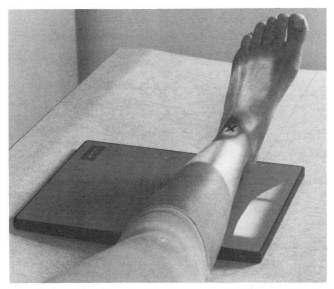

FIGURE 4–29. AP projection of ankle with approximately 10 degrees obliquity for demonstration of the ankle mortise.

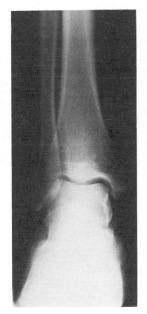

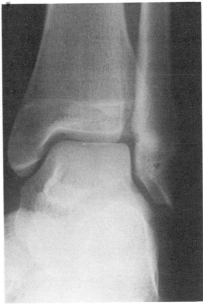

FIGURE 4–30. AP x-ray of right ankle.

FIGURE 4–31. AP x-ray of left ankle with 10 degrees obliquity for demonstration of the ankle mortise. This is a close-up demonstrating the trabecular pattern of the bone.

ANKLE: AP MEDIAL (INTERNAL) OBLIQUE

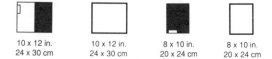

| 10 x 12 in.
24 x 30 cm | 10 x 12 in.
24 x 30 cm | 8 x 10 in.
20 x 24 cm | 8 x 10 in.
20 x 24 cm |

FILM: No grid or table Bucky. Use tabletop only. Collimate to the area of interest.

CR: Perpendicularly, at the anterior, obliqued surface, midankle between the medial and lateral malleoli.

POSITION: The patient is supine on the table.

The plantar surface of the foot is perpendicular to the film's surface, toes up. The foot is dorsiflexed. This moves the calcaneus more inferiorly in order to avoid superimposition of the calcaneus over the distal lateral malleolus.

Rotate the leg by moving the hip, knee, and ankle as a unit 30 to 45 degrees medially (Fig. 4–32). Rotating the ankle 30 degrees usually is enough to open the articular surfaces between the talus and fibula, as well as those between the tibia and fibula.

NOTE: When moving a fractured ankle, support the entire lower leg and foot. Minimize movement of the extremity by sliding the film under the gurney (or bed) sheet. On postreductions of the ankle, only the AP and lateral projections are taken. A wet plaster cast needs more kVp than a dry one. A fiberglass cast generally requires less technique than a plaster cast. Be careful, however, of abnormally thick casts or abnormally thin partial casts or splints, which may throw your techniques off.

STRUCTURES DEMONSTRATED: The distal tibia and fibula particularly, the malleoli free from superimposition (Fig. 4–33).

The greater the degree of dorsiflexion (with no toe extension), the better the visualization of the superior aspect of the talus.

COMMON ERROR: Poor dorsiflexion resulting in a obstructed view of the lateral malleolus. Not including enough long bone on the film may result in a missed spiral fracture diagnosis.

TECHNIQUE

KV _____ MA _____ SECS _____ MAS _____ CALIPER _____ cm

_____ :1 GRID / B / none SCREEN: RE / High / Par / Detail / None

SID: _____ Rm _____ ADULT / CHILD age: _____ mos. / yrs.

HABITUS: Hyper / s / hypo / a   XS   S   M   L   XL   XXL

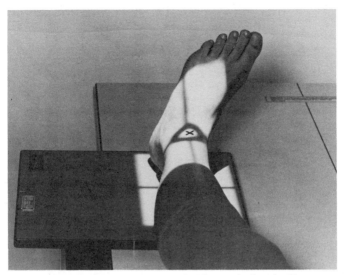

FIGURE 4–32. AP internal (medial) oblique projection of ankle.

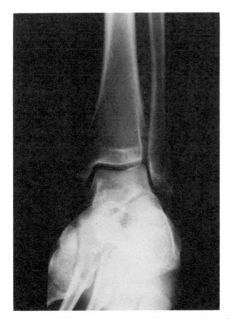

FIGURE 4–33. X-ray of AP internal (medial) oblique projection of left ankle.

ANKLE: LATERAL

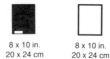

8 x 10 in.   8 x 10 in.
20 x 24 cm   20 x 24 cm

FILM: No grid or table Bucky. Use tabletop only. Collimate to the area of interest.

CR: Perpendicular at 1 inch (2.54 cm) above the lateral malleolus or at the medial malleolus.

POSITION: The patient is recumbent and rolled up toward the side of interest for the mediolateral projection (roll them away from the side of interest for the lateromedial projection of the ankle).

Slightly dorsiflex the foot if the patient tolerates it; otherwise, take as is if the range of motion is impaired.

Place a sponge under the knee to prevent overrotation (Fig. 4–34).

NOTE: A crosstable lateral of the ankle can be taken when fractures are obvious or when the patient is severely debilitated.

STRUCTURES DEMONSTRATED: The tibiotalar articulation in profile.

The lateral malleolus will be seen superimposed over the talus (Fig. 4–35).

NOTE: When moving a fractured ankle, support the entire lower leg and foot. Minimize movement of the extremity by shooting a crosstable lateral. On postreductions of the ankle, only the AP and lateral projections are taken.

COMMON ERROR: Underpenetration. The technique must be sufficient to see the shadow of the lateral malleolus through the talus.

TECHNIQUE

KV _____ MA _____ SECS _____ MAS _____ CALIPER _____ cm

_____ :1 GRID / B / none SCREEN: RE / High / Par / Detail / None

SID: _____ Rm _____ ADULT / CHILD age: _____ mos. / yrs.

HABITUS: Hyper / s / hypo / a XS S M L XL XXL

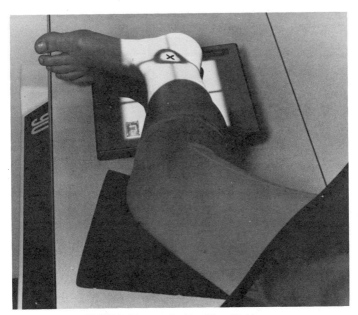

FIGURE 4–34. Lateral ankle with padded knee.

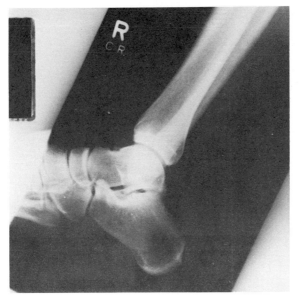

FIGURE 4–35. X-ray of right lateral ankle.

LOWER LEG (TIBIA AND FIBULA): AP

7 x 17 in.
18 x 43 cm

7 x 17 in.
18 x 43 cm

14 x 17 in.
35 x 43 cm

14 x 17 in.
35 x 43 cm

FILM: No grid or table Bucky. Use tabletop only. Collimate to the area of interest.

CR: Perpendicularly at midshaft, equidistant from each articulation.

POSITION: The patient is supine on the table.

The ankle, knee, and hip are in the same longitudinal plane (Fig. 4–36).

The plantar surface of the foot is perpendicular to the film's surface, toes up. The foot and ankle are dorsiflexed. This moves the calcaneus more inferiorly in order to avoid superimposition of the calcaneus over the distal lateral malleolus (Fig. 4–37). Another way to accomplish this is to slightly invert the foot when dorsiflexed slightly.

NOTES:

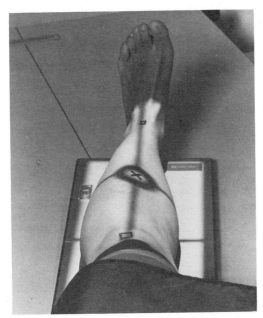

FIGURE 4–36. AP projection of lower leg (tibia and fibula). Knee joint space *(proximal, large square)*. Ankle mortise *(distal, small square)*.

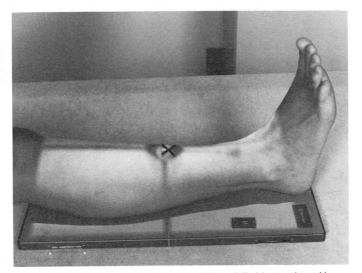

FIGURE 4–37. AP projection of lower leg (tibia and fibula), attention ankle.

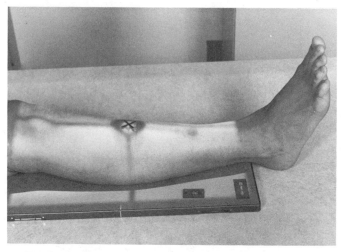

FIGURE 4–38. AP projection of lower leg (tibia and fibula), attention knee.

When positioning the AP lower leg with attention to the knee (Fig. 4–38), use gonadal shielding as the area of interest is relatively near the gonadal area.

NOTE: When moving a fractured leg, support the entire lower leg, ankle, and foot. Minimize movement of the extremity by sliding the film under the gurney (or bed) sheet. On postreductions of the lower leg, only the AP and lateral projections are usually taken. A wet plaster cast needs more kVp than a dry one. A fiberglass cast generally requires less technique than a plaster cast. Be careful, however, of abnormally thick casts or abnormally thin partial casts or splints, which may throw your techniques off.

STRUCTURES DEMONSTRATED: The shafts of the tibia and fibula will show separation along the diaphyses (shafts) with superimposition at their articular aspects (Fig. 4–39).

Both articulations, the knee and the ankle, should be included on the film. Occasionally due to film length limits, only one articulation will be included, that nearest the injury (Figs. 4–37 and 4–38).

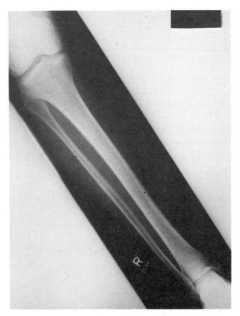

FIGURE 4–39. AP projection of lower leg (tibia and fibula) x-ray using a film cassette diagonally.

The proximal tibiofibular articulation will be slightly superimposed by the lateral condyle of the tibia.

The distal tibiofibular articulation will not be open with this position. The talofibular articulation may be open if the foot was slightly inverted and slightly medially obliqued.

COMMON ERROR: (1) Technique too light for the thicker (proximal) aspect of the lower leg. Bony trabecular markings will not be demonstrated with a technique that is too low. (2) Both articulations are not included. Some technologists increase their 40 inches (or 100 cm) SID slightly in order to include both articulations on the film. Be sure that the knee and ankle joint distance measures less than the length of your film; otherwise, the SID increase won't help anyway—the extremity doesn't fit on your film!

TECHNIQUE

KV _____ MA _____ SECS _____ MAS _____ CALIPER _____ cm

_____ :1 GRID / B / none SCREEN: RE / High / Par / Detail / None

SID: _____ Rm _____ ADULT / CHILD age: _____ mos. / yrs.

HABITUS: Hyper / s / hypo / a   XS   S   M   L   XL   XXL

LOWER LEG (TIBIA AND FIBULA): LATERAL

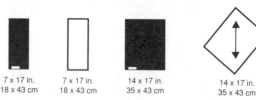

| 7 x 17 in. | 7 x 17 in. | 14 x 17 in. | 14 x 17 in. |
| 18 x 43 cm | 18 x 43 cm | 35 x 43 cm | 35 x 43 cm |

FILM: No grid or table Bucky. Use tabletop only. Collimate to the area of interest.

CR: Perpendicularly at midshaft, equistant from each articulation.

POSITION: The patient is supine on the table. Have the patient roll up on the side of interest in order to lateralize the lower leg.

The lateralized ankle and knee should be in the same longitudinal plane. The knee is flexed slightly.

The plantar surface of the foot is perpendicular to the film's surface.

Sponge the calcaneus to lateralize the knee (Fig. 4–40), or sponge the knee to lateralize the ankle. The articulation nearest the injury needs to be lateralized correctly.

NOTE: A crosstable lateral of the lower leg can be taken when fractures are obvious or when the patient is severely debilitated (Fig. 4–41). As the area of interest is relatively near the pelvic area, use gonadal shielding. When moving a fractured leg, support the entire lower leg, ankle, and foot. Minimize movement of the extremity by sliding the film under the gurney (or bed) sheet. On postreductions of the lower leg, only the AP and lateral projections are usually taken. A wet plaster cast needs more kVp than a dry one. A fiberglass cast generally requires less technique than a plaster cast. Be careful, however, of abnormally thick casts or abnormally thin partial casts or splints, which may throw your techniques off.

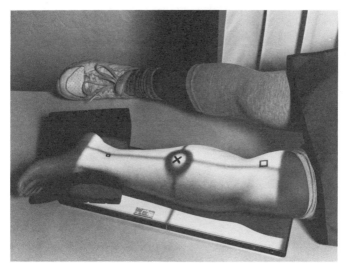

FIGURE 4–40. Lateral lower leg (tibia and fibula) with padded ankle to lateralize knee. Knee joint space *(large square)*. Ankle mortise *(small square)*.

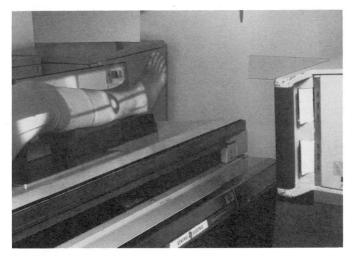

FIGURE 4–41. Crosstable lateral lower leg (tibia and fibula) for trauma patients. Use radiolucent pads only under lower leg.

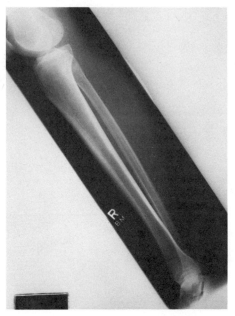

FIGURE 4–42. Lateral lower leg (tibia and fibula) x-ray.

STRUCTURES DEMONSTRATED: Both articulations, the knee and the ankle, should be included on the film (Fig. 4–42).

The proximal tibiofibular articulation will be slightly superimposed by the lateral condyle of the tibia.

The lateral and medial malleoli will be superimposed at the ankle.

Very often the knee joint space will not be opened due to the divergence of the x-ray beam when centered at midshaft.

COMMON ERROR: Both articulations are not included. Some technologists increase their 40 inches (or 100 cm) SID slightly in order to include both articulations on the film. Be sure that the knee and ankle joint distance measures less than the length of your film; otherwise, the SID increase won't help anyway— the extremity doesn't fit on your film!

TECHNIQUE

KV _____ MA _____ SECS _____ MAS _____ CALIPER _____ cm

_____ :1 GRID / B / none SCREEN: RE / High / Par / Detail / None

SID: _____ Rm _____ ADULT / CHILD age: _____ mos. / yrs.

HABITUS: Hyper / s / hypo / a   XS   S   M   L   XL   XXL

KNEE: AP OR PA

| 8 x 10 in. | 8 x 10 in. | 10 x 12 in. | 11 x 14 in. |
| 20 x 24 cm | 20 x 24 cm | 24 x 30 cm | 30 x 35 cm |

FILM: If the part thickness is greater than 3 to 4 inches (8 to 10 cm), use a grid or table Bucky. Collimate to the area of interest.

CR: For the AP, angle 5 to 7 degrees cephalad (proximal) to open the joint space.

Use a perpendicular CR for the PA if the joint space is not of interest, or for long bone detail.

POSITION

AP (Fig. 4–43)**:** The patient is supine on the table for the AP projection.

Place the lower leg in a true AP projection by slightly medially (internally) obliquing the foot 2 to 3 degrees in the AP projection.

The knee should be in extension. The popliteal area of the knee normally will not be in contact with the film.

PA (Fig. 4–44)**:** The patient is pronated on the table for the PA projection.

Rest the foot on the extended toes. This elevates the lower leg so that no CR angle is necessary.[11]

The pelvis should be flat and unobliqued.

The ankle, knee, and hip lie in the same longitudinal plane.

NOTE: As the area of interest is relatively near the pelvic area, use gonadal shielding.

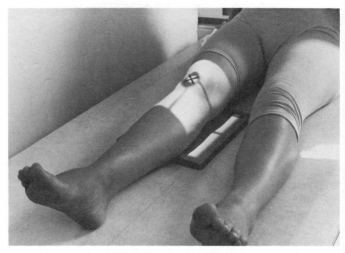

FIGURE 4–43. AP projection of knee.

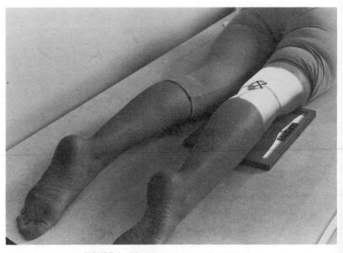

FIGURE 4–44. PA projection of right knee.

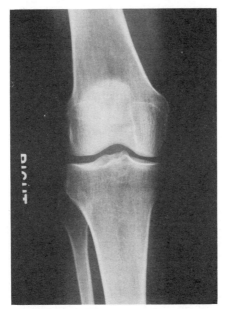

FIGURE 4–45. X-ray of AP projection of right knee.

STRUCTURES DEMONSTRATED: The joint spaces open and equal bilaterally if normal.

The proximal tibiofibular articulation will be partially superimposed by the lateral condyle of the tibia. The fibular head will be partially hidden by the lateral tibial condyle (Fig. 4–45).

The patella will be completely superimposed upon the femur.

All soft tissues of the knee.

COMMON ERROR: The joint space is not centered to the center of the film. The joint space is located ½ to 1 inch (1 to 3 cm) below the inferior border (apex) of the patella.

TECHNIQUE

KV _____ MA _____ SECS _____ MAS _____ CALIPER _____ cm
_____ :1 GRID / B / none SCREEN: RE / High / Par / Detail / None
SID: _____ Rm _____ ADULT / CHILD age: _____ mos. / yrs.
HABITUS: Hyper / s / hypo / a XS S M L XL XXL

KNEE: AP OR PA MEDIAL (INTERNAL) OBLIQUE

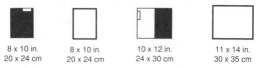

| 8 x 10 in. | 8 x 10 in. | 10 x 12 in. | 11 x 14 in. |
| 20 x 24 cm | 20 x 24 cm | 24 x 30 cm | 30 x 35 cm |

FILM: If the part thickness is greater than 3 to 4 inches (8 to 10 cm), use a grid or table Bucky. Collimate to the area of interest.

CR: Perpendicularly at the highest point of the knee joint or at the thickest point of the obliqued knee along the joint space. Sometimes, a 5-degree cephalic angle[13] or a 5- to 7-degree cephalic angle[14] is used on the AP oblique projection. The joint space is ½ to 1 inch (1 to 3 cm) below the inferior border (apex) of the patella.

POSITION: The patient is supinated for the AP medial oblique (Fig. 4–46) or pronated for the PA medial oblique projection (Fig. 4–47).

Rotate the hip, knee, and ankle as a unit 45 degrees medially or internally.

NOTE: The movement is the same for either the AP oblique or PA oblique projection. The rotation is always described from the anatomical position, or anterior surface movement. The direction of the toes will be toward the medial aspect in either the AP oblique or PA oblique study.

If the patient is debilitated and cannot assist in holding the position, a radiolucent sponge can be used to help the patient hold the obliquity.

Use gonadal shielding.

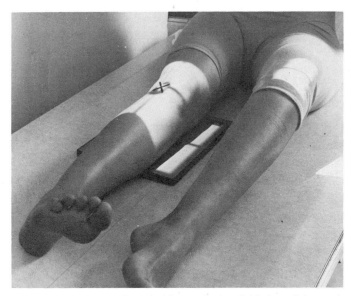

FIGURE 4–46. AP internal (medial) oblique projection of right knee. Point toes in with foot and rotate the lower leg toward the medial aspect.

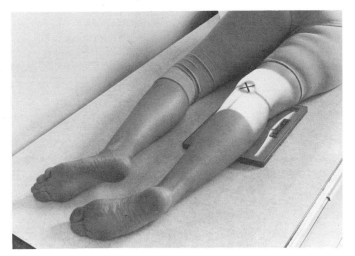

FIGURE 4–47. PA internal (medial) oblique projection of right knee. Toes in with foot rotated to medial aspect.

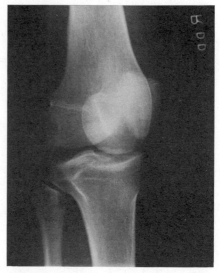

FIGURE 4–48. AP internal (medial) oblique x-ray of right knee.

STRUCTURES DEMONSTRATED: The head and neck of the fibula will be free from superimposition of the lateral tibial condyle (Fig. 4–48).

The lateral tibial plateau in profile.

The lateral femoral and tibia condyles.

The patella's medial margin will be free from superimposition.

NOTE: The AP medial (internal) oblique projection is the same as or analogous to the PA medial (internal) oblique projection. The same structures are demonstrated. The only difference is that certain structures are closer to the film in the PA oblique, which may be an important consideration in order to maximize the detail.

COMMON ERRORS: (1) Not all soft tissue is included. (2) The joint space is not centered to the center of the film.

TECHNIQUE

KV _____ MA _____ SECS _____ MAS _____ CALIPER _____ cm

_____ :1 GRID / B / none SCREEN: RE / High / Par / Detail / None

SID: _____ Rm _____ ADULT / CHILD age: _____ mos. / yrs.

HABITUS: Hyper / s / hypo / a   XS   S   M   L   XL   XXL

KNEE: AP OR PA LATERAL (EXTERNAL) OBLIQUE

8 x 10 in.	8 x 10 in.	10 x 12 in.
20 x 24 cm	20 x 24 cm	24 x 30 cm

FILM: If the part thickness is greater than 3 to 4 inches (8 to 10 cm), use a grid or table Bucky. Collimate to the area of interest.

CR: Perpendicularly at the highest point of the knee joint or at the thickest point of the obliqued knee along the joint space. The joint space is ½ to 1 inch (1 to 3 cm) below the inferior border (apex) of the patella.

POSITION: The patient is supinated for the AP lateral oblique (Fig. 4–49) or pronated for the PA lateral oblique projection (Fig. 4–50).

Rotate the hip, knee, and ankle as a unit 45 degrees laterally or externally.

NOTE: The movement is the same for either the AP oblique or the PA oblique projection. The rotation is always described from the anatomical position, or anterior surface movement. The direction of the toes will be toward the lateral aspect in either the AP oblique or the PA oblique study.

If the patient is debilitated and cannot assist in holding the position, a radiolucent sponge can be used to help the patient hold the obliquity.

Use gonadal shielding.

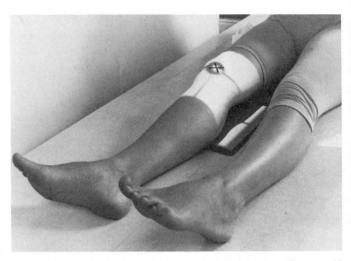

FIGURE 4–49. AP external (lateral) oblique projection of right knee. Toes out with lower leg rotated to lateral aspect.

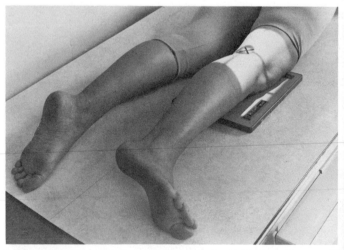

FIGURE 4–50. PA external (lateral) oblique projection of right knee. Toes out with foot rotated to lateral aspect.

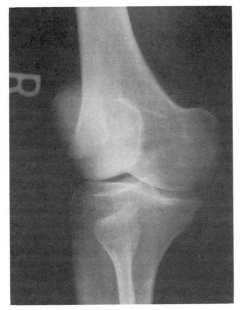

FIGURE 4–51. AP external (lateral) oblique x-ray of knee.

STRUCTURES DEMONSTRATED: The head and neck of the fibula will be superimposed over the lateral tibial condyle (Fig. 4–51).

The medial tibial plateau in profile.

The medial femoral and tibial condyles.

The patella's lateral margin will be free from superimposition.

NOTE: The AP lateral (external) oblique projection is the same as or analogous to the PA lateral (external) oblique projection. The same structures are demonstrated. The only difference is that certain structures are closer to the film in the PA oblique, which may be an important consideration in order to maximize the detail.

COMMON ERROR: Not all soft tissue is included. The joint space is not centered to the center of the film.

TECHNIQUE

KV _____ MA _____ SECS _____ MAS _____ CALIPER _____ cm

_____ :1 GRID / B / none SCREEN: RE / High / Par / Detail / None

SID: _____ Rm _____ ADULT / CHILD age: _____ mos. / yrs.

HABITUS: Hyper / s / hypo / a   XS   S   M   L   XL   XXL

KNEE: LATERAL

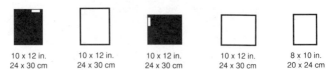

| 10 x 12 in. | 10 x 12 in. | 10 x 12 in. | 10 x 12 in. | 8 x 10 in. |
| 24 x 30 cm | 24 x 30 cm | 24 x 30 cm | 24 x 30 cm | 20 x 24 cm |

FILM: If the part thickness is greater than 3 to 4 inches (8 to 10 cm), use a grid or table Bucky. Collimate to the area of interest.

CR: Perpendicular to midjoint on medial surface or angle 5 degrees cephalad (proximal) at midjoint in order to avoid closure of the joint space from superimposition of the medial condyle. This superimposition is caused by magnification due to an increased object-to-image distance (OID) of the medial condyle to the film.

POSITION: From the supine position, the patient should roll toward the side of interest. The CR enters the medial aspect (Fig. 4–52).

The knee should be flexed from 30 to 45 degrees if the patient tolerates it (if a patellar injury is suspected, do not flex the knee).

Slightly elevate the calcaneus with a small sponge in order to lateralize the knee when recumbent.

Use gonadal shielding.

NOTE: A crosstable lateral of the knee can be taken when fractures are obvious or when the patient is severely debilitated (Fig. 4–53). When the patient is placed supine on the table with his or her head to the technologist's left, the film is positioned against the medial surface of the right knee and the x-ray tube is placed so the central ray enters the knee at its lateral surface. The left knee very often is taken in the mediolateral projection due to the patient's predetermined position on the x-ray table. The crosstable study should include all soft tissue in order to demonstrate fluid levels.

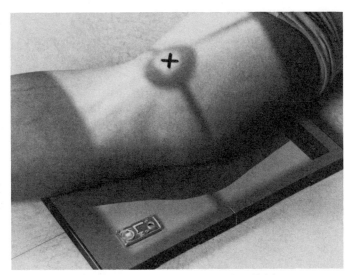

FIGURE 4–52. Left lateral recumbent position of left knee.

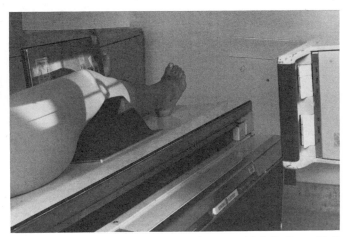

FIGURE 4–53. Crosstable lateral of right knee for trauma. Mark film "crosstable."

STRUCTURES DEMONSTRATED: The femoral condyles will be superimposed.

The patella will be seen in profile free from superimposition (Fig. 4–54).

The head of the fibula will be superimposed by the tibial condyles.

Best demonstration of a fabella (if present) in the gastrocnemius muscle of the lower leg, usually in the popliteal area.

COMMON ERROR: Rotation from the lateral position. Make sure the ankle is padded in order to lateralize the knee when the patient is lateral recumbent. When the patient's knee is taken in the crosstable projection, make sure the hip, knee, ankle, and foot are in the same longitudinal plane.

TECHNIQUE

KV _____ MA _____ SECS _____ MAS _____ CALIPER _____ cm

_____ :1 GRID / B / none SCREEN: RE / High / Par / Detail / None

SID: _____ Rm _____ ADULT / CHILD age: _____ mos. / yrs.

HABITUS: Hyper / s / hypo / a XS S M L XL XXL

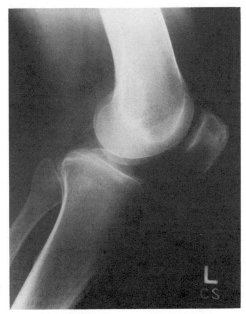

FIGURE 4–54. Lateral knee x-ray.

KNEE: INTERCONDYLAR FOSSA—PA AXIAL
PROJECTION (TUNNEL)

| 10 x 12 in.
24 x 30 cm | 10 x 12 in.
24 x 30 cm | 8 x 10 in.
20 x 24 cm | 8 x 10 in.
20 x 24 cm |

FILM: If the part thickness is greater than 3 to 4 inches (8 to 10 cm), use a grid or table Bucky. Collimate to the area of interest.

CR: Caudal (distal) angle of 30 to 40 degrees with entrance at midpopliteal depression and exit at apex of patella.

The CR angle must match the angle of the long axis of the lower leg with the tabletop. The collimator face must be parallel to and the CR will be perpendicular to the longitudinal line of the lower leg (Fig. 4–55).

NOTE: Do not use the overhead distance indicators to measure the SID. Always use the tape measure along the path of the central ray to measure to the tabletop or film when using a tube angle.

POSITION: The patient is pronated on the table (Fig. 4–55).

The leg of interest is flexed approximately 30 to 40 degrees.

Use the footboard or sponges and sandbags to brace the lower leg.

Use gonadal shielding.

STRUCTURES DEMONSTRATED: The intercondylar fossa is best demonstrated (similar to Fig. 4–57).

The intercondylar eminence (tibial spine) is seen.

COMMON ERROR: Superimposition of the patella within the intercondylar fossa. The apex of the patella should not be seen in the fossa. Make sure the plane of the lower leg and the CR are perpendicular. Flex the knee and support the lower leg to adjust.

TECHNIQUE

KV _____ MA _____ SECS _____ MAS _____ CALIPER _____ cm

_____ :1 GRID / B / none SCREEN: RE / High / Par / Detail / None

SID: _____ Rm _____ ADULT / CHILD age: _____ mos. / yrs.

HABITUS: Hyper / s / hypo / a   XS   S   M   L   XL   XXL

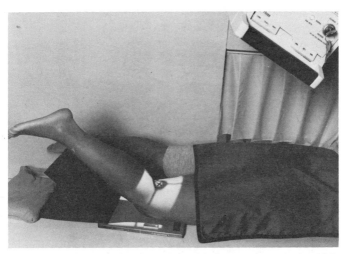

FIGURE 4–55. PA projection of intercondylar fossa (tunnel) knee. The face of the collimator housing should match (be parallel to) the plane of the lower leg.

KNEE: INTERCONDYLOID FOSSA—AP AXIAL PROJECTION (TUNNEL)

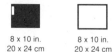

8 x 10 in.
20 x 24 cm

8 x 10 in.
20 x 24 cm

FILM: No grid. Collimate to the area of interest.

CR: Cephalic (proximal) angle usually 30 to 40 degrees to match the angle of the lower leg from the table. The CR enters the knee at apex of the patella (Fig. 4–56).

The CR angle must match the angle of the long axis of the lower leg. The collimator face must be parallel to and the CR will be perpendicular to the longitudinal line of the lower leg.

NOTE: Do not use the overhead distance indicators to measure the SID. Always use the tape measure along the path of the central ray to measure to the tabletop or film when using a tube angle. Whenever a tube angle is directed toward the body, use appropriate lead shielding.

POSITION: The patient is supinated on the table.

The leg of interest is flexed approximately 30 to 40 degrees.

Using the aid of the patient or by padding, place the film under the knee with the film's edge pressed into the soft tissue of the posterior thigh. Sometimes the mass of the thigh will not allow proper centering of the CR to the film. (Lowering the height of the film placement allows better centering but will increase OID.) The image will be centered "high" on the film in those cases.

Use gonadal shielding.

STRUCTURES DEMONSTRATED: The intercondylar fossa is best demonstrated. The intercondylar eminence (tibial spine) is seen (Fig. 4–57).

COMMON ERROR: Superimposition of the patella within the intercondylar fossa. The apex of the patella should not be seen in the fossa. Make sure the angle of the lower leg with the table matches the angle on the tube.

TECHNIQUE

KV _____ MA _____ SECS _____ MAS _____ CALIPER _____ cm

_____ :1 GRID / B / none SCREEN: RE / High / Par / Detail / None

SID: _____ Rm _____ ADULT / CHILD age: _____ mos. / yrs.

HABITUS: Hyper / s / hypo / a XS S M L XL XXL

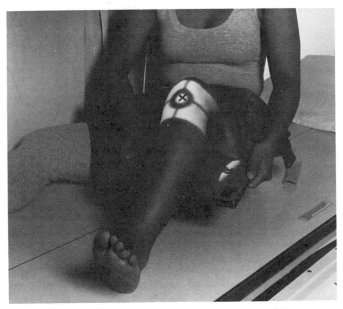

FIGURE 4–56. AP projection of intercondylar fossa (tunnel) knee.

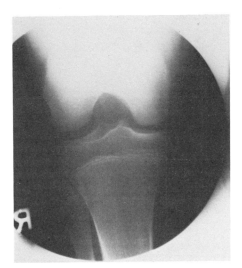

FIGURE 4–57. AP x-ray of intercondylar fossa (tunnel) knee.

PATELLA: POSTEROANTERIOR (PA)

8 x 10 in.
20 x 24 cm

8 x 10 in.
20 x 24 cm

10 x 12 in.
24 x 30 cm

FILM: Use tabletop only if the part thickness is less than 3 to 4 inches (8 to 10 cm). Collimate to the area of interest.

CR: Perpendicularly with entrance at midpopliteal depression (behind the knee), exit at midpatella (Fig. 4–58).

POSITION: The patient is pronated on the table.

If the table Bucky is being used, center the patella to the center of the table.

If the anterior surface of the patella is tender, pad the thigh and lower leg to eliminate pressure on the kneecap.

Rotate the heel 2 to 10 degrees laterally, depending upon the location of the patella, to place the leg in correct anatomical position (the more medial the patella lies in the anatomical position, the less rotation needed).

STRUCTURES DEMONSTRATED: The patella will be super-imposed upon the femur (Fig. 4–59).

The PA projection will detail the patella better than the AP. This is due to the shorter object-film distance in the PA projection. *COMMON ERROR: Underpenetration.*

TECHNIQUE

KV _____ MA _____ SECS _____ MAS _____ CALIPER _____ cm

_____ :1 GRID / B / none SCREEN: RE / High / Par / Detail / None

SID: _____ Rm _____ ADULT / CHILD age: _____ mos. / yrs.

HABITUS: Hyper / s / hypo / a   XS   S   M   L   XL   XXL

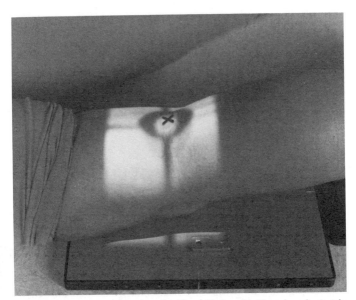

FIGURE 4–58. PA projection of patella. The ankle is padded here in order to take the pressure off of the patella. Notice the lead marker is face down. This will correctly orient the the "L" when the film is read in the anatomical position (see Chapter 10).

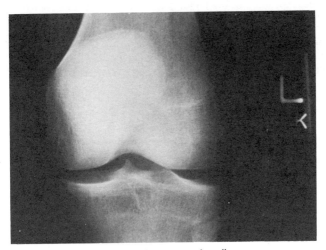

FIGURE 4–59. PA x-ray of patella.

PATELLA: PA OBLIQUES

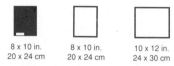

8 x 10 in.   8 x 10 in.   10 x 12 in.
20 x 24 cm   20 x 24 cm   24 x 30 cm

FILM: Grid or table Bucky use. Use tabletop only if the part thickness is less than 3 to 4 inches (8 to 10 cm). Collimate to the area of interest.

CR: Perpendicular to the femoropatellar articulation.

POSITION: The patient is semipronated on the table.

The knee is slightly flexed (do not flex if fracture is suspected). Place a support under the ankle for patient comfort.

Oblique the patient 45 degrees toward the lateral aspect (toes to lateral side) so that the knee will rest on its medial side for the PA lateral oblique (Fig. 4–60).

Oblique the patient 45 degrees toward the medial aspect (toes to medial side) so that the knee of interest will rest on its lateral side for the PA medial oblique (see Fig. 4–47).

Collimate to the part to increase detail.

NOTE: When applying the correct direction for this or for any of the PA oblique knee positions, use the toe direction as an indicator of the correct motion of obliquity. For a PA medial oblique, the toes of the leg of interest will point toward the medial aspect. For a PA lateral oblique, the toes of the leg of interest will point toward the lateral aspect.

STRUCTURES DEMONSTRATED: The PA lateral oblique projection will demonstrate the lateral patellar margin free from superimposition of the femoral condyles. The medial condyles will be isolated (Fig. 4–61).

The opposite oblique, the PA medial, may be taken to demonstrate the medial margin of the patella free from superimposition (similar to Fig. 4–48). The lateral condyles will be isolated.

COMMON ERROR: Lack of collimation to the area of interest.

TECHNIQUE

KV _____ MA _____ SECS _____ MAS _____ CALIPER _____ cm

_____ :1 GRID / B / none SCREEN: RE / High / Par / Detail / None

SID: _____ Rm _____ ADULT / CHILD age: _____ mos. / yrs.

HABITUS: Hyper / s / hypo / a   XS   S   M   L   XL   XXL

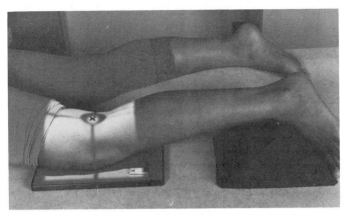

FIGURE 4–60. PA external (lateral) oblique projection of patella.

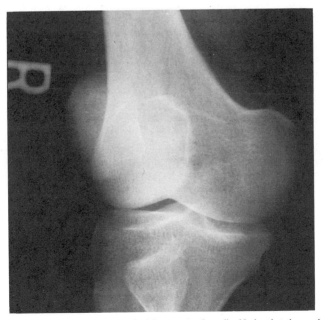

FIGURE 4–61. PA external (lateral) oblique x-ray of patella. Notice that the marker placement is too close to the area of interest.

PATELLA: LATERAL

8 x 10 in. 20 x 24 cm	8 x 10 in. 20 x 24 cm	10 x 12 in. 24 x 30 cm

FILM: Use table Bucky or grid. Use tabletop only if the part thickness is less than 3 to 4 inches (8 to 10 cm). Collimate to the area of interest.

CR: Perpendicular to midpatella. Do not use an angle.

POSITION: Have the recumbent patient lie on side of interest. The CR should enter the medial aspect of the patella (Fig. 4–62).

Lateralize the knee by padding the calcaneus.

Do not flex the knee if fracture is suspected.

Perform crosstable for demonstration of fluid levels.

STRUCTURES DEMONSTRATED: Best demonstration of transverse patellar fractures.

The femoropatellar articulation is open (Fig. 4–63).

COMMON ERROR: The hip, knee, and foot must be in the same longitudinal plane for a crosstable study. Sometimes the femoropatellar joint space is not opened in a true lateral position due to the patella sometimes being located on the more medial aspect of the knee. Check the AP or PA film to determine if the patella is more lateral or medial; slightly overrotate from the lateral position for the medial patella. Underrotate it if the patella lies on the lateral aspect on the AP or PA film.

TECHNIQUE

KV _____ MA _____ SECS _____ MAS _____ CALIPER _____ cm

_____ :1 GRID / B / none SCREEN: RE / High / Par / Detail / None

SID: _____ Rm _____ ADULT / CHILD age: _____ mos. / yrs.

HABITUS: Hyper / s / hypo / a   XS   S   M   L   XL   XXL

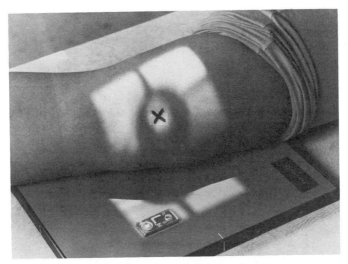

FIGURE 4–62. Mediolateral projection of patella.

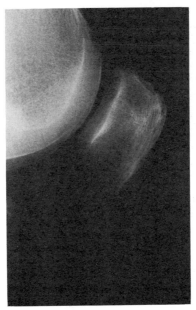

FIGURE 4–63. Lateral patella x-ray, severely collimated. Note the increased detail.

PATELLA: TANGENTIAL (SUNRISE)

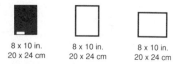

8 x 10 in.   8 x 10 in.   8 x 10 in.
20 x 24 cm   20 x 24 cm   20 x 24 cm

FILM: Tabletop, no Bucky. Collimate to the area of interest.
CR: Adjust the cephalic (proximal) angle to enter the anterior aspect of the femoropatellar joint space (usually 25 to 35 degrees elevated from a horizontal beam).
POSITION: The patient must have good range of motion for this method. The patient is supinated on the table.

The knee is flexed 30 to 45 degrees or better (do not flex if patellar fracture is suspected or if the patient cannot tolerate it).

Place the patient toward the end of the table to allow for the angled tube to travel below the level of the table's surface (Fig. 4–64).

Have the patient hold the tube side of the film against the thigh. Use a 10- to 15-degree angled radiolucent sponge between the thigh and the film. This adjusts the angle of the film from the thigh to match the femoropatellar joint space (measured from a horizontal tube, this is usually a superior, 15- to 25-degree angle). It is particularly difficult to read the amount of tube angle necessary due to the varying degrees of flexion and anatomical differences. The greater the flexion of the knee, the less the tube angle needed (from horizontal). Use less tube angle (closer to horizontal) instead of a greater tube angle to avoid distortion. Use gonadal shielding and have patients turn their face away from the beam.

Collimate closely and place your marker on the lateral aspect in order to provide correct film orientation.

NOTE: Do not use the overhead distance indicators to measure the SID. Always use the tape measure along the path of the central ray to measure to the tabletop or film when using a tube angle.
STRUCTURES DEMONSTRATED: This position will best demonstrate vertical fractures of the patella.

The femoropatellar joint space is open (Fig. 4–65).
COMMON ERROR: Closure of the femoropatellar joint space. Distortion of the patella's trabecular pattern. Usually the angle is too extreme and adds distortion. The more the knee is flexed by the patient, the less the need for the tube to be angled. The tube angle that is lessened will approach horizontal.

TECHNIQUE
KV _____ MA _____ SECS _____ MAS _____ CALIPER _____ cm
_____ :1 GRID / B / none SCREEN: RE / High / Par / Detail / None
SID: _____ Rm _____ ADULT / CHILD age: _____ mos. / yrs.
HABITUS: Hyper / s / hypo / a   XS   S   M   L   XL   XXL

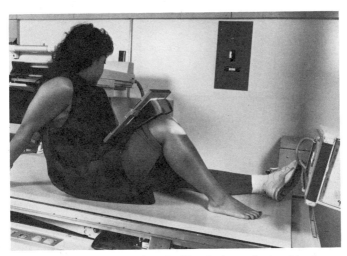

FIGURE 4–64. Tangential (sunrise) patella. Use a lead apron for gonadal and upper torso radiation protection. Have the patient look away from the tube.

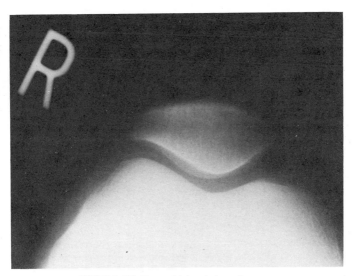

FIGURE 4–65. Tangential (sunrise) patella x-ray.

FEMUR: AP

    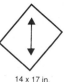

7 x 17 in.	7 x 17 in.	14 x 17 in.	14 x 17 in.	14 x 17 in.
18 x 43 cm	18 x 43 cm	35 x 43 cm	35 x 43 cm	35 x 43 cm

FILM: Use a grid or table Bucky if the part is greater than 3 to 4 inches (8 to 10 cm). Collimate to the area of interest.

CR: Perpendicularly at midshaft, equidistant from each articulation.

NOTE: When using radiographic equipment suspended from an overhead crane and if the patient has a suspected fracture, place the patient on the x-ray table so that the side of injury is on the side of the table away from the technologist (the back side of the table). This will allow more working area for the trauma method using horizontal beam for the next position, the lateral. If using radiographic equipment of a tube stand design, place the patient on the x-ray table so that the side of injury is on the side of the table closest to the technologist. This is particularly important for the accompanying projection for the trauma patient, the crosstable lateral.

POSITION: The patient is supine on the table.

The ankle, knee, and hip are in the same longitudinal plane.

The lower leg, knee, and hip are rotated 15 degrees internally (medially) (Fig. 4–66). This will correct for anteversion of the hip joint, a posterior angle of the anterior surface of the femoral head, neck, and greater trochanter, which is accentuated when the recumbent patient's lower extremities are relaxed with the toes pointing out.

NOTE: As the area of interest is near the pelvic area, use gonadal shielding but do not obstruct the area of interest.

STRUCTURES DEMONSTRATED: Both articulations should be included (Fig. 4–67). For tabletop filming, use the film diagonally in order to accommodate both joints on the film.

The femoral head and neck should be seen in their entirety and not foreshortened.

The greater trochanter will be in profile on the lateral aspect, and the lesser trochanter will be partially superimposed by the shaft (diaphysis) at the medial aspect.

COMMON ERROR: (1) Underpenetration of the hip area. Use a hip technique rather than a knee technique. (2) Both articulations are not included on initial films. Subsequent films for fracture healing assessment will only include one joint, the articulation involving the injury. (3) Foreshortening of the femoral head and neck due to improper positioning of the leg. The leg must be internally (medially) rotated to overcome the posterior angle of the head and neck of the femur (anteversion). If the lesser

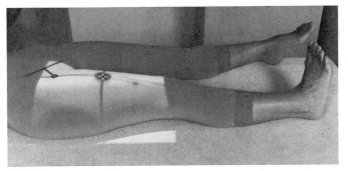

FIGURE 4–66. AP projection of femur using the table Bucky.

trochanter is not partially hidden or superimposed, anteversion of the hip has not been eliminated.

TECHNIQUE

KV _____ MA _____ SECS _____ MAS _____ CALIPER _____ cm
_____ :1 GRID / B / none SCREEN: RE / High / Par / Detail / None
SID: _____ Rm _____ ADULT / CHILD age: _____ mos. / yrs.
HABITUS: Hyper / s / hypo / a   XS   S   M   L   XL   XXL

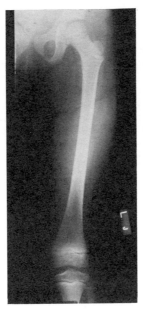

FIGURE 4–67. AP x-ray of femur.

FEMUR: LATERAL

  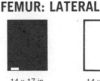

| 7 x 17 in.
18 x 43 cm | 7 x 17 in.
18 x 43 cm | 14 x 17 in.
35 x 43 cm | 14 x 17 in.
35 x 43 cm | 14 x 17 in.
35 x 43 cm |

FILM: Use a grid or table Bucky if the part is greater than 3 to 4 inches (8 to 10 cm). Collimate to the area of interest.

CR

Methods A and B: Perpendicularly at midshaft, equidistant from each articulation.

Method C: Crosstable at the level of the femoral neck. Perpendicular to the plane of the femoral head, neck, and greater trochanter.

POSITION

Method A (Nontrauma when knee is joint of interest—Fig. 4–68): Only used when a fracture is *not* suspected.

The patient is supine on the table. Have the patient roll up on the side of interest in order to lateralize the leg.

The knee is slightly flexed.

The calcaneus is padded in order to lateralize the knee.

Place the opposite, uninjured leg either forward or behind the injured leg to remove it from the area of interest.

The bottom of the film should include the knee joint, at least 2 inches or 5 cm below the apex of the patella.

Method B (Nontrauma when hip is joint of interest—Fig. 4–69): Only used when a fracture is *not* suspected.

The knee of the side of interest is flexed and the leg is then abducted slowly to assess range of motion at the hip.

Abduct the leg until the leg rests upon its lateral surface or simply reaches the end of the range of motion in this direction. This is commonly called a frog-leg position. Place a radiolucent sponge to support the knee. For additional patient comfort, have the patient roll up slightly toward the side of interest. Obliquing the pelvis will help relieve the stress on the hip joint.

The plantar surface of the foot of the side of interest can be braced against the other, uninjured leg, which has not been abducted.

When the table Bucky and a smaller film such as a 10 × 12 inch (24 × 30 cm) film are used, center the femur longitudinally to the center of the table. If this is not convenient, center the hip to the center of the table and simply match the orientation of the film in the Bucky tray to the longitudinal axis of the femur. (Usually this axis will lie diagonally across the center of the table.) Unlock the film holder of the Bucky tray; open it as wide as possible. Place the film diagonally to match the patient's position and lock again without exerting pressure on the film (or tape to secure). Do not use phototiming for this method.

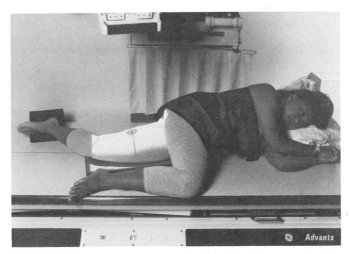

FIGURE 4–68. Lateral nontrauma femur for knee.

Method C (Trauma): Use a crosstable or horizontal beam with a grid. Perform a lateromedial projection when the knee is the only articulation of interest (Fig. 4–70).

If your equipment consists of a radiographic unit on an overhead crane, place the patient on the x-ray table so that the side of injury lies on the side of the table away from the technologist (the back

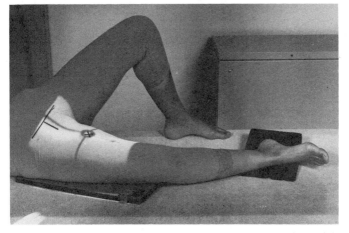

FIGURE 4–69. Lateral nontrauma femur for hip. The pelvis is obliqued toward the side of interest and the hip slightly abducted (frogged).

side of the table). This will allow more working area at the front of the table for the x-ray tube to be used with a horizontal beam.

If your equipment consists of an x-ray tube with a tube stand, you will want to place the patient on the x-ray table with the injured side away from the tube stand.

Use a film holder and place the film and grid against the lateral aspect of the hip and proximal femur. Match the film's plane to the plane of the femoral head, neck, and greater trochanter when that joint is of interest and a smaller film is used (Fig. 4–76). Elevate the opposite, uninjured leg to remove it from the path of the x-ray beam (Fig. 4–71). The mediolateral projection is always used when either the hip or both the hip and knee joints are of interest.

Maintain proper SID. Adjust the central ray so that it is perpendicular to the center of the film. The plane of the collimator face should be parallel to the plane of the film.

NOTE: As the area of interest is relatively near the pelvic area, use gonadal shielding that does not obscure the area of interest.

STRUCTURES DEMONSTRATED

Method A: The knee is seen with the condyles superimposed over each other. The condyle farthest from the film will be magnified due to its greater object-image distance. The hip is obscured by the soft tissue of the opposite thigh.

Method B: The hip joint is seen in abduction. The greater trochanter will be superimposed over the femoral neck in a true lateral position. The lesser trochanter will be slightly superimposed at the posterior aspect of the proximal femur. The proximal shaft of the femur is seen in its lateral aspect.

Method C: The greater trochanter is superimposed over the femoral neck. The lesser trochanter is superimposed over the posterior (lower) aspect of the proximal femur. The proximal shaft of the femur is seen in its lateral aspect (Fig. 4–72).

COMMON ERROR: In method A, loss of detail due to underpenetration of the middle to proximal femur due to superimposition of the soft tissue of the uninjured thigh. In method B, the patient is unable to sufficiently lateralize the femur. In method C, the film must be sufficiently penetrated in order to demonstrate the acetabulum and femoral head and femoral neck (a common fracture site).

TECHNIQUE

KV _____ MA _____ SECS _____ MAS _____ CALIPER _____ cm
_____ :1 GRID / B / none SCREEN: RE / High / Par / Detail / None
SID: _____ Rm _____ ADULT / CHILD age: _____ mos. / yrs.
HABITUS: Hyper / s / hypo / a   XS   S   M   L   XL   XXL

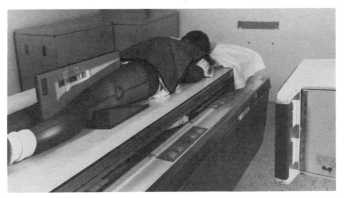

FIGURE 4–70. Crosstable lateral trauma femur for knee using a lateral-to-medial projection.

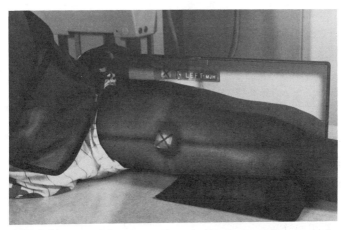

FIGURE 4–71. Crosstable lateral trauma femur for hip using a mediolateral projection. Use gonadal shielding.

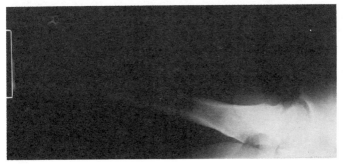

FIGURE 4–72. Lateral femur x-ray. A problem frequently experienced with taking lateral femur x-rays is arriving at a technique sufficient to penetrate the hip while leaving the shaft still readable even if overpenetrated.

HIP: AP

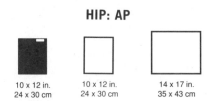

10 x 12 in.
24 x 30 cm

10 x 12 in.
24 x 30 cm

14 x 17 in.
35 x 43 cm

FILM: Grid or table Bucky use, if the part is greater than 3 to 4 inches (8 to 10 cm). Collimate to the area of interest.
CR: Perpendicular and centered to the femoral neck.
POSITION: The patient is supine on the table.

Use the "T" method to locate the femoral head and neck. *(See Chapter 1, Fig. 1–19, on body landmarks for instruction.)*

NOTE: When using radiographic equipment suspended from an overhead crane and if the patient has a suspected fracture, place the patient on the x-ray table so that the side of injury is on the side of the table away from the technologist (the back side of the table). This will allow more working area for the trauma method using a horizontal beam for the next position, the lateral. If using radiographic equipment of a tube stand design, place the patient on the x-ray table so that the side of injury is on the side of the table closest to the technologist. This is particularly important for the accompanying projection, the crosstable lateral.

Nontrauma: The ankle, knee, and hip are in the same longitudinal plane.

The lower leg, knee, and hip are rotated 15 degrees internally (medially) (Fig. 4–73). This will correct for anteversion of the hip joint, a posterior angle of the anterior surface of the femoral head, neck, and greater trochanter, which is accentuated when the recumbent patient's lower extremities are relaxed with the toes pointing out.

Trauma: Take "as is." Do not move the extremity.

NOTE: As the area of interest is near the pelvic area, use gonadal shielding, but do not obstruct the area of interest.

STRUCTURES DEMONSTRATED

Nontrauma: The acetabulum and femoral head and neck should be seen in their entirety and not foreshortened (Fig. 4–74).

The greater trochanter will be in profile on the lateral aspect and the lesser trochanter will be slightly superimposed by the proximal femoral shaft (diaphysis) on its medial aspect.

Trauma: The acetabulum, femoral head and neck, and the proximal shaft should be demonstrated.

The femoral head and neck are usually seen foreshortened due to the relaxed, toes-out position of the leg of the trauma patient. In this case, the lesser trochanter will be profiled on the medial aspect of the femoral shaft (diaphysis).

COMMON ERROR: Foreshortening of the femoral head and neck due to lack of or improper positioning of the leg. In the non-

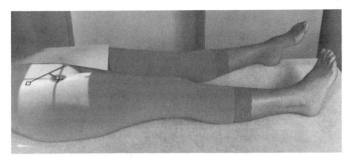

FIGURE 4–73. AP projection of hip with lower leg rotated to overcome the anteversion of the femoral head, neck, and greater trochanter.

trauma position, *the leg must be internally (medially) rotated to overcome the posterior angle of the head and neck of the femur (anteversion). If the lesser trochanter is not superimposed, anteversion of the hip has not been eliminated. In the trauma position, the leg's position is not moved; take it "as is."*

TECHNIQUE

KV _____ MA _____ SECS _____ MAS _____ CALIPER _____ cm

_____ :1 GRID / B / none SCREEN: RE / High / Par / Detail / None

SID: _____ Rm _____ ADULT / CHILD age: _____ mos. / yrs.

HABITUS: Hyper / s / hypo / a XS S M L XL XXL

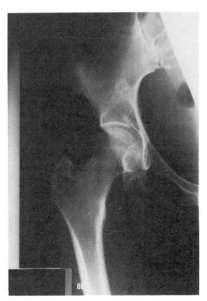

FIGURE 4–74. AP x-ray of hip. (Notice gonadal shield.) (Courtesy of Lorena Mendez, S.R.T.)

HIP: LATERAL

 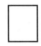

10 x 12 in.   10 x 12 in.   10 x 12 in.   10 x 12 in.   **10 x 12 in.**
24 x 30 cm   24 x 30 cm   24 x 30 cm   24 x 30 cm   **24 x 30 cm.**

FILM: Grid or table Bucky use, if the part is greater than 3 to 4 inches (8 to 10 cm). Collimate to the area of interest.

CR: Method A and B: Perpendicularly at femoral neck.

Method C: Crosstable at the level of the femoral neck. Perpendicular to the plane of the femoral head and neck.

POSITION

Method A (Nontrauma for hip): Only used when a fracture is *not* suspected.

The knee of the side of interest is flexed and the leg is then abducted slowly to assess range of motion.

Abduct the leg until the leg rests upon its lateral surface or simply reaches the end of the range of motion in this direction. This is commonly called a frog-leg position (Fig. 4–75). Place a radiolucent sponge to support the knee. For comfort, have the patient roll up slightly toward the side of interest. Obliquing the pelvis will help relieve the stress on the hip joint.

The plantar surface of the foot of the side of interest can be braced against the other, uninjured, extended leg, which has not been abducted.

When the table Bucky and a smaller film such as a 10 × 12 inch (24 × 30 cm) film are used, center the frogged hip and femur longitudinally to the center of the table. If this is not convenient, center the hip to the center of the table and simply match the orientation of the film in the Bucky tray to the longitudinal axis of the hip and proximal femur of the patient (usually this axis will lie diagonally across the center of the table). Unlock the film holder of the Bucky tray; open it as wide as possible. Place the film diagonally to match the patient's position (Fig. 4–75). Lock again without exerting pressure on the film (or tape to secure). (Do not use phototiming when the collimator housing is changed to match the film placement unless you are able to use the correct cell selection for the hip.)

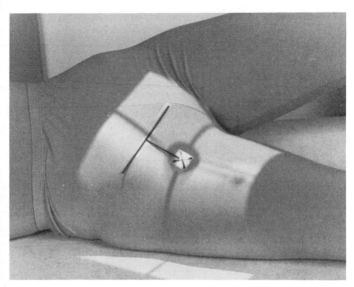

FIGURE 4–75. Lateral nontrauma "frogged" or abducted hip. The collimator housing is turned to match the proximal femur. Phototiming not recommended when collimator used diagonally.

Method B (Daniclius-Miller's method for trauma hip): Use a crosstable or horizontal beam with a grid (Fig. 4–76).

If your equipment consists of a radiographic unit on an overhead crane, place the patient on the x-ray table so that the side of injury lies on the side of the table away from the technologist (the back side of the table). This will allow more working area at the front of the table for the x-ray tube to be used with a horizontal beam.

If your equipment consists of an x-ray tube with a tube stand, you will want to place the patient on the x-ray table with the injured side away from the tube stand.

Use a film holder and place the film and grid against the lateral aspect of the hip and proximal femur. Match the film's plane to the plane of the femoral head, neck, and greater trochanter. (The inferior aspect of the film should be further away from the patient and the superior aspect of the film should be placed touching the patient at the iliac crest.) See Figure 4–76. Use the "T" method to locate the femoral head and neck. *(See Chapter 1, Figs. 1–19 to 1–22, on body landmarks for further instruction on these methods.)*

Use the grid so that the grid lines are parallel to the table.[15]

Elevate the opposite, uninjured leg to remove it from the path of the x-ray beam (Fig. 4–76).

Maintain proper SID. Adjust the central ray so that it is perpendicular to the center of the film. The plane of the collimator face should be parallel to the plane of the film.

Method C (Clements-Nakayama's method for trauma, bilateral hip fractures): Use a crosstable or horizontal beam with a grid.

Your equipment must be able to be placed behind the x-ray table for a study of the side closest to the technologist *and* in front of the x-ray table for the injured side away from the technologist for this procedure (otherwise follow the patient placement advice for method B, knowing the patient will have to be moved after each lateral).

Place the patient's body and side of interest hip as close to the edge of the table as possible without endangering the patient. Place the top of the film and grid at the ASIS. Try to adjust the placement of the film so that its lower edge is below the level of the table. Match the film's plane to the plane of the femoral head and neck. This will result in the inferior aspect of the film angling away from the body. Use the "T" method to locate the femoral head and neck. *(See Chapter 1, Fig. 1–19, on body landmarks for further instruction on these methods.)*

Position the tube horizontally (crosstable) and adjust the CR perpendicularly to the grid and film. Now vertically raise the tube above the level of the thigh closest to the tube. Now adjust the tube to angle inferiorly 15 degrees from horizontal. This angle allows the tube to bypass the opposite thigh and avoid most superimposition.

Maintain proper SID. Adjust the central ray so that it is placed at the center of the film. Use the grid vertically to avoid grid

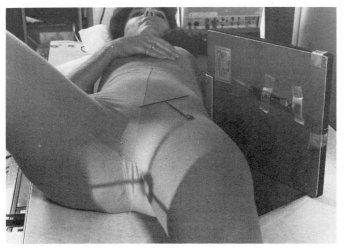

FIGURE 4–76. Crosstable lateral trauma hip.

cutoff. Place the grid lines perpendicularly to the tabletop, gurney, or bed. Perform both laterals.

NOTE: As the area of interest is relatively near the pelvic area, use gonadal shielding that does not obscure the area of interest.

STRUCTURES DEMONSTRATED

Method A: The hip joint is seen in abduction (Fig. 4–77). The greater trochanter will be superimposed over the femoral neck in a true lateral position. The lesser trochanter is seen on the medial aspect. The proximal shaft of the femur is seen in its lateral aspect.

Method B: The greater trochanter is superimposed over the femoral neck. The lesser trochanter is located at the posterior aspect of the proximal femur. The proximal shaft of the femur is seen in its lateral aspect (Fig. 4–78).

Method C: The greater trochanter is partially superimposed over the femoral neck. The lesser trochanter is slightly superimposed over the posterior aspect of the proximal femur. The proximal shaft of the femur is seen in its lateral aspect (similar to Fig. 4–78). The image is distorted due to the use of the two tube angles.

COMMON ERROR: In method A, the patient is unable to sufficiently lateralize the femur. In methods B and C, the film must be sufficiently penetrated in order to demonstrate the acetabulum and femoral head and femoral neck (a common fracture site). Grid cutoff is common in method C. Rest grid on its short side.

TECHNIQUE

KV _____ MA _____ SECS _____ MAS _____ CALIPER _____ cm

_____ :1 GRID / B / none SCREEN: RE / High / Par / Detail / None

SID: _____ Rm _____ ADULT / CHILD age: _____ mos. / yrs.

HABITUS: Hyper / s / hypo / a   XS   S   M   L   XL   XXL

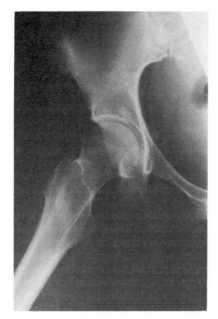

FIGURE 4–77. Lateral frogged hip x-ray.

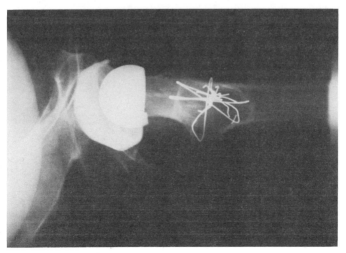

FIGURE 4–78. Crosstable lateral hip x-ray.

PELVIS: AP

14 x 17 in.
35 x 43 cm

14 x 17 in.
35 x 43 cm

FILM: Collimate to the area of interest.

CR: Perpendicular at the center of the film when the top of the film is placed 1 inch (2 to 3 cm) above the iliac crest.

POSITION: The patient is supinated upon the table.

Center the midsagittal plane of the patient to the center of the table or grid cassette.

Place a sponge under the knees to take the pressure off of the lower back of the patient.

Rotate the legs 15 degrees medially (internally) (Fig. 4–79). This places the hips so that the head, neck, and greater trochanter lie in the same plane (corrects anteversion and eliminates foreshortening).

Have the patient place his or her hands upon the chest with elbows resting at the side.

Make sure the pelvis is flat and the patient is not favoring one side or the other.

Make the exposure at the end of full expiration.

STRUCTURES DEMONSTRATED: The pelvic girdle is seen in its entirety (Fig. 4–80).

The femoral head and neck are not foreshortened.

The ilia are seen in an obliqued position.

The proximal femurs are demonstrated.

The 4th and 5th lumbar vertebrae are seen.

Both obturator foramina should be equal in size and shape.

COMMON ERROR: (1) Asymmetry of the ilia. Check to see if the ilia are equal in size. If they are not, the patient's pelvis is not flat. (2) The femoral head and neck are foreshortened. Make sure the patient's legs are rotated 15 degrees medially to correct for anteversion of the hips.

TECHNIQUE

KV _____ MA _____ SECS _____ MAS _____ CALIPER _____ cm

_____ :1 GRID / B / none SCREEN: RE / High / Par / Detail / None

SID: _____ Rm _____ ADULT / CHILD age: _____ mos. / yrs.

HABITUS: Hyper / s / hypo / a XS S M L XL XXL

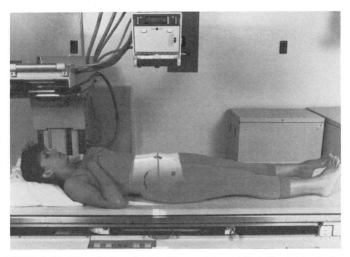

FIGURE 4–79. AP projection of pelvis. Iliac crest *(curved line)*. Greater trochanter *(square)*.

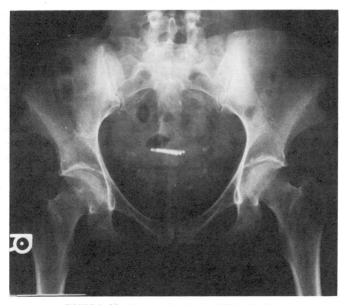

FIGURE 4–80. AP x-ray of pelvis for IUD localization.

SI JOINTS: AP OBLIQUES

8 x 10 in.
20 x 24 cm

8 x 10 in.
20 x 24 cm

FILM: Collimate to the area of interest.

CR: Perpendicularly at the longitudinal level of ASIS, and transversely at 1 inch (2.5 cm) medially from the ASIS of the side up. A 20- to 25-degree cephalic angle may also be used; enter along the longitudinal plane one inch (2.5 cm) medially from the ASIS of the side up; exit through the ASIS of the side up.*

POSITION: The patient is semisupinated on the table. Oblique the patient 30 degrees from the table using a radiolucent sponge for patient comfort (Fig. 4–81). Hint: If *not* using a floating tabletop and with the patient supinated on the table, in order to demonstrate the right side, pull the patient toward you first, and then oblique the patient away from you. This will place the obliqued patient closer to the correct and final position at the center of the x-ray table (and save your back).

Center the point to the x-ray table on the side up that is at 1 inch (2.5 cm) medially from the ASIS.

STRUCTURES DEMONSTRATED: The side up will be the side demonstrated on posterior obliques (RPO and LPO) (Fig. 4–82).

COMMON ERROR: The patient is obliqued too much so that the ilium superimposes the sacroiliac joint.

TECHNIQUE

KV _____ MA _____ SECS _____ MAS _____ CALIPER _____ cm

_____ :1 GRID / B / none SCREEN: RE / High / Par / Detail / None

SID: _____ Rm _____ ADULT / CHILD age: _____ mos. / yrs.

HABITUS: Hyper / s / hypo / a   XS   S   M   L   XL   XXL

With the cephalic tube angle, the transverse mark of the CR (where it strikes the table) will be found significantly higher than the actual level of the ASIS. Center the film to the transverse CR mark.

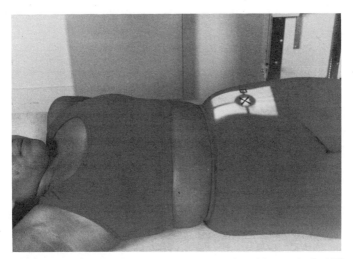

FIGURE 4–81. AP oblique projection of SI joint. Side up demonstrated. ASIS *(square)*.

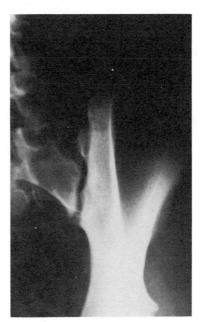

FIGURE 4–82. AP oblique x-ray of SI joint.

SI JOINTS: PA OBLIQUES

8 x 10 in.
20 x 24 cm

8 x 10 in.
20 x 24 cm

FILM: Collimate to the area of interest.

CR: Perpendicularly 1 inch (2.5 cm) medially from the ASIS. A 20- to 25-degree caudal angle may also be used. Exit through the longitudinal level of the ASIS and 1 inch (2.5 cm) medially from the ASIS.*

POSITION: The patient is semipronated. The unaffected side is elevated 30 degrees from the table. The side down is studied (Fig. 4–83).

Center the ASIS of the side down to the center of the x-ray table.

Flex the patient's knees for stability.

STRUCTURES DEMONSTRATED: The side down will be the side demonstrated on anterior obliques (similar to Fig. 4–82). The right side will be demonstrated for the RAO and the left side for the LAO position.

COMMON ERROR: The patient is obliqued too much so that the ilium superimposes the sacroiliac joint.

TECHNIQUE

KV _____ MA _____ SECS _____ MAS _____ CALIPER _____ cm

_____ :1 GRID / B / none SCREEN: RE / High / Par / Detail / None

SID: _____ Rm _____ ADULT / CHILD age: _____ mos. / yrs.

HABITUS: Hyper / s / hypo / a   XS   S   M   L   XL   XXL

With the caudal tube angle, the transverse mark of the CR (where it strikes the table) will be found significantly lower than the actual level of the ASIS. Center the film to the transverse CR mark.

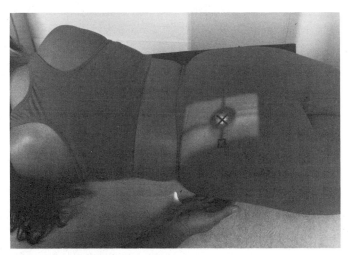

FIGURE 4–83. PA oblique projection of SI joint with patient semipronated. Side down demonstrated. ASIS level *(square)*. Reach under patient to palpate.

NOTES:

CERVICAL SPINE: AP

8 x 10 in.
20 x 24 cm

8 x 10 in.
20 x 24 cm

FILM: Use table Bucky or grid. Collimate to the area of interest.
CR: Entrance at C-5, exit at C-4 with a 15- to 20-degree cephalic angle (use the thyroid cartilage at C-5 to locate C-4).
POSITION: Patient is supinated on the x-ray table. Remove all head and neck jewelry and removable dental work.

Center the midsagittal plane to the center of the table.

Place the bottom of the film just above the jugular (sternal) notch, or center the center of the film to the transverse CR indicator on the tabletop (see CR, above).

NOTE: For trauma patients, perform a crosstable lateral (with patient as is) first to determine fracture. A radiologist will determine the permissible movement of the patient for the remaining x-ray procedure. *Do not move the patient until the radiologist makes an assessment!*

Slightly extend the head to remove the mandible from the area of interest (Fig. 5–1).

You can properly adjust the extension of the head and neck by temporarily centering the angled CR at the inferior edge of the occipital bone of the skull. If you have trouble palpating the base of the occipital bone, follow the line of the occipital bone from the mastoid area (see Figs. 1–3 and 1–8). Adjust flexion (or extension) to align both the mentum and occiput along the path of the CR. This method will superimpose the mandible over the occipital base and maximize the visualization of the upper cervical area. Don't forget to recenter the central ray at C-4.

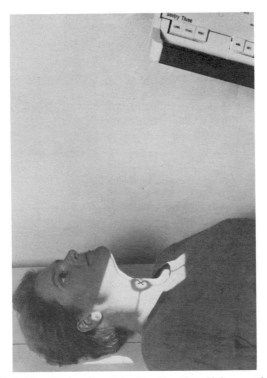

FIGURE 5–1. AP projection of cervical spine with a 15- to 20-degree cephalic angle used to open the intervertebral joint spaces.

STRUCTURES DEMONSTRATED: The cephalic angle will open the intervertebral disk spaces (Fig. 5–2).

The lower five cervical and upper one or two thoracic vertebrae.

The interpediculate spaces.

The superimposed transverse, spinous, and articular processes.

COMMON ERROR: *The mandible superimposed over the upper two cervical vertebrae. Adjust the flexion of the neck to correctly place the lower border of the mandible to be superimposed over the lower border of the occipital bone.*

TECHNIQUE

KV _____ MA _____ SECS _____ MAS _____ CALIPER _____ cm

_____ :1 GRID / B / none SCREEN: RE / High / Par / Detail / None

SID: _____ Rm _____ ADULT / CHILD age: _____ mos. / yrs.

HABITUS: Hyper / s / hypo / a   XS   S   M   L   XL   XXL

NOTES:

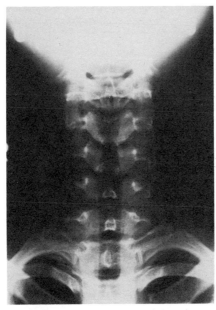

FIGURE 5–2. AP x-ray of cervical spine.

CERVICAL SPINE: AP DENS (OPEN MOUTH)

8 x 10 in.	8 x 10 in.	8 x 10 in.
20 x 24 cm	20 x 24 cm	20 x 24 cm

FILM: Use table Bucky or grid. Collimate to the area of interest.
CR: Perpendicularly at the center of the open mouth. Center the film to the mastoid tips. (Refer to Fig. 1–3.)
POSITION: The patient is supinated on the table. Remove all head and neck jewelry and removable dental work.

Set exposures before positioning.

Center the midsagittal plane to the center of the table.

Place the upper incisors at the level of the mastoid tips by flexing or extending the patient's head and neck. Check this alignment after instructing the patient to open the mouth as wide as possible by dropping the lower jaw (Fig. 5–3). Be careful that the patient does not throw the head back (extend) upon opening the mouth. Also check that the inferior edge of the occipital bone is positioned at the lower edge of the upper incisors. This is essential in order to avoid superimposition of the occipital bone over C-1 and C-2.

To avoid patient fatigue and drift, make the exposure as soon as you verify the baselines after the patient opens his or her mouth.
STRUCTURES DEMONSTRATED: The dens (odontoid process) should be free from superimposition of the occipital bone (Fig. 5–4). Do not mistake the lighter demarcation of the rings of C-1 for the occipital bone. The occipital bone will be scalloped and more dense.

The articular surfaces of C-1 and C-2 (the atlanto-occipital area) are demonstrated.

COMMON ERROR: Unnecessary repeats when the odontoid is superimposed. If the shadows of the upper incisors are directly superimposed over the inferior margin of the occipital bone, the head and neck position cannot be further corrected to avoid superimposition over the odontoid. A 3- to 5-degree cephalic angle may help in this case.

TECHNIQUE

KV _____ MA _____ SECS _____ MAS _____ CALIPER _____ cm
_____ :1 GRID / B / none SCREEN: RE / High / Par / Detail / None
SID: _____ Rm _____ ADULT / CHILD age: _____ mos. / yrs.
HABITUS: Hyper / s / hypo / a   XS   S   M   L   XL   XXL

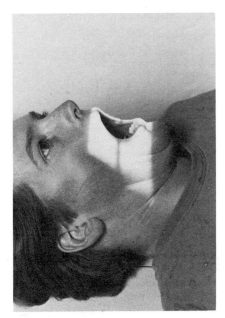

FIGURE 5–3. AP projection, open mouth (dens).

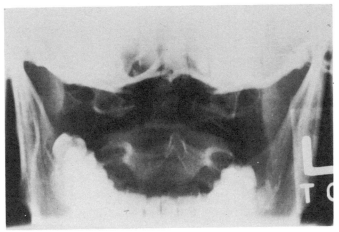

FIGURE 5–4. AP x-ray of open mouth.

CERVICAL SPINE: AP OBLIQUES (RPO AND LPO POSITIONS)

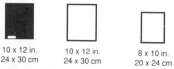

10 x 12 in.
24 x 30 cm

10 x 12 in.
24 x 30 cm

8 x 10 in.
20 x 24 cm

FILM: Use table Bucky or grid. Collimate to the area of interest.
CR: With 15- to 20-degree cephalic angle, exit at level of C-4 just lateral to the trachea (Fig. 5–5). (Use the thyroid cartilage at C-5 to locate the level of C-4).

POSITION: Remove all head and neck jewelry and any removable dental work. For the supinated, recumbent position, have the patient lie on his or her back and roll up for the first position to either the right or left (always take both obliques). Slightly pad the skull to keep the head in midsagittal alignment with the rest of the body.

The patient should be obliqued 45 degrees by moving the head, neck, shoulders, and torso as a unit (Fig. 5–5). However, if you find yourself having trouble opening the upper foramina, rotate the patient's head slightly toward the film.

Extend (tilt back) the head to avoid superimposition of the mandibular angles over the upper cervical area.

The patient, if capable, may also be standing (Fig. 5–6) or seated for this exam.

Remember to oblique the head, neck, shoulders, and torso as a unit.

Perform both obliques for comparison.

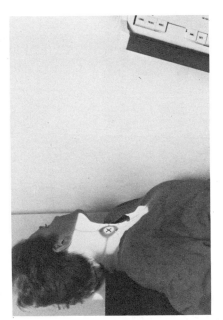

FIGURE 5–5. AP oblique of cervical spine (LPO position). Side up (right), side demonstrated.

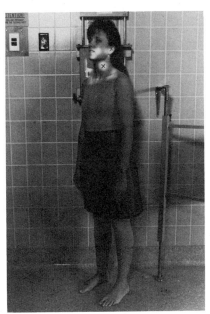

FIGURE 5–6. Upright AP oblique of cervical spine (RPO position). Side up (left), side demonstrated.

STRUCTURES DEMONSTRATED: Best demonstration of the intervertebral foramina further away from the film (Fig. 5–7). The RPO demonstrates the left intervertebral foramina and the LPO the right.

The pedicles of the cervical vertebrae away from the film.

COMMON ERRORS: (1) Superimposition of the mandibular angles over the upper cervical area. Slightly extend (tilt back) the head to avoid superimposition. Do not hyperextend as this will cause superimposition of the base of the skull. (2) Closure of the upper intervertebral foramina. This occurs with an incorrect cephalic angle of the tube, or when a recumbent patient's head and neck are extended or turned excessively. Slightly pad the upper skull with a small sponge in order to maintain the midsagittal alignment.

TECHNIQUE

KV _____ MA _____ SECS _____ MAS _____ CALIPER _____ cm

_____ :1 GRID / B / none SCREEN: RE / High / Par / Detail / None

SID: _____ Rm _____ ADULT / CHILD age: _____ mos. / yrs.

HABITUS: Hyper / s / hypo / a   XS   S   M   L   XL   XXL

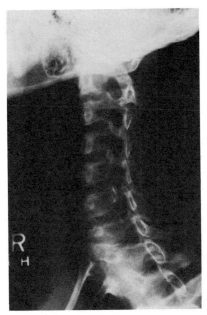

FIGURE 5–7. Right AP oblique x-ray (RPO) of cervical spine.

CERVICAL SPINE: PA OBLIQUES (RAO AND LAO POSITIONS)

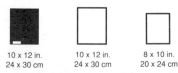

| 10 x 12 in. | 10 x 12 in. | 8 x 10 in. |
| 24 x 30 cm | 24 x 30 cm | 20 x 24 cm |

FILM: Use table Bucky or grid. Collimate to the area of interest.

CR: With 15- to 20-degree caudal angle, exit mid-neck at level of C-4 (use the thyroid cartilage at C-5 to locate the level of C-4).

POSITION: Remove all head and neck jewelry and any removable dental work. For the pronated, recumbent position, have the patient lie on the stomach and roll up to either the right or left (always take both obliques). Turn the patient's head toward the elevated side of each oblique.

For the RAO position (Fig. 5–8), have the patient place the right arm down by the side; for the LAO, the left arm is placed down by the side.

The patient should be obliqued 45 degrees by obliquing the head, neck, shoulders, and torso as a unit. Some technologists position the patient's head in a "no" position without padding for the head. Try this as an alternate when you have difficulty opening the upper foramina.

Extend (tilt back) the head to avoid superimposition of the mandibular angles over the upper cervical area.

The patient, if capable, may also be standing or seated for this exam.

Perform both obliques for comparison.

STRUCTURES DEMONSTRATED: Best demonstration of the intervertebral foramina closest to the film (Fig. 5–9). The RAO demonstrates the right intervertebral foramina, and the LAO, the left.

The pedicles of the cervical vertebrae closest to film.

COMMON ERRORS: (1) Superimposition of the mandibular angles over the upper cervical area. Extend (tilt back) the head to avoid superimposition. (2) Closure of the upper intervertebral foramina. This occurs with an incorrect caudal angle of the tube, or when a recumbent patient's head and neck are extended excessively.

TECHNIQUE

KV _____ MA _____ SECS _____ MAS _____ CALIPER _____ cm

_____ :1 GRID / B / none SCREEN: RE / High / Par / Detail / None

SID: _____ Rm _____ ADULT / CHILD   age: _____ mos. / yrs.

HABITUS: Hyper / s / hypo / a   XS   S   M   L   XL   XXL

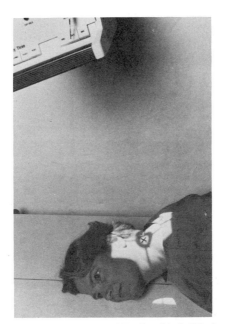

FIGURE 5–8. PA oblique of cervical spine (RAO position). Side down (right), side demonstrated.

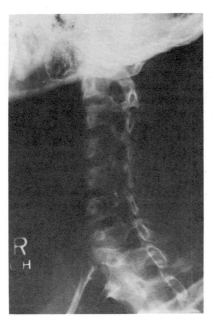

FIGURE 5–9. PA oblique x-ray (LAO) of cervical spine.

CERVICAL SPINE: LATERAL (NONTRAUMA)

10 x 12 in.   10 x 12 in.
24 x 30 cm   24 x 30 cm

FILM: Grid or no grid. Collimate to the area of interest.

CR: Perpendicularly, 72 inches (183 cm) mid-neck at C-4. Use the thyroid cartilage at C-5 to locate the level of C-4.

POSITION: Remove any head and neck jewelry and any removable dental work. With the patient either sitting or standing at the chest board or film holder, center the coronal plane through the cervical spine to the center of the film. The patient should be in a true lateral position with the shoulder closest to the film touching the film or holder for stabilization.

The shoulders are even and should be placed directly over the hips.

The head and neck should be first placed in the neutral position (between flexion and extension), with the head tilted slightly back or the mandible slightly elevated to avoid superimposition of the mandibular angles over the anterior aspect of the cervical vertebrae.

If the patient is hypersthenic or large shouldered, use equal weights in each hand in order to lower the shoulders for visualization of the lower cervical area (Fig. 5–10).

Palpate the vertebra prominens (C-7 spinous process); make sure it is included on the bottom of the film.

The exposure should be made at the end of exhalation in order to lower the shoulders.

STRUCTURES DEMONSTRATED: All seven cervical vertebrae in the lateral aspect (Fig. 5–11).

The best demonstration of the zygapophyseal joints (apophyses and articular facets) of the cervical vertebrae.

The spinous processes of C-2 through C-7 (vertebra prominens).

The posterior tubercle of C-1.

COMMON ERRORS: (1) Superimposition of the mandibular angles over the upper cervical area. Extend (tilt back) the head to avoid superimposition. Do not hyperextend to avoid superimposition of the base of the skull. (2) Lack of inclusion of the body of C-7. Sometimes the swimmer's position is used in order to demonstrate C-7 and T-1 when the lateral fails to do so.

TECHNIQUE

KV _____ MA _____ SECS _____ MAS _____ CALIPER _____ cm

_____ :1 GRID / B / none SCREEN: RE / High / Par / Detail / None

SID: _____ Rm _____ ADULT / CHILD age: _____ mos. / yrs.

HABITUS: Hyper / s / hypo / a   XS   S   M   L   XL   XXL

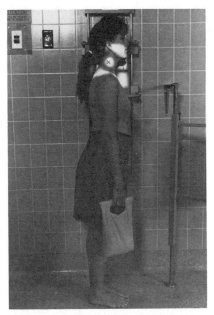

FIGURE 5–10. Upright lateral cervical spine (nontrauma).

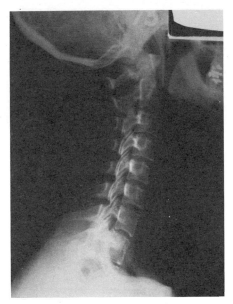

FIGURE 5–11. Lateral cervical spine x-ray.

CERVICAL SPINE: CROSSTABLE LATERAL FOR TRAUMA PATIENTS

10 x 12 in.
24 x 30 cm

10 x 12 in.
24 x 30 cm

FILM: Grid or no grid. Collimate to the area of interest.

CR: Perpendicularly, 72 inches (183 cm) source-image distance (SID) mid-neck at C-4. Use the thyroid cartilage at C-5 to locate the level of C-4.

POSITION: The patient should be recumbent and supine on the table (Fig. 5–12).

Shoulders should be relaxed and at the same level and the hands at the hips if the patient's condition permits; avoid excessive movement of the patient.

Remove any necklaces or earrings without moving the patient's head and neck.

Do not correct the placement of the head; take as is.

Place the film to include the shoulder. The bottom of the film should include the sternal notch (T-2 or T-3), and the top of the film should include the mastoid tip (C-1).

A grid is not necessary due to the air gap between the neck and film. The SID will correct the magnification caused by the increased object-image distance (OID).

The exposure should be made at the patient's full expiration.

STRUCTURES DEMONSTRATED: All seven cervical vertebrae in the lateral aspect (Fig. 5–13).

The best demonstration of the zygapophyseal joints (apophyses and articular facets) of the cervical vertebrae.

The spinous processes of C-2 through C-7. The posterior tubercle of C-1.

COMMON ERROR: Lack of inclusion of the body of C-7. NOTE: When the lateral fails to demonstrate C-7 and T-1 on trauma patients, never use the swimmer's position unless you confer with a radiologist.

TECHNIQUE

KV _____ MA _____ SECS _____ MAS _____ CALIPER _____ cm

_____ :1 GRID / B / none SCREEN: RE / High / Par / Detail / None

SID: _____ Rm _____ ADULT / CHILD age: _____ mos. / yrs.

HABITUS: Hyper / s / hypo / a   XS   S   M   L   XL   XXL

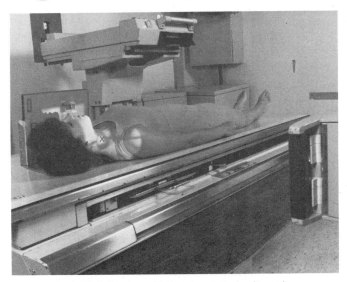

FIGURE 5–12. Crosstable lateral cervical spine (trauma).

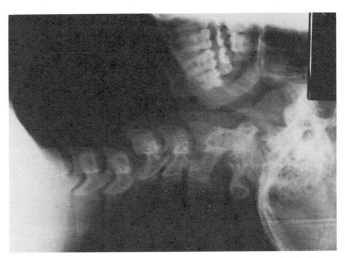

FIGURE 5–13. Crosstable lateral cervical spine x-ray with severe anterior displacement at C-4.

CERVICAL SPINE: FLEXION LATERAL
(NONTRAUMA)

| 10 x 12 in. | 10 x 12 in. | 10 x 12 in. | 10 x 12 in. |
| 24 x 30 cm | 24 x 30 cm | 24 x 30 cm | 24 x 30 cm |

FILM: Grid or no grid. Collimate to the area of interest.

CR: Perpendicularly, 72 inches (183 cm) mid-neck at C-4. Use the thyroid cartilage at C-5 to locate the level of C-4.

POSITION: Remove all head and neck jewelry. With the patient either sitting or standing at the chest board or film holder, center the coronal plane through the posterior cervical area to the center of the film (Fig. 5–14). The patient should be in a true lateral position with the shoulder closest to the film touching the film or holder for stabilization.

The shoulders are even and should be placed over the hips.

NOTE: Do not perform this position if trauma is suspected; always confer with the radiologist before performing this exam.

The head and neck should be placed in the extreme forward position (flexed) with the chin as close to touching the chest as possible. This position should not cause undue pain or discomfort to the patient. Place only the head and neck in flexion so far as the patient is comfortable.

If the patient is hypersthenic or large shouldered, use equal weights in each hand in order to lower the shoulders for visualization of the lower cervical area.

The exposure should be made at the end of exhalation in order to lower the shoulders.

STRUCTURES DEMONSTRATED: All seven cervical vertebrae extremely flexed in the lateral aspect (Fig. 5–15).

The best demonstration of the zygapophyseal joints (apophyses and articular facets) of the cervical vertebrae.

The flared, spinous processes of C-2 through C-7.

The posterior tubercle of C-1.

COMMON ERROR: The upper cervical (or lower cervical) vertebrae are clipped or not included on the film. Make sure in this position that the film includes all cervical vertebrae. You may have to place the film crosswise depending on the patient's ability to flex the head and neck.

TECHNIQUE

KV _____ MA _____ SECS _____ MAS _____ CALIPER _____ cm

_____ :1 GRID / B / none SCREEN: RE / High / Par / Detail / None

SID: _____ Rm _____ ADULT / CHILD age: _____ mos. / yrs.

HABITUS: Hyper / s / hypo / a XS S M L XL XXL

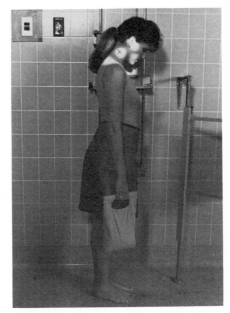

FIGURE 5–14. Flexion lateral cervical spine.

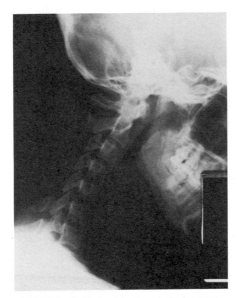

FIGURE 5–15. Flexion lateral cervical spine x-ray.

CERVICAL SPINE: EXTENSION LATERAL
(NONTRAUMA)

10 x 12 in.   10 x 12 in.
24 x 30 cm   24 x 30 cm

FILM: Grid or no grid. Collimate to the area of interest.

CR: Perpendicularly, 72 inches (183 cm) mid-neck at C-4. Use the thyroid cartilage at C-5 to locate the level of C-4.

POSITION: Remove all head and neck jewelry. With the patient either sitting or standing at the chest board or film holder, center the coronal plane through the cervical spine to the center of the film (Fig. 5–16). The patient should be in a true lateral position with the shoulder closest to the film touching for stabilization.

The shoulders are even and should be placed over the hips.

NOTE: Do not perform this position if trauma is suspected; always confer with the radiologist before performing this exam.

The head and neck should be placed in the extreme posterior position (extension). This position should not cause undue pain or discomfort to the patient. Only place the head and neck in extension so far as the patient is comfortable.

If the patient is hypersthenic or large shouldered, use equal weights in each hand in order to lower the shoulders for visualization of the lower cervical area.

The exposure should be made at the end of exhalation in order to lower the shoulders.

STRUCTURES DEMONSTRATED: All seven cervical vertebrae extended, in the lateral aspect (Fig. 5–17).

The best demonstration of the superior and inferior articular processes and zygapophyseal joints (apophyses) of the cervical vertebrae.

The compressed, spinous processes of C-2 through C-7. The posterior tubercle of C-1.

COMMON ERROR: *The upper cervical (or lower cervical) vertebrae are clipped or not included on the film. Make sure in this position that the film includes all cervical vertebrae. You may have to place the film crosswise depending on the patient's ability to extend the head and neck.*

TECHNIQUE

KV _____ MA _____ SECS _____ MAS _____ CALIPER _____ cm

_____ :1 GRID / B / none SCREEN: RE / High / Par / Detail / None

SID: _____ Rm _____ ADULT / CHILD age: _____ mos. / yrs.

HABITUS: Hyper / s / hypo / a   XS   S   M   L   XL   XXL

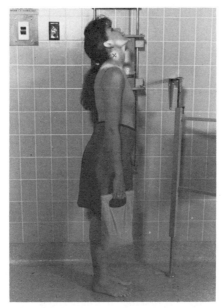

FIGURE 5–16. Extension lateral cervical spine.

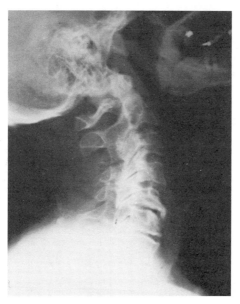

FIGURE 5–17. Extension lateral cervical spine x-ray.

CERVICOTHORACIC SPINE (C-7 TO T-1): LATERAL (SWIMMER'S)

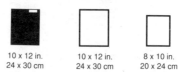

10 x 12 in.
24 x 30 cm

10 x 12 in.
24 x 30 cm

8 x 10 in.
20 x 24 cm

FILM: Use table Bucky or grid. Collimate to the area of interest.
CR: Perpendicular to C-7 or T-1. If upper shoulder cannot be depressed, use a 5-degree caudal angle.
POSITION: Remove all neck jewelry. The patient can be either recumbent, Pawlow method[16] (Fig. 5–18), or upright, Twining method[17] (Fig. 5–19). Use the upright for ambulatory patients. Use the recumbent for disabled or trauma patients. For trauma patients that cannot be lateralized, use a crosstable projection, with a dorsal decubitus position of the patient (Fig. 5–20).

Elevate the arm closest to the film.

Relax the shoulder farthest from the film so that it is depressed as much as possible.

Keeping the upper torso in a true, lateral position, rotate one shoulder anteriorly and the other posteriorly. Usually the shoulder of the side down is placed more anteriorly and the side up, inferiorly or posteriorly. Before the patient lies on it, make sure the upper arm is extended away from the body. This will "round" the shoulder and remove the humeral head from the area of interest. The shoulders must be moved in different directions while maintaining the lateral position of the thorax.

It is important to keep the level of the head (and cervical spine) at the same level as the rest of the vertebral column.

Collimate closely to the area of interest.

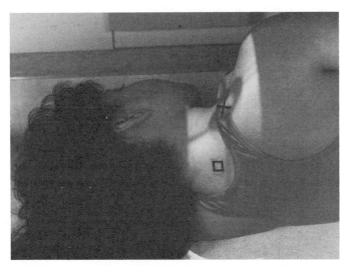

FIGURE 5–18. Recumbent lateral cervicothoracic spine (swimmer's). Vertebral prominens *(square)*. Make sure the head is level with the rest of the vertebral column.

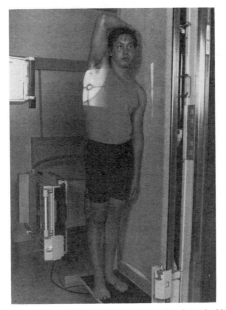

FIGURE 5–19. Alternate, upright cervicothoracic spine lateral. Notice the arm positions can be reversed from the swimmer's method. Sometimes the original method does not result in good separation of the shoulders, or the patient has multiple injuries that preclude elevating the side closest to the film.

STRUCTURES DEMONSTRATED: The lower cervical spine (C-5, C-6, and C-7) and upper thoracic spine (T-1, T-2, and T-3) should be seen in their lateral aspects (Fig. 5–21).

The shoulders should be separated and not directly superimposed upon each other.

COMMON ERRORS: (1) The upper thorax is not lateralized. Make sure the anterior and posterior positions of the shoulders do not pull the upper torso out of lateral alignment. (2) Underpenetration.

TECHNIQUE

KV _____ MA _____ SECS _____ MAS _____ CALIPER _____ cm

_____ :1 GRID / B / none SCREEN: RE / High / Par / Detail / None

SID: _____ Rm _____ ADULT / CHILD age: _____ mos. / yrs.

HABITUS: Hyper / s / hypo / a   XS   S   M   L   XL   XXL

NOTES:

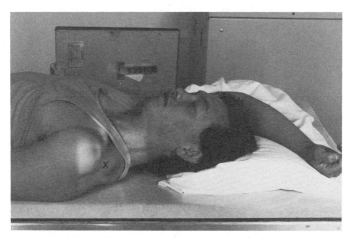

FIGURE 5–20. Crosstable lateral of cervicothoracic spine.

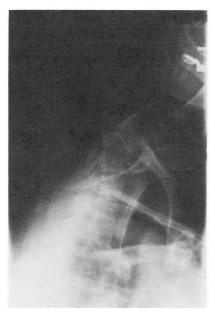

FIGURE 5–21. Lateral cervicothoracic spine x-ray. (Courtesy of T. Abney, S.R.T.)

CERVICAL SPINE: VERTEBRAL ARCH STUDY (AP AXIAL, PILLARS OR LATERAL MASS)

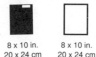

8 x 10 in. 8 x 10 in.
20 x 24 cm 20 x 24 cm

FILM: Collimate to the area of interest.

CR: A 20- to 30-degree caudal angle, enter mid-neck at C-4; exit at approximately C-7. The greater the lordosis of the head and neck, the greater the degree of caudal angle.

POSITION: Remove all head and neck jewelry and any removable dental work. The patient is supinated on the table.

The midsagittal plane is centered to the table.

NOTE: Do not perform this position if trauma is suspected; always confer with the radiologist before performing this exam.

Hyperextend the head and neck of the patient if the patient tolerates it (Fig. 5–22).

Center the film to the transverse CR line indicator on the tabletop (see CR, above). Make sure the top of the film includes the external acoustic meatus (EAM).

Sometimes the patient's head is placed in the "no" position to better demonstrate the upper cervical area for the AP oblique axial projection.[18] Turn the patient's head away from the side of interest. Do both sides for comparison if this method is used.

STRUCTURES DEMONSTRATED: Best demonstration of the posterior portion or vertebral arch of the middle cervical, lower cervical, and upper thoracic vertebrae (Fig. 5–23). The anterior portions are not demonstrated due to the severe caudal angle.

The articular pillars, or lateral masses of both sides, are demonstrated.

The superior and inferior articular processes and zygapophyseal articulations (apophyses) are seen.

The spinous processes are seen in midline.

COMMON ERROR: Underpenetration.

TECHNIQUE

KV _____ MA _____ SECS _____ MAS _____ CALIPER _____ cm

_____ :1 GRID / B / none SCREEN: RE / High / Par / Detail / None

SID: _____ Rm _____ ADULT / CHILD age: _____ mos. / yrs.

HABITUS: Hyper / s / hypo / a XS S M L XL XXL

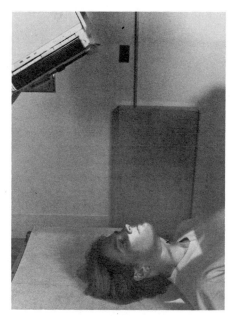

FIGURE 5–22. Vertebral arch study of cervical spine (AP axial projection with caudal angle).

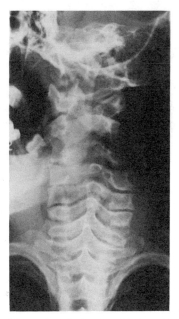

FIGURE 5–23. AP axial x-ray (vertebral arch study) of cervical spine. The patient's head is turned in the "no" position.

THORACIC SPINE: AP

| 7 x 17 in. | 7 x 17 in. | 14 x 17 in. | 14 x 17 in. |
| 18 x 43 cm | 18 x 43 cm | 35 x 43 cm | 35 x 43 cm |

FILM: Collimate to the area of interest.

CR: Perpendicular to T-6.

POSITION: The patient is supine on the x-ray table. Remove all neck jewelry.

The midsagittal plane is centered to the table (Fig. 5–24).

To reduce the kyphotic curve of the thoracic spine do not use excess padding for the head.

Bend the patient's legs at the knee with the feet flat against the table in order to reduce the lordotic curve of the lumbar spine (and ease lower back discomfort).

Use expiration in order to even the density of the thorax.

Occasionally, a wedge filter attached to the collimator housing is used with the thicker side over the thinnest anatomical area (the upper thoracic) in order to even the exposure over the differing thicknesses of the thoracic vertebrae.

STRUCTURES DEMONSTRATED: All twelve vertebral bodies of the thoracic spine (Fig. 5–25).

Some intervertebral spaces will be more open than others due to the kyphotic curvature of the thoracic spine.

The pedicles of the thoracic spine.

COMMON ERROR: The upper thoracic will usually be overpenetrated. Use the anode-heel effect to even the exposure over the entire area (patient's head should be on the technologist's left; when anode is on left side, thicker part should be on the right). Use a collimator-attached filter if available.

TECHNIQUE

KV _____ MA _____ SECS _____ MAS _____ CALIPER _____ cm

_____ :1 GRID / B / none SCREEN: RE / High / Par / Detail / None

SID: _____ Rm _____ ADULT / CHILD age: _____ mos. / yrs.

HABITUS: Hyper / s / hypo / a   XS   S   M   L   XL   XXL

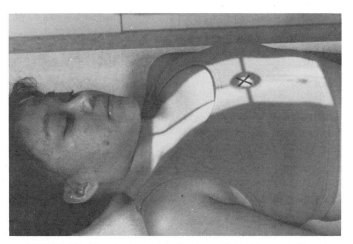

FIGURE 5–24. AP projection of thoracic spine collimated to area of interest.

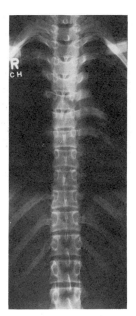

FIGURE 5–25. AP x-ray of thoracic spine. (Note the near clip of T-1.)

THORACIC SPINE: LATERAL

7 x 17 in.
18 x 43 cm

7 x 17 in.
18 x 43 cm

14 x 17 in.
35 x 43 cm

14 x 17 in.
35 x 43 cm

FILM: Collimate to the area of interest.

CR: Perpendicular to T-6; follow the kyphotic curve to find the correct longitudinal (coronal) plane of T-6.

POSITION: Remove all neck jewelry. The patient is in the left lateral, recumbent position (lying on the left side). The pelvis and shoulders should be lateralized equally with the knees bent and on top of each other. Have the patient hold the side of the table for stabilization (Fig. 5–26).

Pad the waist in order to straighten the thoracic spine and place it in the same horizontal plane. If no padding is available, you may angle the central ray 10 to 15 degrees cephalad in order to correct the horizontal plane of the thoracic spine.

Center the midaxillary (slightly posterior to the midcoronal)[19] plane to the center of the table. If the patient has an excessive kyphotic curve, center the levels of T-3 and T-9 to the center of the table. A quiet breathing technique may be used, or just make the exposure at the end of patient exhalation.

STRUCTURES DEMONSTRATED: The thoracic vertebrae in their lateral aspect. The upper thoracic vertebrae are frequently obscured due to the bulk of the shoulders (Fig. 5–27).

The intervertebral spaces are open.

The thoracic bodies are seen in profile.

The intervertebral thoracic foramina are demonstrated.

The posterior ribs should be superimposed, with the right posterior ribs slightly magnified when performing a left lateral.

COMMON ERROR: Uneven density. Adjust your technique for type of respiration—less air, higher technique; more air, less technique.

TECHNIQUE

KV _____ MA _____ SECS _____ MAS _____ CALIPER _____ cm

_____ :1 GRID / B / none SCREEN: RE / High / Par / Detail / None

SID: _____ Rm _____ ADULT / CHILD age: _____ mos. / yrs.

HABITUS: Hyper / s / hypo / a   XS   S   M   L   XL   XXL

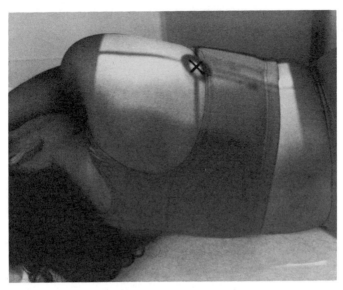

FIGURE 5–26. Lateral thoracic spine.

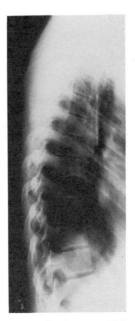

FIGURE 5–27. Lateral thoracic spine x-ray with breathing technique.

UPPER THORACIC: LATERAL (SWIMMER'S POSITION)

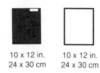

10 x 12 in.   10 x 12 in.
24 x 30 cm   24 x 30 cm

FILM: Use table Bucky or grid. Collimate to the area of interest.
CR: Perpendicular to C-7 or T-1. If upper shoulder cannot be depressed, use a 5-degree caudal angle.
POSITION: Remove all neck jewelry. The patient can be either recumbent, Pawlow method (see Fig. 5–18), or upright, Twining method (see Fig. 5–19). Use the upright for ambulatory patients. Use the recumbent for disabled or trauma patients. For trauma patients that cannot be lateralized, use a crosstable projection, with a dorsal decubitus position of the patient (see Fig. 5–20).

Elevate the arm closest to the film.

Relax the shoulder farthest from the film so that it is depressed as much as possible.

Keeping the upper torso in a true, lateral position, rotate one shoulder anteriorly and the other inferiorly or posteriorly. Usually the shoulder of the side down is rotated anteriorly and the side up inferiorly or posteriorly. The shoulders must be moved in different directions while maintaining the lateral position.

It is important to keep the level of the head (and cervical spine) at the same level as the rest of the vertebral column.

STRUCTURES DEMONSTRATED: The lower cervical spine (C-5, C-6, and C-7) and upper thoracic spine (T-1, T-2, and T-3) should be seen in their lateral aspects (see Fig. 5–21).

The shoulders should be separated, and not directly superimposed upon each other.

COMMON ERRORS: (1) The upper thorax is not lateralized. Make sure the anterior and inferior or posterior position of the shoulders does not pull the upper torso out of lateral alignment. (2) Underpenetration. Frequently, the technique necessary to penetrate the shoulders and upper thorax is underestimated.

TECHNIQUE

KV _____ MA _____ SECS _____ MAS _____ CALIPER _____ cm
_____ :1 GRID / B / none SCREEN: RE / High / Par / Detail / None
SID: _____ Rm _____ ADULT / CHILD age: _____ mos. / yrs.
HABITUS: Hyper / s / hypo / a   XS   S   M   L   XL   XXL

LUMBAR SPINE: AP OR PA

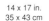
14 x 17 in.
35 x 43 cm

14 x 17 in.
35 x 43 cm

7 x 17 in.
18 x 43 cm

11 x 14 in.
30 x 35 cm

10 x 12 in.
24 x 30 cm

FILM: Use table Bucky or grid. Collimate to the area of interest.
CR: Perpendicularly at the level of L-4 at the midsagittal plane.
L-4 is found at midline, at the level of the iliac crest.
POSITION: The midsagittal plane of the patient should be centered to the center of the x-ray table.

The shoulders should be in the same plane.
AP: The patient should be supinated for the AP projection.

Place the arms upon the chest for the AP or away from the body at the side (Fig. 5–28).

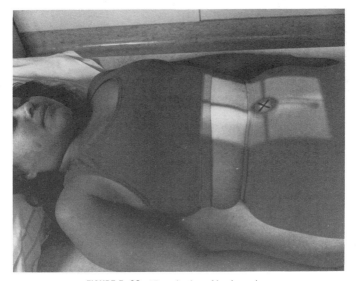

FIGURE 5–28. AP projection of lumbar spine.

Reduce the patient's discomfort and lumbar lordosis in the supine position by flexing the knees with a pad. This takes the pressure off of the lumbar area and flattens the back against the x-ray table.
PA: The patient should be pronated for the PA projection.

For the PA, place the arms in the same positions, either up by the pillow, or down by the sides (Fig. 5–29). Do not use the PA projection for a patient with a large abdomen.

Use a gonadal shield when it does not obscure the area of interest.

STRUCTURES DEMONSTRATED: The lumbar bodies, transverse processes, and the intervertebral disk spaces will be demonstrated (Fig. 5–30).

The spinous processes will be seen in the midsagittal plane.

The vertebral arch components, the laminae, and interpediculate areas will be seen superimposed over the vertebral bodies.

The intervertebral disk spaces will be more completely opened on the PA projection than on the AP. The space between L-5 and S-1 will not be well demonstrated by either the AP or PA.

The PA projection will decrease the lordotic curve of the lumbar spine.

NOTES:

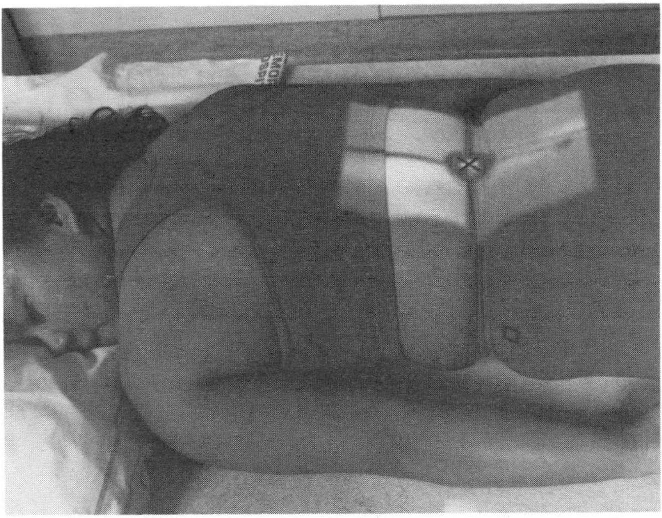

FIGURE 5–29. PA projection of lumbar spine. Iliac crest *(square)*.

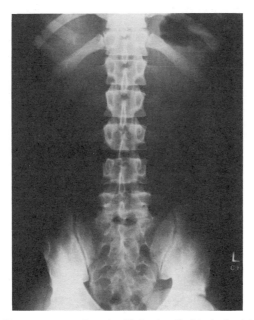

FIGURE 5–30. PA x-ray of lumbar spine. Notice that all of the lumbar intervertebral disk spaces are opened.

An upright study of the complete spine is sometimes preferred by orthopedic physicians and chiropractors (Fig. 5–31).
COMMON ERROR: The midsagittal plane is not centered to the center of the x-ray table.

TECHNIQUE

KV _____ MA _____ SECS _____ MAS _____ CALIPER _____ cm
_____ :1 GRID / B / none SCREEN: RE / High / Par / Detail / None
SID: _____ Rm _____ ADULT / CHILD age: _____ mos. / yrs.
HABITUS: Hyper / s / hypo / a   XS   S   M   L   XL   XXL

NOTES:

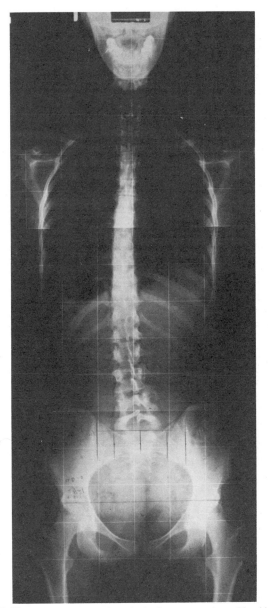

FIGURE 5–31. Full body AP x-ray of vertebral column commonly used for chiropractic study. (Courtesy of C. Rangel, D.C.)

LUMBAR SPINE: LATERAL

      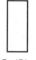

| 14 x 17 in. | 14 x 17 in. | 7 x 17 in. | 7 x 17 in. | 11 x 14 in. |
| 35 x 43 cm | 35 x 43 cm | 18 x 43 cm | 18 x 43 cm | 30 x 35 cm |

FILM: Use table Bucky or grid. Collimate to the area of interest.
CR: Perpendicular to L-3 when the waist is padded with a radio-lucent sponge. L-3 is found 2 to 3 inches (5 to 8 cm) above the level of the iliac crest. Use a 5- to 8-degree caudal angle if no waist pad is used (5 for male patients and 8 for female patients).
POSITION: The patient is recumbent on the left side (left lateral recumbent) (Fig. 5–32).

Center the midaxillary (slightly behind the midcoronal [see Fig. 1–2]) plane of the patient to the center of the x-ray table.

Pad the waist with a radiolucent sponge in order to level the lumbar spine. This will open the lumbar disk spaces evenly.

The knees should be flexed equally. Pad between the knees if the patient's upper hip still leans slightly anteriorly after making an attempt to adjust.

Shield the gonads when it will not obscure the areas of interest.
STRUCTURES DEMONSTRATED: The lateral aspect of the intervertebral disk spaces (Fig. 5–33).

The intervertebral foramina of L-1 to L-4 are best demonstrated.
The spinous processes are seen in profile.

For the demonstration of the intervertebral foramen of L-5, use a 70-degree obliquity measured from the table with the patient semipronated. A 35-degree caudal tube angle entering at the level of the iliac crest may be used. Side up is demonstrated.
COMMON ERRORS: (1) Underpenetration of the lower lumbar area. (2) Uneven intervertebral disk spaces due to unpadded waist area.

TECHNIQUE
KV _____ MA _____ SECS _____ MAS _____ CALIPER _____ cm
_____ :1 GRID / B / none SCREEN: RE / High / Par / Detail / None
SID: _____ Rm _____ ADULT / CHILD age: _____ mos. / yrs.
HABITUS: Hyper / s / hypo / a   XS   S   M   L   XL   XXL

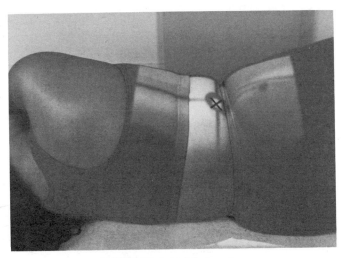

FIGURE 5–32. Lateral lumbar spine.

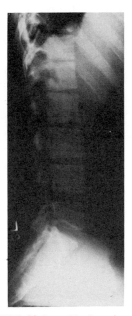

FIGURE 5–33. Lateral lumbar spine x-ray.

LUMBAR SPINE: LATERAL SPOT OF L-5 AND S-1

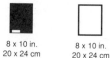

8 x 10 in.
20 x 24 cm

8 x 10 in.
20 x 24 cm

FILM: Use table Bucky or grid. Collimate to the area of interest.
CR: If waist is sponged, perpendicular to L5-S1. If not, use an 8-degree caudal angle for female patients, and a 5-degree caudal angle for males.
POSITION: After taking the lateral lumbar film with the patient still in the left lateral recumbent position, center the point 2 inches (5 cm) posterior to the midcoronal plane at the level of the ASIS to the center of the table (Fig. 5–34).

NOTE: Many technologists use the "L" shape of their right thumb and index finger to locate L5-S1 (see Fig. 1–24).

Depending on the body habitus or lordosis of the lumbar spine, you may have to move the patient anteriorly from the centerline of the table (about 1 to 2 inches or 3 to 4 cm) while still in the lateral lumbar position. The greater the lordosis, the more the anterior placement in order to center L5-S1 to the center of the table and film.

Extend the hips slightly, flex the knees equally, and pad them if necessary.

Shield the gonads when shielding will not obscure the areas of interest.

Collimate severely in order to reduce the scattered radiation effects on the film (increased overall grayness).
STRUCTURES DEMONSTRATED: The lateral aspect of L5-S1 closely collimated (Fig. 5–35).

The intervertebral disk space must be opened.
COMMON ERRORS: (1) The area of interest is not centered to the center of the film. (2) Underpenetration. (3) The joint space is not open. Sometimes changing the patient to the opposite lateral recumbent position will open the L5-S1 disk space.

TECHNIQUE

KV _____ MA _____ SECS _____ MAS _____ CALIPER _____ cm
_____ :1 GRID / B / none SCREEN: RE / High / Par / Detail / None
SID: _____ Rm _____ ADULT / CHILD age: _____ mos. / yrs.
HABITUS: Hyper / s / hypo / a   XS   S   M   L   XL   XXL

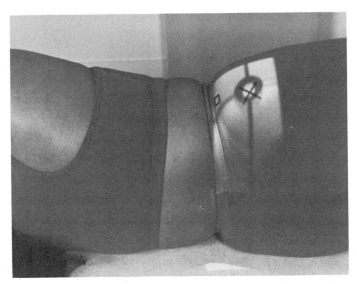

FIGURE 5–34. Lateral spot of L5-S1 joint. Iliac crest *(square)*.

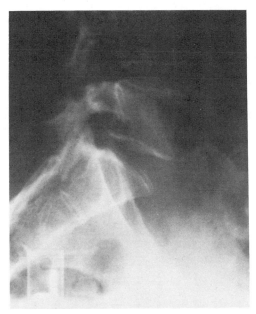

FIGURE 5–35. Lateral L5-S1 joint x-ray.

LUMBAR SPINE: AP OR PA OBLIQUES

11 x 14 in.   11 x 14 in.   10 x 12 in.   10 x 12 in.   14 x 17 in.
30 x 35 cm   30 x 35 cm   24 x 30 cm   24 x 30 cm   35 x 43 cm

FILM: Collimate to the area of interest.

CR: Perpendicular to the level of L-3.

POSITION: Use a 45-degree obliquity of the patient for L-1 to L-4. Make sure the entire body is obliqued as a unit.

NOTE: For the demonstration of the superior and inferior articular processes and zygapophyseal joint of L5-S1, use an obliquity of 30 degrees from the table, or supine position.

AP Obliques: The patient should be semisupinated for the AP oblique projections (Fig. 5–36).

The surface longitudinal (coronal) plane that intersects the ASIS in the oblique position represents the location of the lumbar spinous processes. Use the point 2 inches or 5 cm medial to this imaginary surface line to center the obliqued bodies of the lumbar spine (see PA Obliques) to the center of the table.

For AP obliques (RPO and LPO positions), pad the patient's back with a 45-degree radiolucent sponge for comfort.

PA Obliques: The patient should be semipronated for the PA oblique projections (Fig. 5–37).

For PA obliques (RAO and LAO positions), palpate the spinous processes in order to center 2 inches (5 cm) anterior from the spinous processes, that is, the midline of the obliqued lumbar spine, to the center of the x-ray table. (Some technologists use the "V" position of their 2nd and 3rd digits to estimate this for centering.)

Shield the gonads when shielding will not obscure the areas of interest.

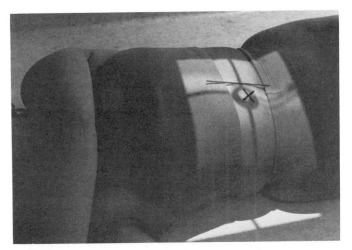

FIGURE 5–36. AP oblique (RPO position) of the lumbar spine. Line on anterior surface marks posterior location of the lumbar spinous processes.

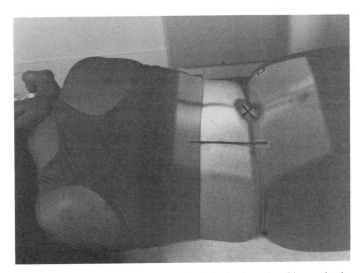

FIGURE 5–37. PA oblique (LAO position) of the lumbar spine. Line marks the location of the lumbar spinous processes. Iliac crest *(square)*.

STRUCTURES DEMONSTRATED: With a 45-degree obliquity, the superior and inferior articular processes and zygapophyseal articulations of L-1 through L-4 will be best demonstrated (Fig. 5–38).

For the demonstration of the inferior articular process of L-5, the superior articular process of S-1, and the L5-S1 zygapophyseal articulation, an obliquity of 30 degrees from either the supine or prone position is used.

The AP oblique projections (RPO and LPO positions) will best demonstrate the superior and inferior articular processes and zygapophyseal joints of the side down.

The PA oblique projections (RAO and LAO) will best demonstrate the superior and inferior articular processes and zygapophyseal joints of the side up (Fig. 5–38).

Sometimes radiologists like to have the SI joints included on the oblique films. Use the film with the blocker up if this is the case and include 1 to 2 inches (2.5 to 5 cm) below the ASIS.

COMMON ERRORS: (1) The lumbar spine (L-1 or L-5) is clipped. After centering the film to L-3, make sure the bottom of the film just includes the transverse plane of the ASIS. (2) The obliquity is not equal throughout the length of the lumbar vertebrae. To correct this, make sure the entire torso—shoulders and pelvis—is obliqued equally at 45 degrees.

TECHNIQUE

KV _____ MA _____ SECS _____ MAS _____ CALIPER _____ cm

_____ :1 GRID / B / none SCREEN: RE / High / Par / Detail / None

SID: _____ Rm _____ ADULT / CHILD age: _____ mos. / yrs.

HABITUS: Hyper / s / hypo / a XS   S   M   L   XL   XXL

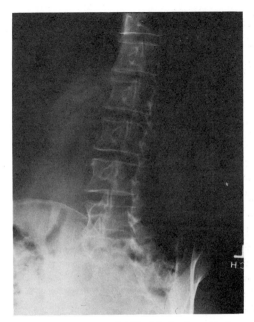

FIGURE 5–38. Left PA oblique x-ray (LAO) of the lumbar spine demonstrating the side up (right).

NOTES:

L5-S1: SEMI-AXIAL AP

| 8 x 10 in. 20 x 24 cm | 8 x 10 in. 20 x 24 cm | 8 x 10 in. 20 x 24 cm |

FILM: Collimate to the area of interest.

CR: For the AP projection, use a 30- to 35-degree cephalic angle. Enter the midsagittal plane at the level of the ASIS. The CR will exit at the level of L-4.

For the PA projection, use a caudal angle of 35 degrees. Enter the midsagittal plane at the level of L-4, and exit at the transverse plane of the ASIS.

POSITION: The patient is supinated on the x-ray table (Fig. 5–39).

Center the midsagittal plane to the center of the table.

Make sure that the patient's hips and shoulders are flat and in like positions.

Flex the patient's knees with feet flat on the tabletop.

Shield the gonads when shielding will not obscure the areas of interest.

Collimate severely to L5-S1.

STRUCTURES DEMONSTRATED: The angle of the central ray will demonstrate the open intervetebral disk space between L-5 and S-1 (Fig. 5–40).

COMMON ERROR: Underpenetration. When using a severe angle and severe collimation, one must significantly increase the technique from the routine AP lumbar study.

TECHNIQUE

KV _____ MA _____ SECS _____ MAS _____ CALIPER _____ cm

_____ :1 GRID / B / none SCREEN: RE / High / Par / Detail / None

SID: _____ Rm _____ ADULT / CHILD age: _____ mos. / yrs.

HABITUS: Hyper / s / hypo / a   XS   S   M   L   XL   XXL

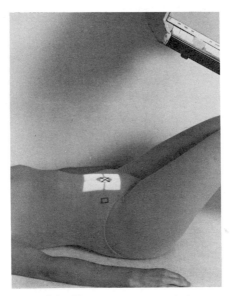

FIGURE 5–39. AP axial projection of L5-S1.

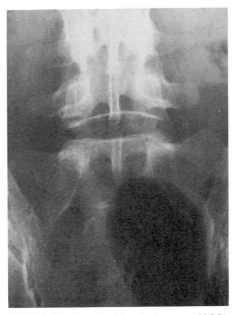

FIGURE 5–40. AP semi-axial projection x-ray of L5-S1.

LUMBAR SPINE: AP (RIGHT AND LEFT BENDING)

14 x 17 in.
35 x 43 cm

14 x 17 in.
35 x 43 cm

FILM: Use table Bucky or grid. Collimate to the area of interest.
CR: Perpendicularly at the level of L-4 at the midsagittal plane.
L-4 is found at midline, at the level of the iliac crest.
POSITION: The patient should be supinated and upright.

The midsagittal plane of the pelvis should be centered to the center of the x-ray table. Have the patient bend as far as possible left for one exposure (Fig. 5–41) and then right for another (Fig. 5–42) using a fresh second film.

The shoulders should be in the same plane during the bend.

The pelvis should remain flat against the table. Do not allow the pelvis to be rotated or moved from centerline.

NOTES:

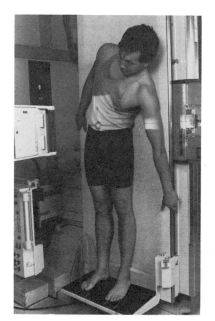

FIGURE 5–41. Left bending AP projection of lumbar spine. Arm positions to help make patient feel secure (make sure Bucky tray is locked).

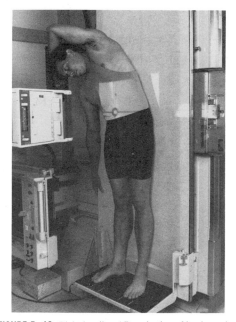

FIGURE 5–42. Right bending AP projection of lumbar spine.

STRUCTURES DEMONSTRATED: The range of motion (ROM) of the five lumbar vertebrae (Fig. 5–43).

The lumbar bodies, transverse processes, and the intervertebral disk spaces will be seen.

Localization of a herniated disk by demonstrating limited ROM. *COMMON ERROR: The pelvis shifts during bending and does not remain centered to the center of the x-ray table or is rotated slightly upon bending.*

TECHNIQUE

KV _____ MA _____ SECS _____ MAS _____ CALIPER _____ cm

_____ :1 GRID / B / none SCREEN: RE / High / Par / Detail / None

SID: _____ Rm _____ ADULT / CHILD age: _____ mos. / yrs.

HABITUS: Hyper / s / hypo / a   XS   S   M   L   XL   XXL

NOTES:

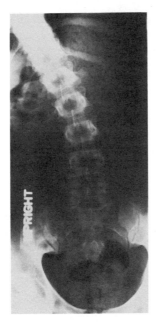

FIGURE 5–43. Right bending AP x-ray of lumbar spine. (Courtesy of C. Rangel, D.C.)

LUMBAR SPINE: LATERAL (FLEXION AND EXTENSION)

14 x 17 in.
35 x 43 cm

14 x 17 in.
35 x 43 cm

FILM: Use table Bucky or grid. Collimate to the area of interest.
CR: Perpendicular to L-3, which is found 2 to 3 inches (5 to 8 cm) above the level of the iliac crest.
POSITION: The patient is recumbent or upright with the left side next to the table.

Center the midaxillary plane (slightly behind the midcoronal plane)[20] of the patient to the center of the x-ray table.
Flexion: Have the patient bend forward (flex) while the pelvis is centered to the film or slightly posterior from center (Fig. 5–44).
Extension: Have the patient bend back (extend) while the pelvis is centered to the film or slightly anterior from center (Fig. 5–45).

NOTES:

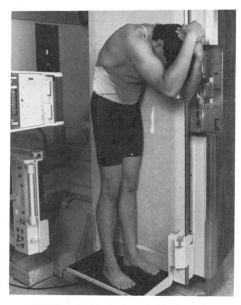

FIGURE 5–44. Flexion lateral of lumbar spine.

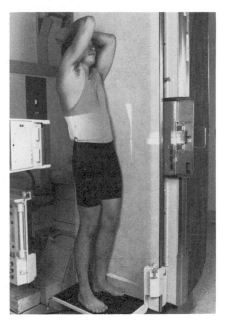

FIGURE 5–45. Extension lateral of lumbar spine.

STRUCTURES DEMONSTRATED: The range of motion of the five lumbar vertebrae (Fig. 5–46).

The lateral aspect of the intervertebral disk spaces.

COMMON ERROR: Misalignment due to the shift of the pelvis upon flexion or extension. Keep the pelvis fixed in place, or return it to the center of the film upon flexion or extension.

TECHNIQUE

KV _____ MA _____ SECS _____ MAS _____ CALIPER _____ cm

_____ :1 GRID / B / none SCREEN: RE / High / Par / Detail / None

SID: _____ Rm _____ ADULT / CHILD age: _____ mos. / yrs.

HABITUS: Hyper / s / hypo / a　XS　S　M　L　XL　XXL

NOTES:

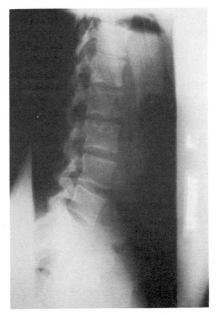

FIGURE 5–46. Extension lateral x-ray of lumbar spine. (Courtesy of C. Rangel, D.C.)

NOTES:

SACRUM: ANGLED AP OR PA

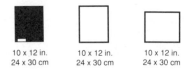

| 10 x 12 in. | 10 x 12 in. | 10 x 12 in. |
| 24 x 30 cm | 24 x 30 cm | 24 x 30 cm |

FILM: Collimate to the area of interest.

CR: For the AP, use a 15- to 20-degree cephalic angle. Enter at the midsagittal plane at the midpoint between the ASIS and the symphysis pubis (Fig. 5–47).

For the PA, use a 15- to 20-degree caudal angle. Enter at the midsagittal plane at the level of the ASIS.

POSITION: Center the midsagittal plane to the center of the table. Make sure the pelvis is flat.

For the AP, the patient is supinated. Pad under the knees if the patient is made more comfortable. This will vary as to the injury.

If the patient is unable to tolerate the supine position, use the pronated. This, however, is not optimal due to the increased OID.

For the PA, the patient is pronated.

STRUCTURES DEMONSTRATED: The sacrum will be free from the foreshortening of the sacral curvature (Fig. 5–48).

The sacrum and sacroiliac joints are seen in their entirety.

The obturator foramina will be open and the symphysis pubis will be broadened with this tube angle.

COMMON ERROR: The sacrum is obscured by bowel contents. Sometimes a bowel prep is necessary. The physician will order if necessary; check with the radiologist.

TECHNIQUE

KV _____ MA _____ SECS _____ MAS _____ CALIPER _____ cm

_____ :1 GRID / B / none SCREEN: RE / High / Par / Detail / None

SID: _____ Rm _____ ADULT / CHILD age: _____ mos. / yrs.

HABITUS: Hyper / s / hypo / a   XS   S   M   L   XL   XXL

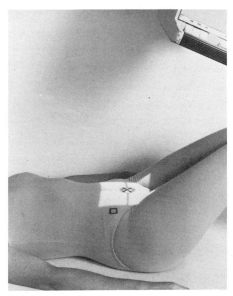

FIGURE 5–47. Semi-axial AP projection of sacrum. ASIS *(square)*.

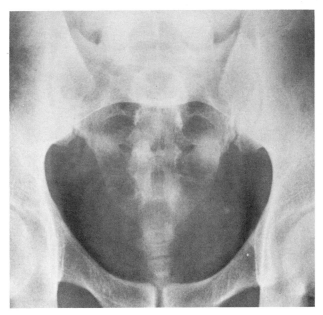

FIGURE 5–48. Semi-axial AP x-ray of sacrum.

SACRUM: LATERAL

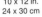

10 x 12 in.
24 x 30 cm

10 x 12 in.
24 x 30 cm

FILM: Collimate to the area of interest.

CR: Perpendicular to S-2 (at level of ASIS).

POSITION: The patient is in the left lateral recumbent position.

Extend the hips slightly; flex the knees equally and pad them if the patient's upper hip still leans slightly anteriorly after attempting to correct.

Center the point on the patient, 3 inches posterior to the midcoronal plane at the level of the ASIS, to the center of the x-ray table (Fig. 5–49).

Center the film and Bucky tray to the ASIS.

Shield the gonads when shielding will not obscure the areas of interest.

Collimate to slightly less than the size of the film in order to reduce the scattered radiation effects on the film (increased overall grayness). Sometimes a lead strip is placed on the table near the posterior margin in order to reduce the effects of scattered radiation on the film.

STRUCTURES DEMONSTRATED: The lateral aspect of the sacrum in its entirety (Fig. 5–50).

COMMON ERROR: Sometimes the sacrum is clipped due to its excessive curvature and the resultant diagonal placement on the film. Adjust the longitudinal axis of the sacrum to the longitudinal plane of the x-ray table centerline (see Fig. 5–53).

TECHNIQUE

KV _____ MA _____ SECS _____ MAS _____ CALIPER _____ cm

_____ :1 GRID / B / none SCREEN: RE / High / Par / Detail / None

SID: _____ Rm _____ ADULT / CHILD age: _____ mos. / yrs.

HABITUS: Hyper / s / hypo / a   XS   S   M   L   XL   XXL

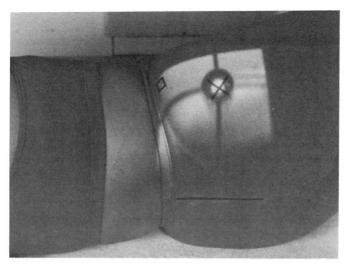

FIGURE 5—49. Lateral sacrum. Iliac crest *(square)*. Posterior border of sacrum *(line)*. Place this line in a longitudinal plane to the table to avoid diagonal placement of the sacrum on the film (and potential clipping or superimposition of sacrum over the identification blocker of film).

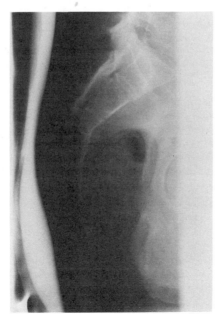

FIGURE 5—50. Lateral sacrum x-ray. Notice that the L5-S1 joint space is clipped by collimation. This was not repeated because this patient also had lumbar spine x-rays ordered as well. You must include the L5-S1 joint on a sacrum study.

COCCYX: AP OR PA

8 x 10 in. 20 x 24 cm	8 x 10 in. 20 x 24 cm	8 x 10 in. 20 x 24 cm

FILM: Use table Bucky or grid. Collimate to the area of interest.
CR: For the AP, use a 10-degree caudal angle. Enter at the midsagittal plane just above the midpoint between the ASIS and the symphysis pubis (Fig. 5–51).

For the PA, use a 10-degree cephalic angle. Enter at the midsagittal plane at the symphysis pubis.
POSITION: The patient is supinated for the AP and pronated for the PA.

If the patient is unable to tolerate the supine position, use the pronated. This, however, is not optimal due to the increased OID.

For the AP, pad under the knees if it will make the patient more comfortable. This varies depending on the injury.

Center the midsagittal plane to the center of the table.

Center the film and Bucky tray to the midpoint between the ASIS and symphysis pubis.

Make sure the pelvis is flat.
STRUCTURES DEMONSTRATED: The anterior aspect of the coccygeal vertebrae corrected for its curvature (Fig. 5–52).

The obturator foramina will be closed and the symphysis pubis will be narrowed (or seen on edge) with this tube angle.
COMMON ERRORS: (1) Overpenetration. (2) The coccyx is obscured by bowel contents. Sometimes a bowel prep is necessary. The physician will order if necessary; check with the radiologist. For an example of the excellent detail acquired with a bowel preparation, refer to the IVP bladder spot (see Fig. 7–20).

TECHNIQUE

KV _____ MA _____ SECS _____ MAS _____ CALIPER _____ cm

_____ :1 GRID / B / none SCREEN: RE / High / Par / Detail / None

SID: _____ Rm _____ ADULT / CHILD age: _____ mos. / yrs.

HABITUS: Hyper / s / hypo / a   XS   S   M   L   XL   XXL

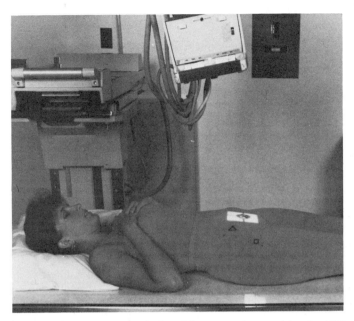

FIGURE 5–51. Semi-axial AP projection of the coccyx using a caudal angle. ASIS *(triangle)*. Greater trochanter *(square)* to demonstrate the level of the symphysis pubis.

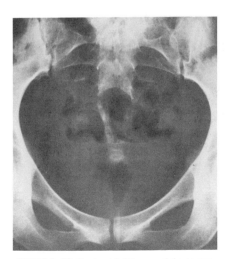

FIGURE 5–52. Semi-axial AP x-ray of the coccyx.

COCCYX: LATERAL

| 8 x 10 in. | 8 x 10 in. | 8 x 10 in. |
| 20 x 24 cm | 20 x 24 cm | 20 x 24 cm |

FILM: Use table Bucky or grid. Collimate to the area of interest.
CR: Perpendicular to the coccyx.
POSITION: The patient is in the left lateral recumbent position.

Extend the hips slightly; flex the knees equally and pad them if necessary.

Center the point on the patient, 3 inches posterior to the midcoronal plane at the midpoint between the ASIS and the symphysis pubis, to the center of the x-ray table (Fig. 5–53).

Center the film and Bucky tray to the area between the ASIS and symphysis pubis.

Shield the gonads when shielding will not obscure the areas of interest.

Collimate to less than the size of the film in order to reduce the scattered radiation effects on the film (increased overall grayness). Sometimes a lead strip is placed on the table near the posterior margin in order to reduce the effects of scattered radiation on the film.

STRUCTURES DEMONSTRATED: The lateral aspect of the coccyx (Fig. 5–54).

The right ischium and the left ischium should be superimposed.
COMMON ERROR: Overpenetration. The technique is significantly lower than that of the lateral sacrum.

TECHNIQUE

KV _____ MA _____ SECS _____ MAS _____ CALIPER _____ cm
_____ :1 GRID / B / none SCREEN: RE / High / Par / Detail / None
SID: _____ Rm _____ ADULT / CHILD   age: _____ mos. / yrs.
HABITUS: Hyper / s / hypo / a   XS   S   M   L   XL   XXL

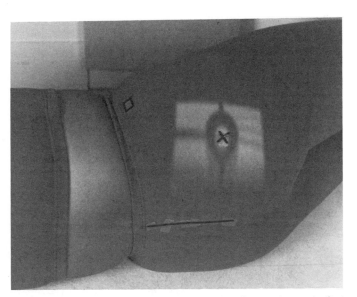

FIGURE 5–53. Lateral coccyx. Iliac crest *(square)*. Place the posterior margin *(line)* in alignment with a longitudinal plane to the center of the table.

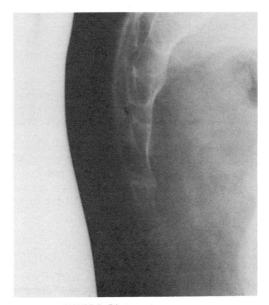

FIGURE 5–54. Lateral coccyx x-ray.

MYELOGRAPHY: VENTRAL DECUBITUS

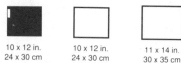

10 x 12 in.
24 x 30 cm

10 x 12 in.
24 x 30 cm

11 x 14 in.
30 x 35 cm

FILM: Use a grid or grid cassette. Collimate severely to the area of interest.

CR: Perpendicularly using a horizontal CR at the midaxillary (slightly posterior to the midcoronal [see Fig. 1–2]) plane at the fluid level of contrast media indicated by the physician. Usually the x-ray table will be tilted in order to place the contrast at the area of interest.

POSITION: The patient is pronated in the ventral recumbent position. The footboard, footstraps, and shoulder board are in place for the fluoroscopy study (Fig. 5–55).

After the fluoroscopy study, a horizontal (crosstable) beam is used for the ventral decubitus projection. Due to the thickness of part, a grid and close collimation are necessary to reduce scattered radiation and its resultant grayness on the finished radiograph.

The horizontal beam will be directed to the vertebral area of interest indicated by the physician.

As with any contrast study, do not leave the patient unattended. Some myelography studies are performed with the spinal puncture needle removed (water-soluble contrast) and on occasion it remains in place (oil-based contrast) throughout the entire exam. In this latter case caution must be taken in maintaining the sterile field and avoiding the spinal needle in setting up the film and grid for the decubitus projection. Make sure the grid cassette is stable and will not tilt or fall into the sterile field.

STRUCTURES DEMONSTRATED: A lateral projection of vertebral disk spaces of interest (Fig. 5–56).

This projection usually demonstrates anterior or posterior disk protrusions or space-occupying lesions.

COMMON ERROR: Increased grayness. Due to the thickness of the part and the increased technique used to accommodate that thickness, this film generally ends up being too gray. Collimate as much as you are able while still including the area of interest. Make sure the parameters of the grid you are using are met (SID, kVp range, etc.).

TECHNIQUE

KV _____ MA _____ SECS _____ MAS _____ CALIPER _____ cm

_____ :1 GRID / B / none SCREEN: RE / High / Par / Detail / None

SID: _____ Rm _____ ADULT / CHILD age: _____ mos. / yrs.

HABITUS: Hyper / s / hypo / a   XS   S   M   L   XL   XXL

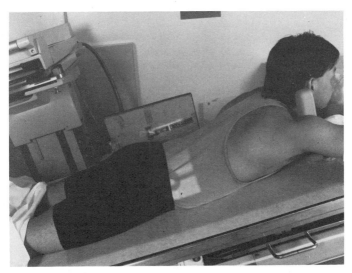

FIGURE 5–55. Ventral decubitus position (lateral projection) for myelography.

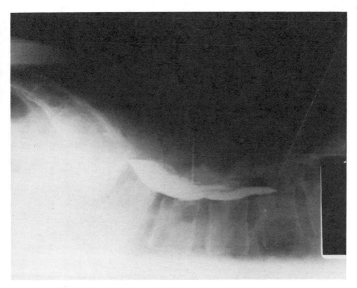

FIGURE 5–56. Ventral decubitus myelography (lateral) x-ray.

Skull

SKULL: SEMI-AXIAL AP (TOWNE'S/GRASHEY)

FILM
Pediatric Patients

8 x 10 in.
20 x 24 cm

8 x 10 in.
20 x 24 cm

Adult Patients

10 x 12 in.
24 x 30 cm

10 x 12 in.
24 x 30 cm

With the table Bucky. Use a stationary grid for portable or gurney patients. Collimate to or slightly less than the size of the film.

CR: Use a caudal tube angle of 30 degrees with the orbitomeatal line (OML) (Fig. 6–1) or 37 degrees with the infraorbitomeatal line (IOML) perpendicular to the tabletop (Fig. 6–2). Exit the base of the skull for a general survey film. (See Fig. 1–8.)

Another method when using the OML is to have the CR exit the level of the sella turcica, at approximately the level of the external auditory meatus (EAM).[21, 22] Place the transverse centering light so that it enshadows or bisects the EAM (usually for cone-down views of petrous pyramids).

Center to the MSP transversely and longitudinally over the rami for the mandible. Use the OML.

Center to the MSP transversely and then longitudinally bisect the zygomatic arches for the arches. Use the OML.

NOTE: Whenever an angle is used that is directed toward the lower axial skeleton, lead shielding should be provided to the patient. Do not use the overhead distance indicators to measure the source-to-image distance (SID) for any tube angle. Always use the tape measure along the path of the central ray to measure to the tabletop when using a tube angle.

POSITION: The patient is supinated upon the table.

Remove hearing aids, eyeglasses, hairpins, necklaces, earrings,

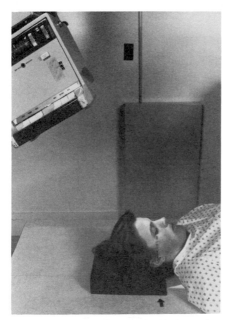

FIGURE 6–1. Semi-axial AP projection (Towne's/Grashey) using OML with 30-degree caudal angle of tube. A radiolucent sponge is used to help the patient hyperflex.

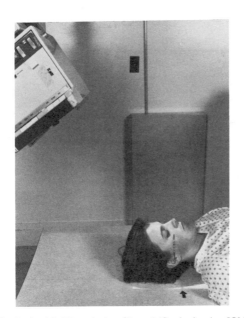

FIGURE 6–2. Semi-axial AP projection (Towne's/Grashey) using IOML with 37-degree caudal angle of tube.

and clothing around neck. Ask the patient to remove dentures or removable dental bridges.

Center the midsagittal plane (MSP) to the center of the table.

The chin is depressed in order to place the OML or IOML perpendicular to the tabletop. The selection of OML versus IOML will depend upon the amount of angle used (see CR, above). The IOML is the least stressful of the two. If the patient's limited range of motion prohibits adjustment of the OML or the IOML, use a small-angle sponge to elevate the vertex of the skull.

Check midsagittal centering again after chin is adjusted.

Recheck all baselines before making an exposure.

NOTE: The reverse Towne's or PA semi-axial (Haas) is positioned with the patient prone. It demonstrates similar structures to those seen on the AP semi-axial or Towne's.

STRUCTURES DEMONSTRATED: Symmetrical petrous pyramids.

The occipital bone.

The posterior aspect of the foramen magnum with the dorsum sellae and posterior clinoid processes projected within its shadow (Fig. 6–3).

The posterior aspect of the parietal bones.

The elongated, mandibular rami when the CR exits the level of the rami (use OML).

The elongated, overpenetrated, zygomatic arches lateral to the mandibular rami when the CR exits the level of the arches (use OML).

With the use of the IOML and when the CR exits the sella turcica just above the level of the EAM, use a severely collimated, 30-degree caudal tube angle for the anterior clinoid processes, dorsum and tuberculum sellae to be projected through occipital bone. Use a 37-degree caudal tube angle for the posterior clinoids and dorsum sellae, which will be demonstrated within the foramen magnum. The internal auditory canals of the petromastoid area are well visualized with severe collimation and when the CR passes through the planes of the EAM.

COMMON ERRORS: (1) Top of head is clipped. Position the top of film at the vertex (top) of the skull. The angulation will throw the vertex lower on the film and allow for proper spacing at the top of the resultant x-ray or the CR is too low. (2) Underpenetration. Of the entire skull series, this projection requires the highest technique. Make sure your technique is greater than that of a nonangled AP or angled PA skull. (3) Rotation. Check for rotation on the finished radiograph by measuring a right-sided structure's distance to the lateral margin and comparing that distance with the same measurement on the left side. The petrous pyramids should be symmetrical on the finished x-ray. Always recheck the MSP, just before exposure.

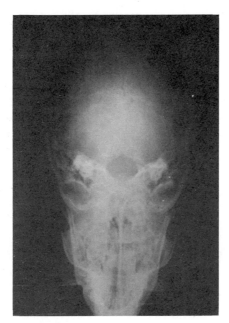

FIGURE 6–3. Semi-axial AP x-ray of skull.

TECHNIQUE

KV _____ MA _____ SECS _____ MAS _____ CALIPER _____ cm

_____ :1 GRID / B / none SCREEN: RE / High / Par / Detail / None

SID: _____ Rm _____ ADULT / CHILD age: _____ mos. / yrs.

HABITUS: Hyper / s / hypo / a   XS   S   M   L   XL   XXL

NOTES:

SKULL: AP

FILM
Pediatric Patients

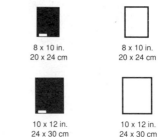

8 x 10 in.
20 x 24 cm

8 x 10 in.
20 x 24 cm

Adult Patients

10 x 12 in.
24 x 30 cm

10 x 12 in.
24 x 30 cm

With the table Bucky. Use a stationary grid for portable or gurney patients. Collimate to or slightly less than the size of the film.

CR: Perpendicularly to the nasion (bridge of nose) when the OML is used (Fig. 6–4). On trauma patients (where the head may be thrown back in a relaxed position and a neck injury prohibits movement), align the CR to the OML. Enter at the nasion.

At a 7-degree caudal angle when the IOML is used (see Fig. 8–6).[23]

Another method is to center to nasion, with the CR forming a 15-degree cephalic angle with the OML.[24, 25] (This in essence is a reverse PA Caldwell.)

Check with your department or facility as to which method is recommended.

NOTE: Whenever an angle is used, do not use the overhead distance indicators to measure the source-to-image distance (SID) for any tube angle. Always use the tape measure along the path of the central ray to measure to the tabletop when using a tube angle.

POSITION: Use this projection when the patient cannot be rotated to the PA because of multiple trauma or patient condition.

The patient is supinated upon the table or gurney.

Remove hearing aids, eyeglasses, hairpins, necklaces, earrings, and clothing around neck. Ask the patient to remove dentures or removable dental bridges.

Center the MSP to the center of the table or grid.

In neck- and skull-injured patients, use the baseline approximate to the patient's pre-existing position and its corresponding tube angulation. *Do not adjust the head or neck*.

The selection of OML versus IOML will depend upon the amount of angle used (see CR above). The chin is depressed (for those without neck injuries) in order to place the OML or IOML perpendicular to the film or tabletop.

Check midsagittal centering again after chin is adjusted.

Recheck all baselines before making an exposure.

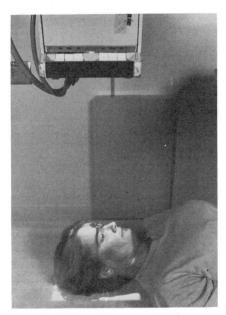

FIGURE 6–4. AP projection of skull.

NOTES:

STRUCTURES DEMONSTRATED: The cranium in its entirety (Fig. 6–5).

The magnified orbits as compared with the PA projection.

With no angulation, the petrous ridges should fill the orbits; with a cephalic angle, they should fill the lower one third of the orbits.

COMMON ERROR: Rotation. Check for rotation on the finished radiograph by measuring a right-sided structure's distance to the lateral margin and comparing that distance with the same distance on the left side. The petrous pyramids should be symmetrical on the finished x-ray. Always recheck the midsagittal plane, just before exposure.

TECHNIQUE

KV _____ MA _____ SECS _____ MAS _____ CALIPER _____ cm

_____ :1 GRID / B / none SCREEN: RE / High / Par / Detail / None

SID: _____ Rm _____ ADULT / CHILD age: _____ mos. / yrs.

HABITUS: Hyper / s / hypo / a XS S M L XL XXL

NOTES:

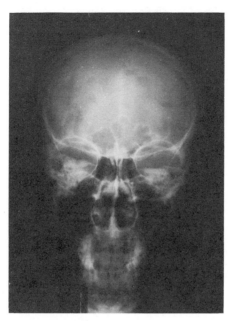

FIGURE 6–5. AP x-ray of skull.

NOTES:

SKULL: PA

FILM
Pediatric Patients

8 x 10 in. ⠀⠀⠀⠀⠀⠀⠀⠀ 8 x 10 in.
20 x 24 cm ⠀⠀⠀⠀⠀⠀⠀⠀ 20 x 24 cm

Adult Patients

10 x 12 in. ⠀⠀⠀⠀⠀⠀⠀⠀ 10 x 12 in.
24 x 30 cm ⠀⠀⠀⠀⠀⠀⠀⠀ 24 x 30 cm

With the table Bucky. Use a stationary grid for portable or gurney patients. Collimate to or slightly less than the size of the film.

CR: Perpendicularly exiting at the nasion.

POSITION: Remove hearing aids, eyeglasses, hairpins, necklaces, earrings, and clothing around neck. Ask the patient to remove dentures or removable dental bridges.

The patient is pronated upon the table. Place the arms up on either side of the patient's head for balance.

Have the patient tuck the chin in order to place the forehead and nose on the center line of the x-ray table.

Center the MSP to the center of the table.

The OML should be perpendicular to the film or tabletop (Fig. 6–6).

Level the skull by assessing the level of each EAM by palpating and leveling the right and left tragi (small flaps partially covering the EAM). They should lie in the same plane (see Common Error below).

Recheck all baselines before making an exposure.

STRUCTURES DEMONSTRATED: Walls of the cranium.

The frontal bone and superior parietals.

The perpendicular tube PA will demonstrate the posterior ethmoidal air cells. The petrous pyramids will fill the entire orbital areas. The cristi galli is seen superimposed by the dorsum sellae. The inferior nasal conchae (turbinates) and anterior, frontal (nasal) spine are demonstrated (Fig. 6–7).

COMMON ERROR: Rotation. Check the positioning of the midsagittal after the chin is tucked. Position the skull by assessing the level of each EAM by palpating the right and left tragi. From the vertex, place your index fingers over the tragi. Rotate the skull slightly to the right and back slightly to the left. Now bring your fingertip level to each other and to the plane of the tabletop. They should be adjusted to lie in the same coronal plane in order to avoid rotation.

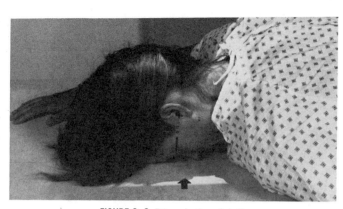

FIGURE 6–6. PA projection of skull.

TECHNIQUE

KV _____ MA _____ SECS _____ MAS _____ CALIPER _____ cm

_____ :1 GRID / B / none SCREEN: RE / High / Par / Detail / None

SID: _____ Rm _____ ADULT / CHILD age: _____ mos. / yrs.

HABITUS: Hyper / s / hypo / a   XS   S   M   L   XL   XXL

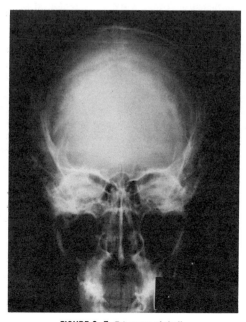

FIGURE 6–7. PA x-ray of skull.

SKULL: SEMI-AXIAL PA (CALDWELL)

FILM
Pediatric Patients

8 x 10 in.
20 x 24 cm

8 x 10 in.
20 x 24 cm

Adult Patients

10 x 12 in.
24 x 30 cm

10 x 12 in.
24 x 30 cm

With the table Bucky. Use a stationary grid for portable or gurney patients. Collimate to or slightly less than the size of the film.

CR: Using the OML perpendicular to the tabletop, a 15-degree caudal angle at the MSP and exiting the nasion (Fig. 6–8). A 23-degree caudal angle may be used with the glabellomeatal line (GML) perpendicular to the tabletop, or no tube angle (see p. 370).

NOTE: Whenever an angle is used, do not use the overhead distance indicators to measure the SID for any tube angle. Always use the tape measure along the path of the central ray to measure to the tabletop when using a tube angle.

POSITION: Remove hearing aids, eyeglasses, hairpins, necklaces, earrings, and clothing around neck. Ask the patient to remove dentures or removable dental bridges.

The patient is pronated upon the table. Place the arms up by the patient's head for balance.

Have the patient tuck the chin in order to place the forehead and nose on the center line of the x-ray table.

Center the MSP to the center of the table.

The OML should be perpendicular to the film or tabletop.

Level the skull by assessing the level of each EAM by palpating the right and left tragus (small flap partially covering the EAM). They should lie in the same transverse plane. (See Common Error below.)

Recheck all baselines before making an exposure.

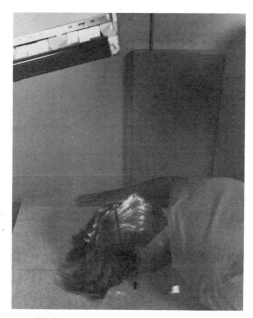

FIGURE 6–8. Semi-axial PA projection (Caldwell).

NOTES:

STRUCTURES DEMONSTRATED: Walls of the cranium.

The frontal bone, lateral and sinuses.

The angled PA (Caldwell) will demonstrate the anterior eth-moidal air cells. The petrous pyramids will fill the lower one third of the orbits (Fig. 6–9). The lesser and greater wings of the sphenoid are projected within the orbits.

COMMON ERROR: Rotation. Check the positioning of the midsag-ittal after the chin is tucked. Position the skull by assessing the level of each EAM by palpating the right and left tragi. From the vertex, place your index fingers over the tragi. Rotate the skull slightly to the right and back slightly to the left. Now bring your fingertip level to each other and to the plane of the tabletop. They should be adjusted to lie in the same coronal plane in order to avoid rotation.

TECHNIQUE

KV _____ MA _____ SECS _____ MAS _____ CALIPER _____ cm

_____ :1 GRID / B / none SCREEN: RE / High / Par / Detail / None

SID: _____ Rm _____ ADULT / CHILD age: _____ mos. / yrs.

HABITUS: Hyper / s / hypo / a   XS   S   M   L   XL   XXL

NOTES:

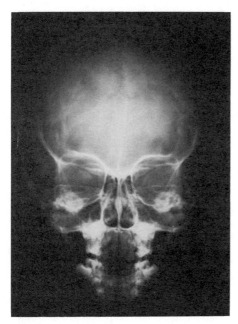

FIGURE 6–9. Semi-axial PA x-ray (Caldwell) of skull.

NOTES:

SKULL: LATERAL

10 x 12 in.
24 x 30 cm

10 x 12 in.
24 x 30 cm

10 x 12 in.
24 x 30 cm

FILM: Use table Bucky.

Portable or Gurney Patients: Use a stationary grid. Collimate to or slightly less than the size of the film (see Fig. 8–7).

CR: Perpendicular to 2 inches (5 cm) above the EAM. For the sella turcica coned-down lateral, center ¾ inch (1.9 cm) anterior to and ¾ inch (1.9 cm) superior to the EAM.

POSITION: Remove hearing aids, eyeglasses, hairpins, necklaces, earrings, and clothing around neck. Ask the patient to remove dentures or removable dental bridges.

Place the recumbent patient in the RAO position for the right lateral and the LAO for the left lateral. Place the arm of the side down at the patient's side. The opposite arm should be up. Have the patient bend the knee of the elevated side in order to relieve strain.

Center the EAM to the center line of the table.

From either the RAO or LAO, adjust the patient's head so that the interpupillary line (IP) is perpendicular to the x-ray table or film. If the patient's limited range of motion prohibits adjustment of the IP, either use a small-angle sponge to raise the vertex of the skull (Fig. 6–10), or reposition the patient again. Instruct the recumbent patient to lay the head down again, touching the top of the lateralized skull to the table first (parietal area) and then following with the shoulders and arms or slightly pad the upper chest area. This will provide more tilt to the skull's position.

The MSP should be parallel to the tabletop or film.

Recenter the EAM to the center line of the table after the IP and MSP adjustments.

Place the IOML so that it is parallel to the top edge of the film by adjusting the flexion or extension of the head and neck.

Collimate slightly less than the size of the film.

Make sure the top of the film (and collimation) includes the top of the skull.

Both laterals are taken for comparison.

Recheck all baselines before making an exposure.

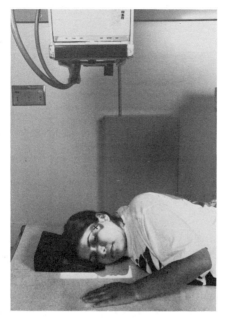

FIGURE 6–10. Lateral skull with sponge adjustment of perpendicular IP line.

NOTES:

A crosstable lateral may be used for multiple-trauma or neck-injured patients (Fig. 6–11). Use a grid.

STRUCTURES DEMONSTRATED: The lateral aspect of the cranium of the side down or closest to the film (Fig. 6–12).

The sella turcica, anterior and posterior clinoid processes, and the dorsum sellae are well demonstrated.

All paranasal sinuses will be demonstrated free of superimposition inferior to the sella turcica.

COMMON ERROR: Rotation or tilt. Tilt is assessed by the superimposition of the orbital roofs on the lateral skull film, rotation by the mandibular rami. Because three baselines are used, when you adjust one, you end up needing to readjust the others. Recheck the midsagittal IOML and IP baselines before making the exposure.

TECHNIQUE

KV _____ MA _____ SECS _____ MAS _____ CALIPER _____ cm

_____ :1 GRID / B / none SCREEN: RE / High / Par / Detail / None

SID: _____ Rm _____ ADULT / CHILD age: _____ mos. / yrs.

HABITUS: Hyper / s / hypo / a   XS   S   M   L   XL   XXL

NOTES:

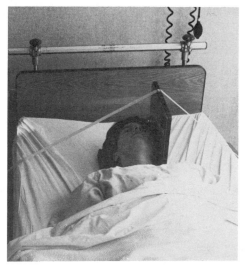

FIGURE 6–11. Crosstable lateral of skull for bedside, trauma patient.

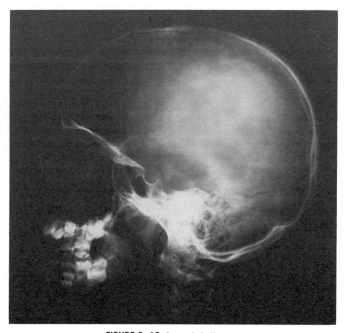

FIGURE 6–12. Lateral skull x-ray.

SKULL: SUBMENTOVERTEX (SMV) BASILAR

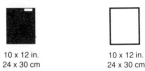

10 x 12 in.
24 x 30 cm

10 x 12 in.
24 x 30 cm

FILM: Use table Bucky. Collimate to or slightly less than the size of the film.

CR: Perpendicular to the IOML, midsagittally at the level of the sella turcica (¾ inch or 1.9 cm anterior and ¾ inch or 1.9 cm superior to the EAM).

NOTE: This position requires excellent mobility of the head and neck.

POSITION: Remove hearing aids, eyeglasses, hairpins, necklaces, earrings, and clothing around neck. Ask the patient to remove dentures or dental bridges.

Recumbent: Load the film into the Bucky tray; mark it. Have the tube readied near the head of the x-ray table with a moderate cephalic angle. Have the technique set. The patient is supinated upon the table or upright with the use of a Bucky or grid. In order to enlist the patient's cooperation, explain what you plan to do.

Use several pillows placed under the back and below the level of the shoulders. Support the head while placing the patient in full neck extension. The vertex should be touching the tabletop. Flex the knees for comfort.

Angle the tube to align perpendicularly to the IOML, a cephalic angle (Fig. 6–13).

Working quickly, center the MSP to the center of the table.

Upright: Load the film; mark it. Have the tube readied near the head of the x-ray table with a cephalic angle. Have the technique set.

The patient should be seated or use a chair, IV pole, etc., for support if standing. Seated is preferred for stability.

With the patient seated with the posterior aspect to the film, support the head while placing the patient in full neck extension. Guide the vertex of the skull to the center of the film. If the full vertex is not touching, the patient is either too far away or too close.

Angle the tube to align perpendicularly to the IOML.

Quickly, center the MSP to the center of the table.

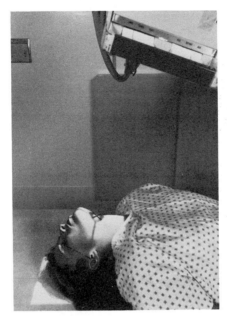

FIGURE 6–13. Submentovertex (SMV) projection of the skull.

NOTES:

STRUCTURES DEMONSTRATED: The basilar portion of the occipital bone (Fig. 6–14).

The symmetrical petrous pyramids.

Mastoid processes.

The foramina ovale and spinosum in the base of the greater wing of the sphenoid bone.

The vomer in midline.

The nasal septum.

The magnified mandible. The mandibular condyles must be anterior to the petrous pyramids.

The maxillary and sphenoid sinuses.

The carotid canals.

The dens (odontoid) within the foramen magnum.

COMMON ERRORS: (1) The mandibular condyles are not anterior to the petrous pyramids. Indicates the head or tube was not sufficiently angled cephalad. Also caused by not angling the tube so that the CR is perpendicular to the IOML. (2) Clipping the occipital area. Depending on the skull classification (i.e., dolichocephalic) when centering to the sella turcica, the CR could end up being positioned at the front third of the length of the skull. If this is the case, the CR must be centered to the middle of the film at about the level of the EAM or the collimation opened wider to avoid clipping the occipital bone.

TECHNIQUE

KV _____ MA _____ SECS _____ MAS _____ CALIPER _____ cm

_____ :1 GRID / B / none SCREEN: RE / High / Par / Detail / None

SID: _____ Rm _____ ADULT / CHILD age: _____ mos. / yrs.

HABITUS: Hyper / s / hypo / a   XS   S   M   L   XL   XXL

NOTES:

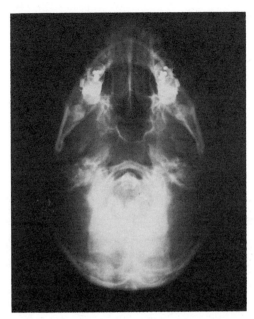

FIGURE 6–14. Submentovertex (SMV) x-ray of the skull.

NOTES:

SKULL: VERTICOSUBMENTAL (VSM) BASILAR

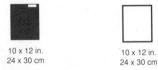

10 x 12 in.
24 x 30 cm

10 x 12 in.
24 x 30 cm

FILM: Use table Bucky. Collimate to or slightly less than the size of the film.

CR: Perpendicular to the IOML, midsagittally at the level of the sella turcica (¾ inch or 1.9 cm anterior to the EAM).

NOTE: This position requires excellent mobility of the head and neck.

POSITION: Remove hearing aids, eyeglasses, hairpins, necklaces, earrings, and clothing around neck. Ask the patient to remove dentures or dental bridges.

Recumbent: Load the film; mark it. Have the tube readied near the head of the x-ray table with a caudal angle. Have the technique set. The patient is pronated upon the table or upright with the use of a Bucky or grid. In order to enlist the patient's cooperation, explain what you plan to do.

Have the patient brace himself or herself by placing the arms up alongside the head. Hyperextend the head and neck. Have the patient resting the head on the chin.

Angle the tube to align perpendicularly to the IOML, a caudal angle (Fig. 6–15).

Quickly, center the MSP to the center of the table.

Upright: Load the film; mark it. Have the tube readied near the head of the x-ray table with a caudal angle. Have the technique set.

Have the patient stand and hold onto the table or film holder for support, or the patient can be seated.

With the patient facing the film, place the patient in full neck extension. Have the patient resting the head on the chin.

Angle the tube to align perpendicularly to the IOML (a caudal angle).

Quickly, center the MSP to the center of the table.

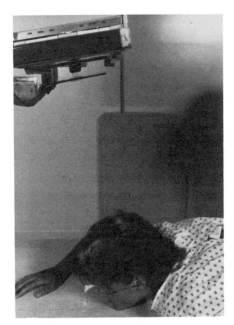

FIGURE 6–15. Verticosubmental (VSM) projection of the skull. (Match IOML to line of collimator face [line].)

NOTES:

STRUCTURES DEMONSTRATED: The basilar portion of the occipital bone (Fig. 6–16).

The symmetrical petrous pyramids.

Mastoid processes.

The foramina ovale and spinosum in the base of the greater wing of the sphenoid bone.

The vomer in midline.

The nasal septum.

The mandible in detail due to its close proximity to the film. The mandibular condyles must be anterior to the petrous pyramids.

The maxillary and sphenoid sinuses.

The carotid canals. The dens (odontoid) within the foramen magnum.

COMMON ERROR: The mandibular condyles are not anterior to the petrous pyramids, which indicates either the patient's head or tube was not sufficiently angled caudad. This can also be caused by not angling the tube so that the CR is perpendicular to the IOML. If x-ray is taken for the entire skull, make sure the collimation includes the occipital bone. The CR level is slightly anterior to the midpoint of the skull's length (especially the dolichocephalic skull). This in turn will force either the collimation to be opened or the CR to be shifted posteriorly in order to accommodate the occipital area.

TECHNIQUE

KV _____ MA _____ SECS _____ MAS _____ CALIPER _____ cm

_____ :1 GRID / B / none SCREEN: RE / High / Par / Detail / None

SID: _____ Rm _____ ADULT / CHILD age: _____ mos. / yrs.

HABITUS: Hyper / s / hypo / a   XS   S   M   L   XL   XXL

NOTES:

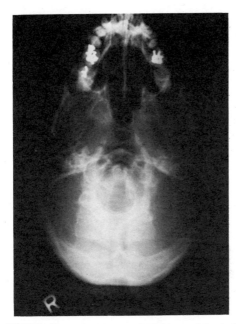

FIGURE 6–16. Verticosubmental (VSM) x-ray of the skull.

NOTES:

SKULL: PA SEMI-AXIAL (HAAS)

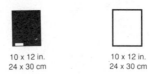

10 x 12 in.
24 x 30 cm

10 x 12 in.
24 x 30 cm

FILM: Use table Bucky. Collimate to or slightly less than the size of the film.

CR: Use a 25-degree cephalic angle. Place the transverse centering light so that it enshadows or bisects the EAM (Fig. 6–17).

POSITION: Remove hearing aids, eyeglasses, hairpins, necklaces, earrings, and clothing around the neck. Ask the patient to remove dentures or removable dental bridges. The patient is pronated upon the x-ray table or an upright Bucky. The recumbent patient's arms are alongside the head for support.

Place the forehead and nose on the center line of the table. Flex the neck to adjust the OML perpendicularly to the table or grid device.

Center the MSP to the center of the tabletop.

Recheck baselines before making the exposure.

STRUCTURES DEMONSTRATED: Symmetrical petrous pyramids (Fig. 6–18).

The occipital bone.

The posterior aspect of the foramen magnum with the dorsum sellae and posterior clinoid processes projected within its shadow.

A portion of the parietal bones.

The temporomandibular fossae.

COMMON ERROR: Rotation. Recheck the midsagittal plane before making the exposure.

TECHNIQUE

KV _____ MA _____ SECS _____ MAS _____ CALIPER _____ cm

_____ :1 GRID / B / none SCREEN: RE / High / Par / Detail / None

SID: _____ Rm _____ ADULT / CHILD age: _____ mos. / yrs.

HABITUS: Hyper / s / hypo / a   XS   S   M   L   XL   XXL

NOTES:

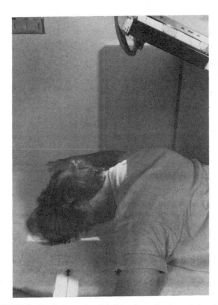

FIGURE 6–17. PA semi-axial (Haas) projection of the skull.

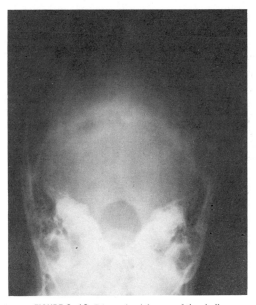

FIGURE 6–18. PA semi-axial x-ray of the skull.

FACIAL BONES: PARIETOACANTHIAL (WATERS')

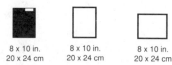

8 x 10 in.   8 x 10 in.   8 x 10 in.
20 x 24 cm   20 x 24 cm   20 x 24 cm

FILM: Use table Bucky. Collimate slightly less than the size of the film.

CR: Perpendicular, exiting the acanthion.

POSITION: Remove hearing aids, eyeglasses, hairpins, necklaces, earrings, and clothing around neck. Ask the patient to remove dentures or removable dental bridges.

The patient is pronated upon the table or upright with a Bucky or grid.

Ask the patient to extend the neck so that the skull rests upon the chin. The OML should measure 37 degrees to the tabletop or grid (Fig. 6–19).[26] Adjust the flexion or extension of the head and neck for this measurement.

Another baseline you can use is the mentomeatal line (MML). Place the MML perpendicular to the tabletop.[27, 28, 29]

Yet another method is to adjust the OML at 45 degrees to the horizontal.[30]

Center the MSP to the center of the table or grid.

Center the film to the acanthion.

Recheck all baselines before making an exposure.

NOTE: For trauma and neck-injured patients, use the reverse Waters' method. With the patient supinated, simply match the angle of the MML with the angle of the tube. The CR enters the acanthion. This method requires no movement (flexion or extension) of the head and neck. Center the MSP to the tabletop or grid if the patient's condition permits.

A modified Waters' method may also be performed. Use a 55-degree OML to the table measurement (Fig. 6–20).

NOTES:

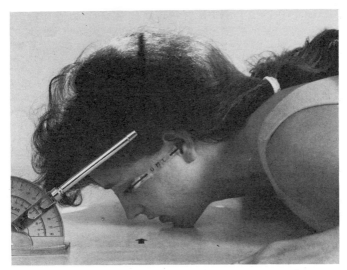

FIGURE 6–19. Parietoacanthial (Waters') projection. Exit level of CR *(arrow).*

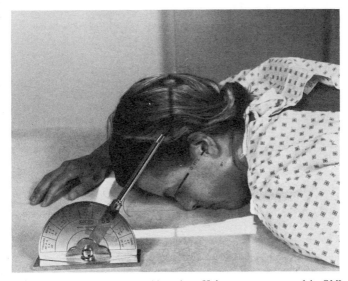

FIGURE 6–20. Modified Waters' position using a 55-degree measurement of the OML from the table.

STRUCTURES DEMONSTRATED: Best demonstration of the orbits, zygomatic bones, zygomatic arches, the maxillae (the upper facial bones), and the maxillary sinuses (Fig. 6–21).

The petrous ridges should be below the maxillary sinuses.

COMMON ERROR: Improper baseline positioning. If your film shows the petrous ridges in the maxillary sinuses, the patient does not have enough extension. If your film shows the rotundum foramina obscured and the petrous ridges well below the maxillary sinuses or in the body of the mandible, your patient has too much extension. (The foramina usually are visible along the medial walls of the maxillary sinuses.)

TECHNIQUE

KV _____ MA _____ SECS _____ MAS _____ CALIPER _____ cm

_____ :1 GRID / B / none SCREEN: RE / High / Par / Detail / None

SID: _____ Rm _____ ADULT / CHILD age: _____ mos. / yrs.

HABITUS: Hyper / s / hypo / a   XS   S   M   L   XL   XXL

NOTES:

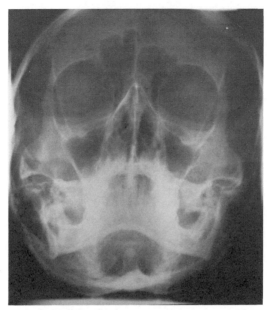

FIGURE 6–21. Parietoacanthial (Waters') x-ray.

NOTES:

FACIAL BONES: LATERAL

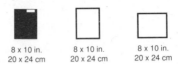

| 8 x 10 in. | 8 x 10 in. | 8 x 10 in. |
| 20 x 24 cm | 20 x 24 cm | 20 x 24 cm |

FILM: Use table Bucky. Collimate to the film or to the area of interest.

CR: Perpendicular to the zygomatic bone (its highest point just below the orbit). Collimate to include the frontal sinuses to the mentum of the mandible and from the nose to the EAM.

POSITION: Remove any hearing aids, eyeglasses, earrings, hairpins, or clips. Ask the patient to remove dentures or removable dental bridges.

Place the recumbent patient in the RAO position for the right lateral and the LAO for the left lateral. Place the arm of the side down at the patient's side. The opposite arm should be up. Have the patient bend the knee of the elevated side in order to relieve strain, or the patient may be upright if able.

Center the zygomatic bone's malar surface of the side down to the center line of the table.

From either the RAO or LAO, adjust the patient's head so that the IP is perpendicular to the x-ray table or film (Fig. 6–22).

The MSP should be parallel to the tabletop or film.

Place the IOML so that it is parallel to the top of the film by adjusting the flexion or extension of the head and neck.

Recenter the zygomatic bone's malar surface to the center line of the table after the baseline adjustments.

Recheck all baselines before making an exposure.

A crosstable lateral may be used for multiple-trauma or neck-injured patients. Use a grid.

NOTES:

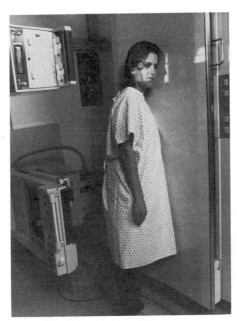

FIGURE 6–22. Lateral projection for facial bones. (Upright will show fluid lines.)

NOTES:

STRUCTURES DEMONSTRATED: The lateral aspect of the facial bones of the side down.

The orbital roofs should be superimposed (Fig. 6–23).

The sphenoid sinus inferior to the sella turcica.

COMMON ERROR: Rotation or tilt. Tilt is assessed by the superimposition of the orbital roofs on the lateral facial bone film, rotation by the mandibular rami. Because three baselines are used, when you adjust one, you end up needing to readjust the others. Recheck the MSP, IP, and IOML before making the exposure.

TECHNIQUE

KV _____ MA _____ SECS _____ MAS _____ CALIPER _____ cm

_____ :1 GRID / B / none SCREEN: RE / High / Par / Detail / None

SID: _____ Rm _____ ADULT / CHILD age: _____ mos. / yrs.

HABITUS: Hyper / s / hypo / a   XS   S   M   L   XL   XXL

NOTES:

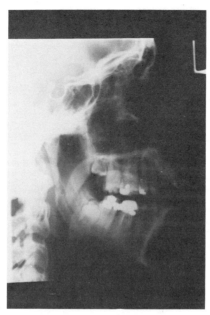

FIGURE 6–23. Lateral facial bone x-ray.

NOTES:

FACIAL BONES: PA OBLIQUE (RHESE)

8 x 10 in.   8 x 10 in.   8 x 10 in.
20 x 24 cm   20 x 24 cm   20 x 24 cm

FILM: Collimate slightly less than the size of the film or to the area of interest.

CR: Perpendicular, exiting the lateral aspect of the infraorbital margin side down (Fig. 6–24).

Another method is to use a 10-degree cephalic angle entering the mastoid tip of the side up.[31]

NOTE: When x-ray is taken for the optic canals (optic foramina), use a cone or collimate severely to the orbit of the side down.

POSITION: Remove hearing aids, eyeglasses, hairpins, necklaces, earrings, and clothing around neck. Ask the patient to remove dentures or removable dental bridges.

The patient is pronated upon the table or upright with a Bucky or grid.

Place the patient's zygoma, nose, and chin on the center line.

Oblique the head 50 to 53 degrees from the tabletop, as measured from the MSP of the posterior skull (Fig. 6–25).[32] Another way to describe the obliquity is to oblique the head 37 to 40 degrees from the CR of the tube (vertical).[33]

Place the acanthomeatal line (AML) parallel to the top edge of the film or grid (transverse axis) by adjusting the flexion or extension of the head and neck (Fig. 6–24).

Center the film to the infraorbital margin of the side down.

Both sides are taken for comparison.

Recheck all baselines before making an exposure.

NOTES:

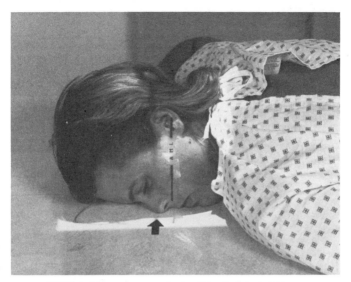

FIGURE 6–24. PA oblique projection (Rhese) of the facial bones.

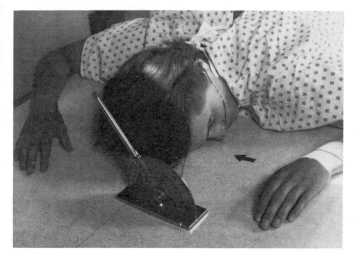

FIGURE 6–25. For the PA oblique facial bone projection, the MSP is positioned at 53 degrees from the tabletop.

NOTE: For trauma, recumbent patients, a reverse Rhese must be performed. The CR will enter the orbit of the side up (Fig. 6–26). The orbit or facial bones of the side up will be demonstrated. **STRUCTURES DEMONSTRATED:** Bilateral study of the obliqued facial bones, each film includes both sides, right and left (Fig. 6–27).

The optic canal (optic foramen) of the side down.

COMMON ERROR: Underpenetration. The side up is easily penetrated. The side down represents a much greater density so that the technique must be increased accordingly.

TECHNIQUE

KV _____ MA _____ SECS _____ MAS _____ CALIPER _____ cm

_____ :1 GRID / B / none SCREEN: RE / High / Par / Detail / None

SID: _____ Rm _____ ADULT / CHILD age: _____ mos. / yrs.

HABITUS: Hyper / s / hypo / a   XS   S   M   L   XL   XXL

NOTES:

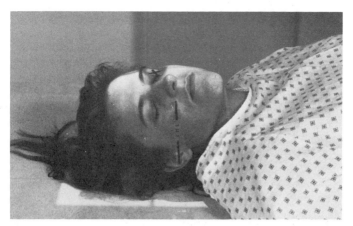

FIGURE 6–26. A reverse Rhese, an AP oblique facial bone projection may be performed for trauma patients unable to be pronated.

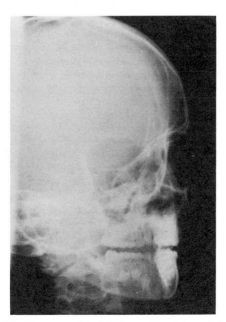

FIGURE 6–27. PA oblique x-ray of the facial bones. Use a lower technique (as shown) to detail the zygoma and lateral orbit of the side up. Notice the optic foramen of the side down located just within the lateral orbital margin.

MANDIBLE: SEMI-AXIAL AP (TOWNE'S, GRASHEY)

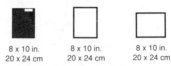

8 x 10 in.   8 x 10 in.   8 x 10 in.
20 x 24 cm   20 x 24 cm   20 x 24 cm

FILM: Use table Bucky. Collimate to the area of interest.

CR: Use a caudal angle of 30 degrees with the OML. Exit slightly inferior to the temporomandibular joints (TMJs) at the MSP (Fig. 6–28).[34]

Another method is to caudally angle 35 degrees with the OML perpendicular to the tabletop. Enter about 3 inches (7 to 8 cm) above the nasion.[35] The transverse center line should enshadow the TMJs (1/2 inch or 1.2 cm anterior to the EAM).

NOTE: Whenever an angle is used that is directed toward the lower axial skeleton, lead shielding should be provided to the patient. Do not use the overhead distance indicators to measure the SID for any tube angle. Always use the tape measure along the path of the central ray to measure to the tabletop when using a tube angle.

POSITION: Remove hearing aids, eyeglasses, hairpins, necklaces, earrings, and clothing around neck. Ask the patient to remove dentures or removable dental bridges.

The patient is supinated upon the table.

Center the MSP to the center of the table.

The chin is depressed in order to place the OML or IOML perpendicular to the tabletop. The selection of OML versus IOML will depend upon the amount of angle selected (see CR above).

Check midsagittal centering again after chin is adjusted.

Recheck all baselines before making an exposure.

NOTE: The reverse Towne's or PA semi-axial (Haas) is positioned with the patient prone. Place the transverse centering light so that it enshadows or bisects the mandibular rami.

STRUCTURES DEMONSTRATED: The elongated, mandibular rami (Fig. 6–29).

The temporomandibular fossae and mandibular condyle.

The elongated, overpenetrated, zygomatic arches lateral to the mandibular rami.

Symmetrical petrous pyramids.

COMMON ERROR: Centering too high and clipping the rami. This projection is centered lower to demonstrate the mandible, not the occipital bone.

TECHNIQUE

KV _____ MA _____ SECS _____ MAS _____ CALIPER _____ cm

_____ :1 GRID / B / none SCREEN: RE / High / Par / Detail / None

SID: _____ Rm _____ ADULT / CHILD age: _____ mos. / yrs.

HABITUS: Hyper / s / hypo / a   XS   S   M   L   XL   XXL

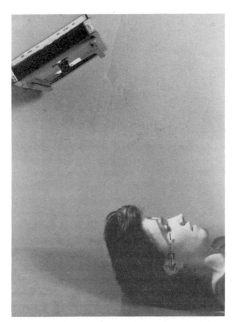

FIGURE 6–28. Semi-axial AP projection for the mandible. Notice the lower transverse centering line placement. TMJ *(square)*. Collimation is opened for demonstration only; collimate to area of interest (see Fig. 6–29).

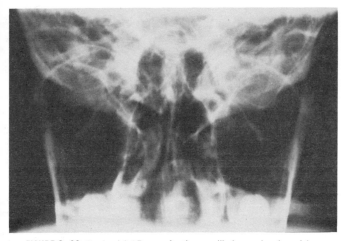

FIGURE 6–29. Semi-axial AP x-ray for the mandibular rami and condyles.

MANDIBLE: PA OR PA SEMI-AXIAL

8 x 10 in.
20 x 24 cm

8 x 10 in.
20 x 24 cm

8 x 10 in.
20 x 24 cm

FILM: Use table Bucky. Collimate to the area of interest.
CR: For the PA, perpendicular at MSP. Exit at the level of the lips.

For the PA semi-axial, a 30-degree cephalic angle may also be used.[36] Exit the acanthion.
POSITION: Remove hearing aids, eyeglasses, hairpins, necklaces, earrings, and clothing around neck. Ask the patient to remove dentures or dental bridges.

The patient is pronated upon the table or upright with the use of a Bucky or grid.

Center the MSP to the center of the table or grid.

Extend the head and neck so that only the lips, nose, and chin (symphysis menti) touch the film (Fig. 6–30).

Recheck the MSP just before making the exposure.

NOTE: For recumbent, trauma patients an AP projection may be performed. Enter at the lips with a perpendicular CR.
STRUCTURES DEMONSTRATED: The perpendicular CR will best demonstrate the mandibular body (Fig. 6–31).

The angled CR will best demonstrate the mandibular rami and mandibular condyles.
COMMON ERROR: Clipping the TMJs. Make sure your collimation includes the TMJs and the mentum.

TECHNIQUE
KV _____ MA _____ SECS _____ MAS _____ CALIPER _____ cm
_____ :1 GRID / B / none SCREEN: RE / High / Par / Detail / None
SID: _____ Rm _____ ADULT / CHILD age: _____ mos. / yrs.
HABITUS: Hyper / s / hypo / a   XS   S   M   L   XL   XXL

NOTES:

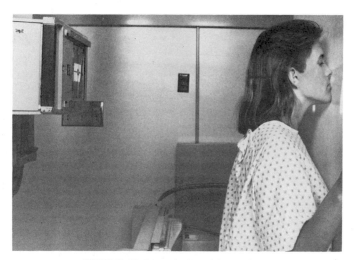

FIGURE 6–30. PA projection of the mandible.

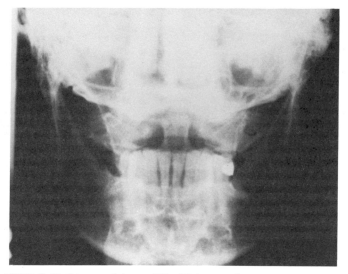

FIGURE 6–31. PA x-ray of the mandible. (Notice near-clip at mentum—use larger film or open collimation slightly.)

MANDIBLE: AXIOLATERALS

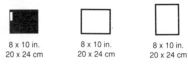

| 8 x 10 in.
20 x 24 cm | 8 x 10 in.
20 x 24 cm | 8 x 10 in.
20 x 24 cm |

FILM: Use tabletop or with Bucky.
CR: Angled 25 degrees cephalad (Fig. 6–32).[37] Enter just below gonion (mandibular angle) of side up.

Another method is a perpendicular CR with a 25-degree head tilt (Fig. 6–33).[38] Enter just below gonion (mandibular angle) of side up.

NOTE: This position requires good mobility of the head and neck. Do not use for neck-injured patients. Instead, employ a crosstable method using the same centering, film size, and CR angled 25 degrees cephalic that does not require moving the head or neck (see below and Fig. 8–11).

POSITION: Remove hearing aids, eyeglasses, hairpins, necklaces, earrings, and clothing around neck. Ask the patient to remove dentures or dental bridges.

The patient is pronated or supinated upon the table or upright with the use of a Bucky or grid.

The patient can be positioned in the RAO/LAO positions for pronated axiolaterals or positioned in the RPO/LPO positions for supinated axiolaterals.

The patient's head is lateralized and/or turned 10 degrees toward the side of interest for a general survey of the side down.

Rotate the head 30 degrees from lateral to demonstrate the body of the mandible.

Rotate the head 45 degrees from lateral to demonstrate the mentum of the mandible.

CR 25 Degrees Cephalic: When using the cephalic angle of 25 degrees, the IP will be perpendicular to the table (see Fig. 6–32). Extend the chin out in order to remove the TMJ of the side down from superimposition. In order not to have to increase tube angle due to head position, avoid head tilt in which the vertex MSP is more elevated than the MSP at the chin; if this is the case, it negates or lessens the 25-degree tube cephalic angle.

Combination Tube Angle and Head Tilt: When the patient is positioned with a head tilt that places the vertex MSP lower than the chin MSP, the 25-degree cephalic tube angle can be reduced by the degree of head tilt. For example, when the angle of the MSP as measured from the table at the vertex is 10 degrees, the necessary tube angle will be 15 degrees. Any combination of 25 can be used with accuracy. This enables a smaller tube angle to be used with hypersthenic patients, or broad-shouldered patients whose side-up shoulder superimposes the area of interest when a

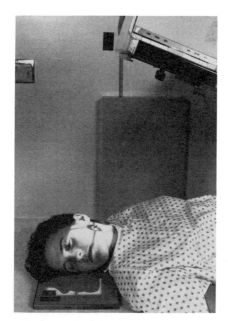

FIGURE 6–32. A tabletop axiolateral mandible position using tube angle only.

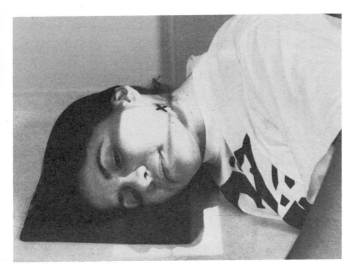

FIGURE 6–33. A Bucky axiolateral mandible position using a perpendicular tube with head tilt only.

25-degree cephalic tube angle is used. The IP will not be perpendicular to the table.

CR Perpendicular: Pad under the recumbent patient's upper torso and shoulders. The head (IP) should tilt approximately 25 degrees with the parietal eminence (vertex) touching the tabletop (Fig. 6–33). The angle from the film to the MSP or glabelloalveolar line (see Fig. 1–7) can be used to measure the 25 degrees. Extend the chin. This method also eliminates superimposition of the shoulder produced by severe cephalic angles.

Recheck all baselines and angles before making an exposure.

STRUCTURES DEMONSTRATED: For the general survey film, the mandible's TMJ, condyle, ramus, body, and mentum of the side down (Fig. 6–34).

Lateralization or a 10-degree rotation of the head will result in a survey film that includes the TMJ of the side down.

Rotation of the head 30 degrees will demonstrate the body.

Rotation of the head 45 degrees will demonstrate the mentum. With this rotation, the side-down TMJ will be superimposed over the cervical spine.

COMMON ERRORS: (1) Excessive elongation or foreshortening of the mandibular structures. Whatever combination of head tilt (vertex down/chin elevated) and tube angle is used, the total amount of angulation should remain within 25 degrees. (2) Overrotation when the TMJ and condyle are of interest. For the TMJ area do not rotate the head. The more you rotate, the more the TMJ of the side down moves posteriorly to be superimposed over the cervical spine.

TECHNIQUE

KV _____ MA _____ SECS _____ MAS _____ CALIPER _____ cm

_____ :1 GRID / B / none SCREEN: RE / High / Par / Detail / None

SID: _____ Rm _____ ADULT / CHILD age: _____ mos. / yrs.

HABITUS: Hyper / s / hypo / a XS S M L XL XXL

NOTES:

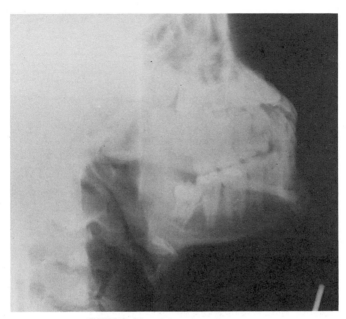

FIGURE 6–34. Axiolateral mandible x-ray.

NOTES:

MANDIBLE: SMV OR VSM

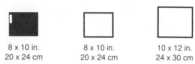

| 8 x 10 in. | 8 x 10 in. | 10 x 12 in. |
| 20 x 24 cm | 20 x 24 cm | 24 x 30 cm |

FILM: Use table Bucky. Collimate severely to the anatomical area of interest.

CR: Perpendicular to the IOML and exiting the body at a point 1 inch (2.54 cm) anterior to the gonion (see Fig. 1–5).

NOTE: This position usually requires excellent mobility of the head and neck. For trauma patients, take as is or omit. Use a greater tube angle to compensate for the patient's inability to flex or extend the head and neck.

SMV POSITION: Remove hearing aids, eyeglasses, hairpins, earrings, or hair clips. Ask the patient to remove dentures or dental bridges.

The patient is supinated upon the table or upright with the use of a Bucky or grid. Explain what you will do in order to enlist the patient's cooperation.

Recumbent: The SMV is commonly used for the multitrauma patient unable to turn for the VSM mandible study. Load the film; mark it. Have the tube readied near the head of the x-ray table with a cephalic angle. Have the technique set. If performing for zygomatic arches, remember that the visualization of the zygomatic arches does not require cranial penetration. Use a much lower technique.

Use several pillows placed under the back and below the level of the shoulders (see Fig. 6–13). Support the head while having the patient in full neck extension. The vertex should be touching the tabletop. Flex the knees.

Angle the tube to align perpendicularly to the IOML (a cephalic angle).

Quickly, center the MSP to the center of the table.

VSM POSITION: The patient is pronated upon the table or upright with the use of a Bucky or grid. In order to enlist the patient's cooperation, explain what you will do.

Remove hearing aids, eyeglasses, hairpins, necklaces, earrings, and clothing around neck. Ask the patient to remove dentures or dental bridges.

Recumbent: Load the film; mark it. Have the tube readied near the head of the x-ray table with a caudal angle. Have the technique set.

Have the patient brace himself or herself by placing the arms up alongside the head. Hyperextend the head and neck. Have the patient resting the head on the chin (see Fig. 6–15).

Angle the tube to align perpendicularly to the IOML (a caudal angle).

Quickly, center the MSP to the center of the table.

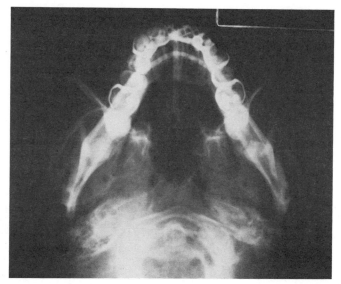

FIGURE 6–35. Verticosubmental x-ray for the mandible.

Upright: Load the film; mark it. Have the tube readied near the head of the x-ray table with a caudal angle. Have the technique set.

Have the patient standing and holding onto the upright table or film holder for support, or the patient can be seated. (Some techs use the table horizontal, with the patient seated at the end, and build up the film to meet the forward-leaning patient.)

With the patient's anterior aspect to the film, place the patient in full neck extension. Have the patient resting the head on the chin.

Angle the tube to align perpendicularly to the IOML (a caudal angle).

Quickly, center the MSP to the center of the table.

STRUCTURES DEMONSTRATED: The basilar aspect of the mandible (Fig. 6–35). The VSM shows the mandibular arch in detail, while the SMV will demonstrate the magnified mandibular arch.

The film includes the condyles, anteriorly to the mentum.

COMMON ERROR: Distortion caused by too much angulation. The CR must be perpendicular to the IOML.

TECHNIQUE

KV _____ MA _____ SECS _____ MAS _____ CALIPER _____ cm

_____ :1 GRID / B / none SCREEN: RE / High / Par / Detail / None

SID: _____ Rm _____ ADULT / CHILD age: _____ mos. / yrs.

HABITUS: Hyper / s / hypo / a   XS   S   M   L   XL   XXL

MANDIBLE: AXIAL TRANSCRANIAL TMJs (OPEN AND CLOSED MOUTH)

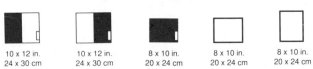

10 x 12 in.
24 x 30 cm

10 x 12 in.
24 x 30 cm

8 x 10 in.
20 x 24 cm

8 x 10 in.
20 x 24 cm

8 x 10 in.
20 x 24 cm

FILM: Use table Bucky. Collimate severely to the anatomical area of interest.

CR: Use a 25-degree caudal angle centered to the TMJ of the side down for an axial transcranial projection. The TMJ is located at the point 1 inch (2.54 cm) anterior to the EAM. Place the CR so that it exits at this point of the side down.

NOTE: An alternate projection to the axial transcranial is a lateral transcranial (Law's method). For details on this method, refer to the axiolateral Law's or lateral transcranial Law's under Mastoids in this chapter.

POSITION: Initially, the patient is pronated upon the table or upright with the use of a Bucky or grid.

Remove any hearing aids, eyeglasses, earrings, hairpins, or clips.

The position of the head will be identical to that of a lateral skull.

Place the recumbent patient in the RAO position for the right TMJ (Fig. 6–36) and/or the LAO for the left TMJ. Place the arm of the side down at the patient's side. The opposite arm should be up. Have the patient bend the knee of the elevated side in order to relieve strain.

Center the point 1 inch (2.54 cm) anterior to the EAM of the side down to the center line of the table.

From either the RAO or LAO, adjust the patient's head so that the IP is perpendicular to the x-ray table or film.

The MSP should be parallel to the tabletop or film.

Place the IOML so that it is parallel to the top of the film by adjusting the flexion or extension of the head and neck.

Recenter the TMJ of the side down after baseline adjustments. Take an exposure of each side with the patient's mouth open (Fig. 6–36), then with it closed. Move the lower jaw only. Use a marker to indicate open mouth positions (or closed) in order to differentiate the positions when pathology is present. An "O" marker is used for open mouth positions (see Fig. 6–38).

Recheck all baselines before making an exposure.

STRUCTURES DEMONSTRATED: The TMJ of the side down with the mouth closed (Fig. 6–37).

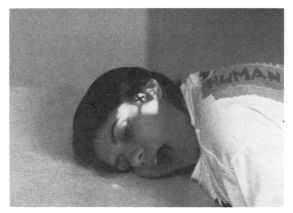

FIGURE 6–36. Open-mouth lateral transcranial projection.

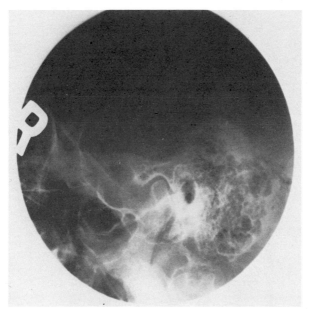

FIGURE 6–37. Closed-mouth right (R) TMJ x-ray.

The TMJ of the side down with the mouth opened (Fig. 6–38).
Both sides are performed for comparison.

COMMON ERROR: Not marking open or closed mouth position or marking right or left side. Sometimes limited range of motion makes an assessment difficult to tell if the radiograph represents one position or the other. This is especially true when you tightly collimate.

TECHNIQUE

KV _____ MA _____ SECS _____ MAS _____ CALIPER _____ cm

_____ :1 GRID / B / none SCREEN: RE / High / Par / Detail / None

SID: _____ Rm _____ ADULT / CHILD age: _____ mos. / yrs.

HABITUS: Hyper / s / hypo / a   XS   S   M   L   XL   XXL

NOTES:

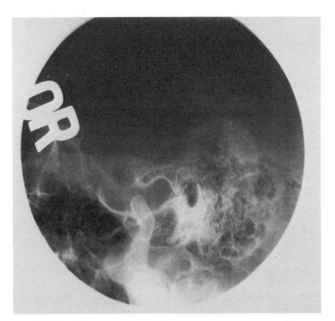

FIGURE 6–38. Open-mouth right (R) TMJ x-ray. Open mouth (O).

NOTES:

NASAL BONES: PARIETOACANTHIAL (WATERS')

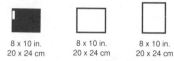

8 x 10 in.   8 x 10 in.   8 x 10 in.
20 x 24 cm   20 x 24 cm   20 x 24 cm

FILM: Use table Bucky. Collimate slightly less than the size of the film.

CR: Perpendicular, exiting the acanthion.

POSITION: The patient is pronated upon the table or upright with a Bucky or grid.

Remove hearing aids, eyeglasses, hairpins, necklaces, earrings, and clothing around neck. Ask the patient to remove dentures or removable dental bridges.

Ask the patient to extend the neck so that the skull rests upon the chin. The OML should measure 37 degrees to the tabletop or grid (Fig. 6–39). Adjust the flexion or extension of the head and neck for this measurement.

Another baseline you can use is the MML. Place the MML perpendicular to the tabletop or grid.

Center the MSP to the center of the table or grid.

Center the film to the acanthion.

Recheck all baselines before making an exposure.

NOTE: For trauma and neck-injured patients, use the reverse Waters' method. With the patient supinated, simply match the angle of the MML with the angle of the tube. The CR enters the acanthion. This method requires no movement (flexion or extension) of the head and neck. Center the MSP to the tabletop or grid if the patient's condition permits.

STRUCTURES DEMONSTRATED: The nasal septum in midline (Fig. 6–40).

The vomer and perpendicular plate of the ethmoid.

The petrous ridges should be below the maxillary sinuses.

COMMON ERROR: Rotation. Check by comparing bilateral structures, e.g., zygomatic arches, maxillary sinuses, or orbits.

TECHNIQUE

KV _____ MA _____ SECS _____ MAS _____ CALIPER _____ cm

_____ :1 GRID / B / none SCREEN: RE / High / Par / Detail / None

SID: _____ Rm _____ ADULT / CHILD age: _____ mos. / yrs.

HABITUS: Hyper / s / hypo / a   XS   S   M   L   XL   XXL

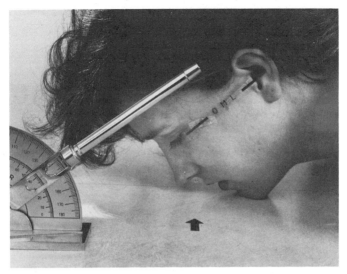

FIGURE 6–39. Parietoacanthial (Waters') OML measurement to table.

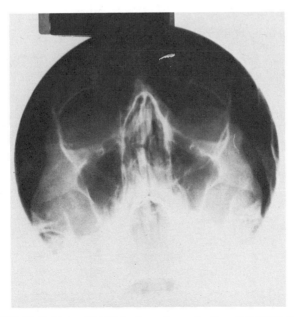

FIGURE 6–40. Parietoacanthial (Waters') x-ray for nasal septum. *Note*: MSP is slightly off center.

NASAL BONES: LATERALS

8 x 10 in.	8 x 10 in.	8 x 10 in.	8 x 10 in.
20 x 24 cm	20 x 24 cm	20 x 24 cm	20 x 24 cm

FILM: Tabletop. Collimate to include base of nasal bone to anterior nasal spine and soft tissue of the nose.

CR: Perpendicular to the nasion (bridge) of the nose. Collimate to include the glabella and anterior nasal (acanthial) spine.

POSITION: The patient is pronated upon the table.

Use the RAO position for the right lateral (Fig. 6–41). Right arm down by the side.

Use the LAO position for the left lateral. Left arm down by the side.

The MSP should be parallel to the film.

The IP is perpendicular to the film.

Place the AML parallel to the top edge of the film or transverse axis of the table.

After any adjustment of the MSP, IP, or AML, you must readjust the other baselines or plane.

Recheck all baselines before making an exposure.

STRUCTURES DEMONSTRATED: The detail of the nasal bone of the side down. Usually both laterals are done for comparison (Fig. 6–42).

Soft tissue of the nose.

The anterior nasal spine (acanthion).

COMMON ERRORS: (1) Underpenetrated. The nasofrontal suture needs to be demonstrated. (2) Not including the anterior nasal spine (acanthion).

TECHNIQUE

KV _____ MA _____ SECS _____ MAS _____ CALIPER _____ cm

_____ :1 GRID / B / none SCREEN: RE / High / Par / Detail / None

SID: _____ Rm _____ ADULT / CHILD age: _____ mos. / yrs.

HABITUS: Hyper / s / hypo / a   XS   S   M   L   XL   XXL

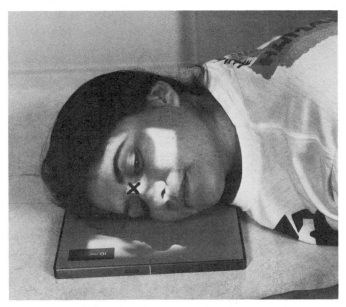

FIGURE 6–41. Lateral off-Bucky position for nasal bones.

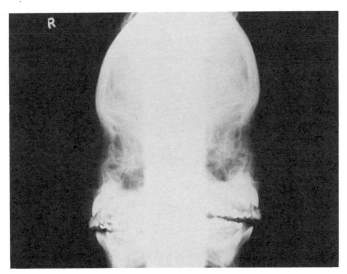

FIGURE 6–42. Lateral nasal bone x-rays (both sides for comparison). It may not be necessary to include more than the nasal bone and acanthion; check your department protocols.

ZYGOMATIC ARCHES: SEMI-AXIAL AP
(TOWNE'S, GRASHEY)

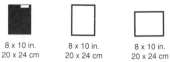

| 8 x 10 in. | 8 x 10 in. | 8 x 10 in. |
| 20 x 24 cm | 20 x 24 cm | 20 x 24 cm |

FILM: Use table Bucky. Use a stationary grid for portable or gurney patients.

CR: Use a caudal angle of 30 degrees with the OML or caudal angle of 37 degrees with the IOML. Enter at the glabella.[39] Exit slightly inferior to the TMJs at the midsagittal plane.[40] Or simply place the transverse line of the CR so that it bisects the zygomatic arch. Keep the CR centered to the table.

NOTE: Whenever an angle is used that is directed toward the lower axial skeleton, lead shielding should be provided to the patient. Do not use the overhead distance indicators to measure the SID for any tube angle. Always use the tape measure along the path of the central ray to measure to the tabletop when using a tube angle.

POSITION: The patient is supinated upon the table.

Remove hearing aids, eyeglasses, hairpins, earrings, necklaces, and clothing around neck. Ask the patient to remove dentures or removable dental bridges.

Center the MSP to the center of the table.

The chin is depressed in order to place the OML or IOML perpendicular to the tabletop (Fig. 6–43). The selection of OML versus IOML will depend upon the amount of angle selected (see CR above).

Check midsagittal centering again after chin is adjusted.

Recheck all baselines before making an exposure.

NOTE: The reverse Towne's or PA semi-axial (Haas) is positioned with the patient prone. It demonstrates similar structures as the AP semi-axial or Towne's.

STRUCTURES DEMONSTRATED: The elongated, zygomatic arches lateral to the mandibular rami (Fig. 6–44).

The elongated, mandibular rami.

The temporomandibular fossae and mandibular condyles.

Symmetrical petrous pyramids.

The occipital bone, but not necessarily in its entirety.

COMMON ERROR: Overpenetration.

TECHNIQUE

KV _____ MA _____ SECS _____ MAS _____ CALIPER _____ cm

_____ :1 GRID / B / none SCREEN: RE / High / Par / Detail / None

SID: _____ Rm _____ ADULT / CHILD age: _____ mos. / yrs.

HABITUS: Hyper / s / hypo / a   XS   S   M   L   XL   XXL

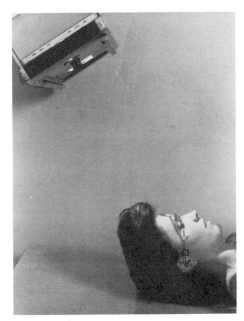

FIGURE 6–43. Semi-axial AP projection (Towne's, Grashey) for zygomatic arches.

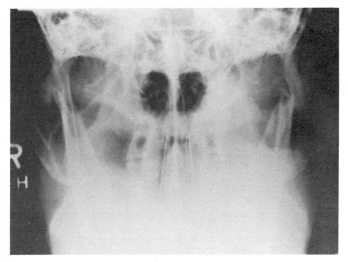

FIGURE 6–44. Semi-axial AP x-ray for zygomatic arches. Marker placement should be extreme up or down—not in the middle area.

ZYGOMATIC ARCHES: PARIETOACANTHIAL (WATERS' POSITION)

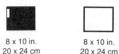

8 x 10 in.
20 x 24 cm

8 x 10 in.
20 x 24 cm

FILM: Use table Bucky. Collimate slightly less than the size of the film or to the area of interest.

CR: Perpendicular, exiting the acanthion.

POSITION: The patient is pronated upon the table or upright facing the film with a Bucky or grid.

Remove hearing aids, eyeglasses, hairpins, earrings, necklaces, and clothing around neck. Ask the patient to remove dentures or removable dental bridges.

Ask the patient to extend the neck so that the skull rests upon the chin. The OML should measure 37 degrees to the tabletop or grid (Fig. 6–45). Adjust the flexion or extension of the head and neck for this measurement.

Another baseline you can use is the MML. Place the MML perpendicular to the tabletop or grid.

Center the MSP to the center of the table or grid.

Center the film to the acanthion.

Collimate slightly less than the size of the film.

Recheck all baselines before making an exposure.

NOTE: For trauma and neck-injured patients, use the reverse Waters' method. With the patient supinated, simply match the angle of the MML with the angle of the tube. The CR enters the acanthion. This method requires no movement (flexion or extension) of the head and neck. Center the MSP to the tabletop or grid if the patient's condition permits.

STRUCTURES DEMONSTRATED: Best demonstration of the orbits, zygomatic bones, zygomatic arches, and the maxillae (the upper facial bones).

The zygomatic arches will be foreshortened (Fig. 6–46).

The petrous ridges should be below the maxillary sinuses.

COMMON ERROR: Overpenetration.

TECHNIQUE

KV _____MA _____SECS _____MAS _____CALIPER _____cm

_____ :1 GRID / B / none SCREEN: RE / High / Par / Detail / None

SID: _____ Rm _____ ADULT / CHILD age: _____ mos. / yrs.

HABITUS: Hyper / s / hypo / a   XS   S   M   L   XL   XXL

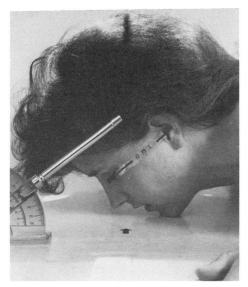

FIGURE 6–45. Parietoacanthial (Waters') projection.

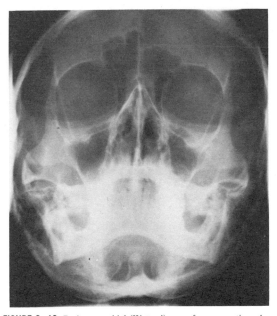

FIGURE 6–46. Parietoacanthial (Waters') x-ray for zygomatic arches.

ZYGOMATIC ARCHES: TANGENTIAL (MAY'S)

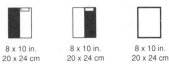

8 x 10 in.   8 x 10 in.   8 x 10 in.
20 x 24 cm   20 x 24 cm   20 x 24 cm

FILM: Tabletop. No grid is necessary due to the low bone density of the arches. Collimate longitudinally, from nose to EAM, and transversely, 2 inches (5 cm).

CR: Bilaterally, perpendicularly to the IOML at each zygomatic arch (bisect the IOML).

POSITION: The patient is pronated upon the table or upright.

Remove hearing aids, eyeglasses, earrings, hairpins, or hair clips.

Recumbent: Place the film on top of the table; mark it. Have the tube readied near the head of the x-ray table with a caudal angle. Have the technique set. Remember that the visualization of the zygomatic arches does not require cranial penetration. Use a much lower technique than that of the skull or sinuses.

Have the patient extend the head and neck in order to rest upon the chin.

Angle the tube to align perpendicularly to the IOML (a caudal angle).

Rotate the anterior aspect of the head (the face) approximately 15 degrees *toward* the side of interest (the occipital area of the skull will move *away* from the side of interest) or until the zygomatic arch is free from superimposition (Fig. 6–47).

If this movement does not free the arch from superimposition of the parietal eminence, use a tilt of 15 degrees of the MSP or the glabelloalveolar line (GAL) from vertical (Fig. 6–47). The MSP or GAL will form a 15-degree angle with the CR or as measured from vertical. (The superior aspect of the skull moves away from the CR or vertical while the chin is relatively fixed).

Quickly, center the unilateral arch to the center of one side of the film.

HINT: Since facial structure varies widely, place a straight edge or ruler standing on end on the film. Adjust the obliquity and/or the tilt of the head so that when approaching the face with the ruler still based on the film, the first contact should be made with the zygoma.

NOTE: Since most patients may have limited extension range of motion and will not be able to tolerate the VSM study, use the SMV projection. The increased object-image distance (OID) will actually aid in opening the zygomatic arches.

Recheck all baselines before making an exposure.

Take both sides for comparison.

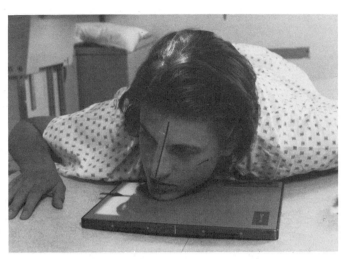

FIGURE 6–47. Tangential projection (May's method) for zygomatic arches. Notice the two angles in use: the MSP 15-degree rotation toward the side of interest and the tilt of the glabelloalveolar baseline (see line) to free the arch from the parietal eminence.

NOTES:

STRUCTURES DEMONSTRATED: The zygomatic arch of interest without superimposition (Fig. 6–48).

A bilateral study of each zygomatic arch.

The technique will not be sufficient to penetrate the cranium.

COMMON ERROR: Superimposition. If the positioning described above still presents superimposition of both arches, either the baselines were off, or the patient's facial structure necessitates alteration of the 15-degree rotation (as well as 15-degree tilt) of the head.

TECHNIQUE

KV _____ MA _____ SECS _____ MAS _____ CALIPER _____ cm

_____ :1 GRID / B / none SCREEN: RE / High / Par / Detail / None

SID: _____ Rm _____ ADULT / CHILD   age: _____ mos. / yrs.

HABITUS: Hyper / s / hypo / a   XS   S   M   L   XL   XXL

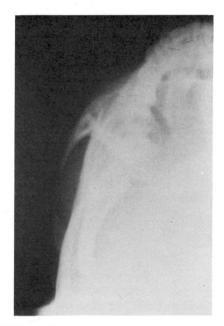

FIGURE 6—48. Tangential x-ray for the zygomatic arch.

BILATERAL ZYGOMATIC ARCHES: SMV OR VSM (BASILAR)

| 10 x 12 in. | 10 x 12 in. | 8 x 10 in. | 8 x 10 in. |
| 24 x 30 cm | 24 x 30 cm | 20 x 24 cm | 20 x 24 cm |

FILM: Use table Bucky. No grid is necessary because of the low bone density of the arches.

CR: Perpendicularly to the IOML at the midsagittal plane. Place it at the point that will bisect the length of the IOML. Collimate to include the EAM, the nose, the right and left zygomatic bones.

NOTE: This position usually requires excellent mobility of the head and neck. For trauma patients, take as is. Use a greater tube angle to compensate for the patient's inability to flex or extend the head and neck.

SVM POSITION: Remove hearing aids, eyeglasses, earrings, hairpins, or hair clips. Ask the patient to remove dentures or dental bridges.

The patient is supinated upon the table or upright with the use of a Bucky or grid. Explain what you will do in order to enlist the patient's cooperation.

NOTE: The SMV is recommended over the VSM for a bilateral study of the arches because of the ease of demonstration due to their magnification by increased OID.

Recumbent: Load the film; mark it. Have the tube readied near the head of the x-ray table with a cephalic angle (Fig. 6–49). Have the technique set. Remember that the visualization of the zygomatic arches does not require cranial penetration. Use a much lower technique.

Use several pillows placed under the back and below the level of the shoulders. Support the head while having the patient in full neck extension. The vertex should be touching the tabletop. Flex the knees.

Angle the tube to align perpendicularly to the IOML (a cephalic angle).

Quickly, center the MSP to the center of the table.

Upright: Load the film, mark it. Have the tube readied near the head of the x-ray table with a cephalic angle. Have the technique set.

Have the patient sit down or use a chair, IV pole, etc., for support if standing. Seated is preferred for stability.

With the patient seated with the posterior aspect to the film, support the head while placing the patient in full neck extension. Guide the vertex of the skull to the center of the film. If the full vertex is not touching, the patient is either too far away or too close.

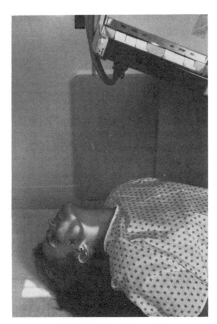

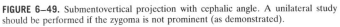

FIGURE 6–49. Submentovertical projection with cephalic angle. A unilateral study should be performed if the zygoma is not prominent (as demonstrated).

Angle the tube to align perpendicularly to the IOML.

Quickly, center the MSP to the center of the table.

VSM POSITION: (Use only for dolichocephalic patients.) Remove hearing aids, eyeglasses, hairpins, earrings, necklaces, and clothing around neck. Ask the patient to remove dentures or dental bridges.

The patient is pronated upon the table or upright with the use of a Bucky or grid. Explain what you will do in order to enlist the patient's cooperation.

Recumbent: Load the film; mark it. Have the tube readied near the head of the x-ray table with a caudal angle. Have the technique set.

Have the patients brace themselves by placing their arms up alongside their head. Hyperextend the head and neck. Have the patients resting their head on their chin (Fig. 6–50).

Angle the tube to align perpendicularly to the IOML (a caudal angle).

Quickly, center the MSP to the center of the table.

Upright: Load the film; mark it. Have the tube readied near the head of the x-ray table with a caudal angle. Have the technique set.

Have the patient standing and holding onto the table or film holder for support, or the patient can be seated.

With the anterior aspect to the film, place the patient in full neck extension. Have the patient resting the head on the chin.

Angle the tube to align perpendicularly to the IOML (a caudal angle).

Quickly, center the MSP to the center of the table.

STRUCTURES DEMONSTRATED: The bilateral, zygomatic arches (Fig. 6–51).

The soft tissue of the anterior cranium. Due to the lower technique, no cranial bony detail will be demonstrated.

COMMON ERRORS: (1) The zygomatic arches are not symmetrical. Check your baselines carefully. However, a right and left unilateral study may be necessary due to the prominence of the parietal eminences. The head tilt and/or rotation will control the opening or closing of the arches (see the tangential May's method). Sometimes the injured side will not be open due to a compressed fracture. (2) The arches are elongated. The CR was not perpendicular to the IOML.

TECHNIQUE

KV _____ MA _____ SECS _____ MAS _____ CALIPER _____ cm

_____ :1 GRID / B / none SCREEN: RE / High / Par / Detail / None

SID: _____ Rm _____ ADULT / CHILD age: _____ mos. / yrs.

HABITUS: Hyper / s / hypo / a   XS   S   M   L   XL   XXL

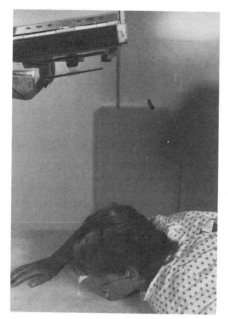

FIGURE 6–50. Verticosubmental projection for bilateral, zygomatic arches.

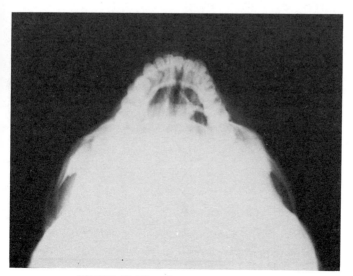

FIGURE 6–51. Bilateral, zygomatic arches x-ray.

PARANASAL SINUSES: PA

8 x 10 in. 20 x 24 cm	8 x 10 in. 20 x 24 cm	8 x 10 in. 20 x 24 cm

FILM: Table Bucky. Collimate slightly less than the size of the film or to the area of interest.

CR: Perpendicular with the CR exiting at the nasion. Use a cylinder cone or collimate to the area of interest, the sinuses.

POSITION: Remove hearing aids, eyeglasses, hairpins, earrings, necklaces, and clothing around neck. Ask the patient to remove dentures or removable dental bridges.

The patient is upright for the exam and for 10 minutes prior to the exam.

Have the patient tuck the chin in order to place the forehead and nose on the center line of the upright x-ray table or head unit (Fig. 6–52).

Use a horizontal beam.

Center the MSP to the center of the table.

Rotate the skull into position while assessing the level of each EAM by palpating the right and left tragus (small flap partially covering the EAM). They should lie in the same transverse plane.

Recheck all baselines before making an exposure.

STRUCTURES DEMONSTRATED: Demonstration of the posterior ethmoidal air cells projected above the anterior cells.

The petrous pyramids will fill the orbits (Fig. 6–53).

COMMON ERROR: Rotation. Check the positioning of the midsagittal after the chin is tucked for the OML placement.

TECHNIQUE

KV _____ MA _____ SECS _____ MAS _____ CALIPER _____ cm

_____ :1 GRID / B / none SCREEN: RE / High / Par / Detail / None

SID: _____ Rm _____ ADULT / CHILD age: _____ mos. / yrs.

HABITUS: Hyper / s / hypo / a XS S M L XL XXL

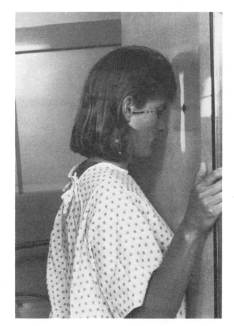

FIGURE 6–52. Upright PA projection.

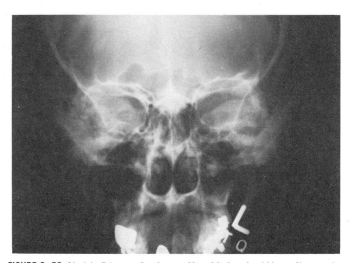

FIGURE 6–53. Upright PA x-ray for sinuses. *Note*: Marker should be at film margin.

PARANASAL SINUSES: SEMI-AXIAL PA
(CALDWELL)

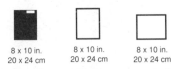

8 x 10 in.
20 x 24 cm

8 x 10 in.
20 x 24 cm

8 x 10 in.
20 x 24 cm

FILM: Table Bucky. Use a cylinder cone or collimate to the area of interest, the sinuses.

CR: A 15-degree caudal tube angle exiting the nasion. The OML should be perpendicular to the film.

A common modification is to avoid the use of a tube angle by using a horizontal beam that exits the nasion. Begin from a position where the OML is perpendicular to the film.[41] Extend the head and neck to the point that the OML is elevated 15 degrees. You may approximate this distance by extending the head and neck twice the distance measured between the distal OML and IOML (7 degrees multiplied twice = 14 degrees). Elevating the OML 15 degrees instead of using a tube angle will demonstrate true air fluid lines without the image distortion normally produced by tube angulation (Fig. 6–54).

A perpendicular CR with a horizontal beam may be used when the film is angled 15 degrees (see positioning note).

NOTE: Whenever an angle is used, do not use the overhead distance indicators to measure the SID for any tube angle. Always use the tape measure along the path of the central ray to measure to the tabletop when using a tube angle.

POSITION: Remove hearing aids, eyeglasses, hairpins, earrings, necklaces, and clothing around neck. Ask the patient to remove dentures or removable dental bridges.

The patient is upright and facing the table or grid device. Have the patient tuck the chin in order to place the forehead and nose on the center line of the upright x-ray table or head unit.

NOTE: If you are working with a head unit, the film may be angled instead of the tube. The top edge (vertex) of the film will be closer to the patient (15 degrees) than the bottom. Use a horizontal beam.

Center the MSP to the center of the table.

The OML should be perpendicular to the film or tabletop (except when using a head unit, it will be 15 degrees or the modification described under CR above).

Rotate the skull into position while assessing the level of each EAM by palpating the right and left tragi (small flap partially covering the EAM). They should lie in the same coronal plane.

Recheck all baselines before making an exposure.

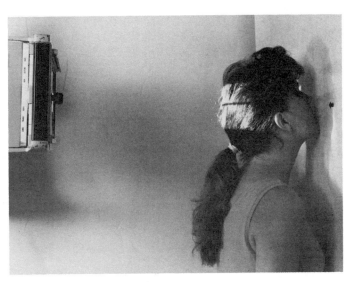

FIGURE 6–54. Upright modified method of PA (Caldwell) projection for sinuses. The OML is elevated 15 degrees with a perpendicular CR.

NOTES:

STRUCTURES DEMONSTRATED: The frontal and ethmoidal sinuses.

Demonstration of the anterior ethmoidal air cells.

The petrous pyramids will fill the lower third of the orbits (Fig. 6–55).

COMMON ERROR: Rotation. Check the positioning of the midsagittal after the chin is tucked. Position the skull by assessing the level of each EAM by palpating the right and left tragi. They should be adjusted to lie in the same transverse (coronal) plane.

TECHNIQUE

KV _____ MA _____ SECS _____ MAS _____ CALIPER _____ cm

_____ :1 GRID / B / none SCREEN: RE / High / Par / Detail / None

SID: _____ Rm _____ ADULT / CHILD age: _____ mos. / yrs.

HABITUS: Hyper / s / hypo / a XS S M L XL XXL

NOTES:

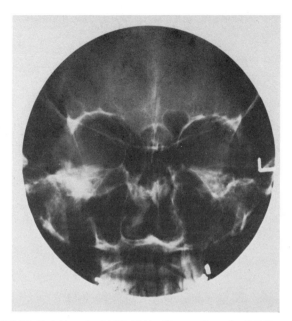

FIGURE 6–55. Upright semi-axial PA (Caldwell) x-ray. Generally, fluid lines should be more easily demonstrated with a moderately penetrating technique.

PARANASAL SINUSES: PARIETOACANTHIAL (WATERS')

8 x 10 in.	8 x 10 in.	8 x 10 in.
20 x 24 cm	20 x 24 cm	20 x 24 cm

FILM: Table Bucky. Use a cylinder cone or collimate to the area of interest, the sinuses.

CR: Perpendicular, exiting the acanthion. Use a cylinder cone or collimate to the area of interest, the sinuses.

POSITION: The patient is upright and facing the table or grid device.

Remove hearing aids, eyeglasses, hairpins, necklaces, earrings, and clothing around neck. Ask the patient to remove dentures or removable dental bridges.

Ask the pronated patient to extend the neck so that the skull rests upon the chin. The OML should measure 37 degrees to the tabletop or grid (Fig. 6–56). Adjust the OML by flexing or extending the head and neck.

An alternate baseline you may use is the MML. Place the MML (see Fig. 1–6) perpendicular to the tabletop or grid.

Center the MSP to the center of the table or grid.

Center the film to the acanthion.

Recheck all baselines before making an exposure.

STRUCTURES DEMONSTRATED: Best demonstration of the maxillary sinuses.

The petrous ridges should be below the maxillary sinuses (Fig. 6–57).

COMMON ERROR: *Improper baseline positioning. If your film shows the petrous ridges in the maxillary sinuses, the patient does not have enough extension. If your film shows the rotundum foramina obscured and the petrous ridges well below the maxillary sinuses in the body of the mandible, your patient has too much extension.*

TECHNIQUE

KV _____ MA _____ SECS _____ MAS _____ CALIPER _____ cm

_____ :1 GRID / B / none SCREEN: RE / High / Par / Detail / None

SID: _____ Rm _____ ADULT / CHILD age: _____ mos. / yrs.

HABITUS: Hyper / s / hypo / a XS S M L XL XXL

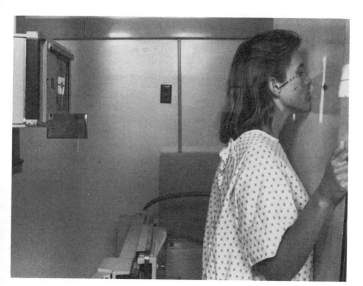

FIGURE 6–56. Upright parietoacanthial projection (Waters') for sinuses.

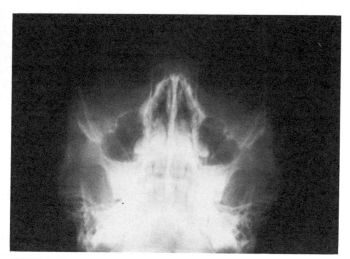

FIGURE 6–57. X-ray of upright parietoacanthial projection (Waters') for sinuses.

PARANASAL SINUSES: LATERAL

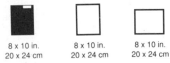

8 x 10 in.   8 x 10 in.   8 x 10 in.
20 x 24 cm   20 x 24 cm   20 x 24 cm

FILM: Use table Bucky. Use a cylinder cone or collimate to the area of interest, the sinuses.

CR: Perpendicular to surface of zygomatic bone just lateral to infraorbital margin. Collimate longitudinally to include the frontal sinuses to the mentum of the mandible and transversely from the nose to the EAM.

POSITION: The patient is upright with the use of a Bucky or grid (Fig. 6–58).

Remove any hearing aids, eyeglasses, earrings, hairpins, or clips. Ask the patient to remove dentures or removable dental bridges.

Place the upright patient in the RAO position for the right lateral or the LAO for the left lateral. (Usually only one lateral is taken. A bilateral study is not necessary.)

Center the zygomatic bone's anterior surface of the side down to the center line of the table.

From either the RAO or LAO, adjust the patient's head so that the IP is perpendicular to the x-ray table or film.

The MSP should be parallel to the tabletop or film.

Place the IOML so that it is parallel to the top of the film by adjusting the flexion or extension of the head and neck.

After any adjustment of the MSP, IP, or IOML, you must readjust the other baselines or plane.

Recenter the zygomatic bone's malar surface to the center line of the table after the baseline adjustments.

Recheck all baselines before making an exposure.

A crosstable lateral may be used for multiple-trauma or neck-injured patients. Use a grid.

STRUCTURES DEMONSTRATED: All paranasal sinuses in their lateral aspect (Fig. 6–59).

All are superimposed except the sphenoidal sinus.

COMMON ERROR: Rotation. Check the rotation by the alignment of the orbital ridges. If not superimposed, the IP needs adjustment.

TECHNIQUE

KV _____ MA _____ SECS _____ MAS _____ CALIPER _____ cm

_____ :1 GRID / B / none SCREEN: RE / High / Par / Detail / None

SID: _____ Rm _____ ADULT / CHILD age: _____ mos. / yrs.

HABITUS: Hyper / s / hypo / a   XS   S   M   L   XL   XXL

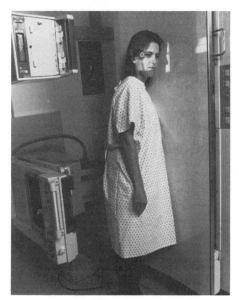

FIGURE 6–58. Upright lateral for sinuses.

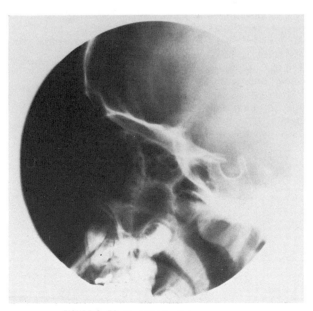

FIGURE 6–59. Upright lateral sinuses x-ray.

PARANASAL SINUSES: PA TRANSORAL
(OPEN MOUTH WATERS')

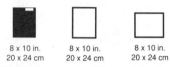

| 8 x 10 in. | 8 x 10 in. | 8 x 10 in. |
| 20 x 24 cm | 20 x 24 cm | 20 x 24 cm |

FILM: Use a cylinder cone or collimated to the area of interest, the sinuses. Use table Bucky.

CR: Perpendicular, exiting the open mouth.

POSITION: The patient is facing the film and upright with the use of a Bucky or grid.

Remove hearing aids, eyeglasses, hairpins, earrings, necklaces, and clothing around neck. Ask the patient to remove dentures or dental bridges.

The patient's head should rest on chin and nose. Have the patient's arms up in order to brace themselves. The OML should be approximately 37 to 45 degrees from the tabletop.

Center the MSP to the center of the table or grid.

Have the patient open the mouth as wide as is comfortable (Fig. 6–60).

Center the CR through the open mouth.

Center the film to the level of the open mouth.

Recheck all baselines before making an exposure.

NOTE: Sometimes the patient will be instructed to softly phonate the sound "ah." This lowers and immobilizes the tongue.[42]

STRUCTURES DEMONSTRATED: The sphenoidal sinus projected through the open mouth (Fig. 6–61).

The nasal septum.

The maxillary sinuses.

COMMON ERROR: The sphenoidal sinus is obscured by the upper teeth. The head and neck are not extended sufficiently due to patient fatigue (see Fig. 6–60).

TECHNIQUE

KV _____ MA _____ SECS _____ MAS _____ CALIPER _____ cm

_____ :1 GRID / B / none SCREEN: RE / High / Par / Detail / None

SID: _____ Rm _____ ADULT / CHILD age: _____ mos. / yrs.

HABITUS: Hyper / s / hypo / a   XS   S   M   L   XL   XXL

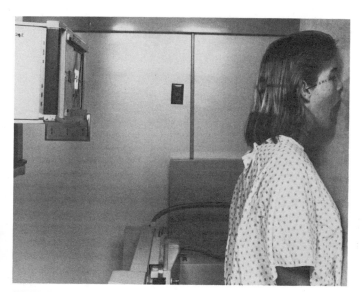

FIGURE 6–60. Upright PA transoral projection for sinuses. Notice the level of the open mouth is slightly lower than the CR due to patient fatigue. Always recheck before making the exposure.

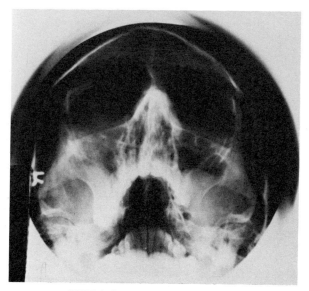

FIGURE 6–61. Upright PA transoral x-ray.

PETROMASTOIDS: SEMI-AXIAL PA (STENVER'S)

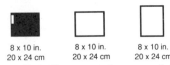

8 x 10 in.	8 x 10 in.	8 x 10 in.
20 x 24 cm	20 x 24 cm	20 x 24 cm

FILM: Table Bucky. Collimate to the area of interest or use a cone.

CR: A 12-degree cephalic angle (Fig. 6–62).

Collimate closely for the petromastoid portion or slightly larger to include the orbit.

Use both the side-up and side-down EAM to assess the projectory of the CR. Use the EAM of the side up to assess the CR entrance. Enter at the point 2 inches (5 cm) posterior and ½ inch (1.25 cm) inferior to the side-up EAM. This should result in the CR exiting the point 1 inch (2.54 cm) anterior to the EAM of the side down. The exit point is the more accurate of the two CR assessments due to the possibility of an obliquity positioning error, which will change the entrance coordinates of the CR.

POSITION: Remove hearing aids, eyeglasses, hairpins, earrings, necklaces, and clothing around neck. Ask the patient to remove dentures or dental bridges.

The patient is pronated and recumbent on the x-ray table or upright at a Bucky or grid device.

Rotate the head's MSP 45 degrees. The side down is demonstrated.

Place the head to rest upon the forehead, nose, and cheek. This will form a three-point landing area for the skull. (Sometimes the chin will also be in contact depending on the facial structure.)

For petromastoid area, have the head already placed in the 45-degree obliquity of the MSP and center the point 1 inch (2.54 cm) anterior to the EAM of the side down on the center line of the table or device. Do this as the patient's head meets the table.

For orbits, when already in a 45-degree obliquity of the MSP, center the orbit to the center line of the table or device.

For mastoid tips, adjust the obliquity so that the mastoid tip is the most lateral aspect of the obliqued skull. (Assess this by using a straight edge or ruler on end resting on the table's surface. Bring it toward the skull at the level of the mastoid; if the obliquity is correct, the edge of the ruler will contact the mastoid tip first. If it contacts the zygomatic arch, there has been too much obliquity, or if contact occurs at the occipital bone, there is not enough obliquity.)

The IOML is parallel to the top of the table or film (the transverse axis).

Both sides are taken for comparison.

Recheck all baselines before making an exposure.

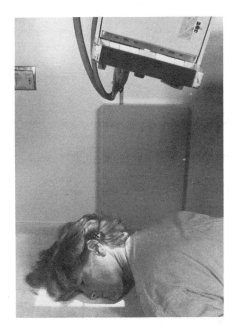

FIGURE 6–62. Semi-axial PA (Stenver's) projection for petromastoid portion or orbit of side down.

STRUCTURES DEMONSTRATED: The petrous portion of the side down.

The petrous portion will lie in a transverse axis, that is, parallel to the top edge of the film (Fig. 6–63).

The internal acoustic canal (IAC) of the side down.

The mastoid tip (process) of the side down (if a lighter technique is used).

The orbit of the side down.

COMMON ERRORS: (1) Improper obliquity. Check for proper rotation by assessing the following (if collimation permits): The mandibular condyle should be projected over the first cervical vertebra; the posterior aspect of the mandibular ramus should be superimposed over the lateral border of the cervical vertebrae; the length of the right and left petrous portions should be equal on the radiographs. (2) Improper CR angulation. The mastoid process should be projected below the cranium.

TECHNIQUE

KV _____ MA _____ SECS _____ MAS _____ CALIPER _____ cm

_____ :1 GRID / B / none SCREEN: RE / High / Par / Detail / None

SID: _____ Rm _____ ADULT / CHILD age: _____ mos. / yrs.

HABITUS: Hyper / s / hypo / a   XS   S   M   L   XL   XXL

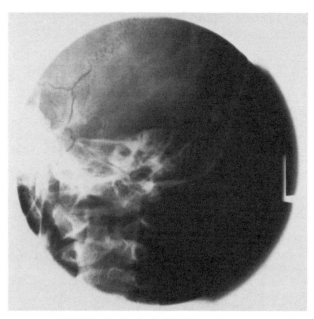

FIGURE 6–63. Semi-axial PA (Stenver's) x-ray.

PETROMASTOIDS: SEMI-AXIAL AP (ARCELIN)—
REVERSE STENVER'S

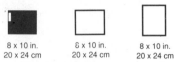

8 x 10 in.   8 x 10 in.   8 x 10 in.
20 x 24 cm   20 x 24 cm   20 x 24 cm

FILM: Table Bucky. Use a stationary grid for portable or gurney patients.

CR: A 10- to 12-degree caudal angle. Enter the orbit of the side up to demonstrate the orbit (Fig. 6–64) or enter the point 1 inch (2.54 cm) anterior to the EAM of the side up to demonstrate the petrous area. Collimate or cone closely to the petromastoid portion.

NOTE: The Arcelin method demonstrates the same structures as the Stenver's method. The object-film distance increases 2 cm, which results in negligible magnification.[43]

POSITION: Remove hearing aids, eyeglasses, hairpins, earrings, necklaces, and clothing around neck. Ask the patient to remove dentures or dental bridges.

The patient is supinated and recumbent on the x-ray table or upright at a Bucky or grid device.

Rotate the head's MSP 45 degrees. The side up is demonstrated (Fig. 6–64).

Center the point 1 inch (2.54 cm) anterior to the EAM of the side up to the center line of the table or device.

The IOML is parallel to the top of the table or film (the transverse axis).

Both sides are taken for comparison.

Recheck all baselines before making an exposure.

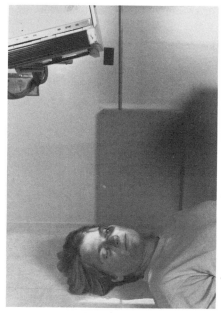

FIGURE 6–64. Semi-axial AP Arcelin's (reverse Stenver's) projection for orbit side up.

STRUCTURES DEMONSTRATED: The petrous portion of the side up.

The petrous portion will lie in a transverse axis (parallel) to the film (Fig. 6–65).

The IAC of the side up.

The mastoid tip (process) of the side up.

The orbit of the side up.

COMMON ERRORS: (1) Improper obliquity. Check for proper rotation by assessing the following (if collimation permits): The mandibular condyle should be projected over the first cervical vertebra; the posterior aspect of the mandibular ramus should be superimposed over the lateral border of the cervical verte-brae; the length of the right and left petrous portions should be equal on the radiographs. (2) Improper CR angulation. The mastoid process should be projected below the cranium.

TECHNIQUE

KV _____ MA _____ SECS _____ MAS _____ CALIPER _____ cm

_____ :1 GRID / B / none SCREEN: RE / High / Par / Detail / None

SID: _____ Rm _____ ADULT / CHILD age: _____ mos. / yrs.

HABITUS: Hyper / s / hypo / a   XS   S   M   L   XL   XXL

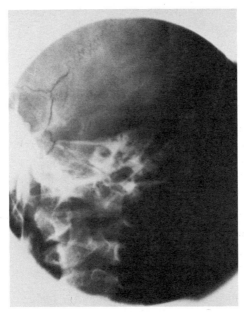

FIGURE 6–65. Semi-axial AP Arcelin's x-ray.

PETROMASTOIDS: SEMI-AXIAL AP OBLIQUE
(MAYER; OWEN)

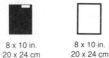

8 x 10 in.   8 x 10 in.
20 x 24 cm   20 x 24 cm

FILM: Table Bucky. Collimate closely or cone to the area of interest.

CR: A 45-degree caudal angle exiting through the EAM side down. The CR light will strike the table 2 to 3 inches (5 to 8 cm) lower than the level of the EAM of the side down due to the elevation of the EAM from the tabletop when using **45-degree obliquity**.

The CR should bisect the point 1 inch (2.54 cm) anterior to the EAM of the side down to the center line of the table or device when using a **30-degree obliquity** from the table.

POSITION: Remove hearing aids, eyeglasses, hairpins, earrings, necklaces, and clothing around neck. Ask the patient to remove dentures or dental bridges.

The patient is supinated and recumbent on the x-ray table or upright at a Bucky or grid device.

Rotate the head's MSP 45 degrees for the Mayer method[48] and 30 degrees for the Owen method[49] (Fig. 6–66). The side down is demonstrated.

The IOML is parallel to the transverse axis of the top of the table or film.

The auricles of the ears may be taped forward.

Both sides are taken for comparison.

Recheck all baselines before making an exposure.

STRUCTURES DEMONSTRATED: The tympanic cavity, acoustic ossicles, attic, auditus, antrum, and the EAM of the side down (Fig. 6–67).

COMMON ERRORS: (1) Off centered. Center the EAM of the side down to the center line. (2) Incorrect obliquity. Use a 54-degree obliquity of the MSP for a brachycephalic skull. Use a 45-degree obliquity of the MSP for a mesocephalic skull. Use a 40-degree obliquity of the MSP for a dolichocephalic skull (see Fig. 6–66).[44] The TMJ should be seen anterior to the EAM.[45]

TECHNIQUE

KV _____ MA _____ SECS _____ MAS _____ CALIPER _____ cm

_____ :1 GRID / B / none SCREEN: RE / High / Par / Detail / None

SID: _____ Rm _____ ADULT / CHILD age: _____ mos. / yrs.

HABITUS: Hyper / s / hypo / a   XS   S   M   L   XL   XXL

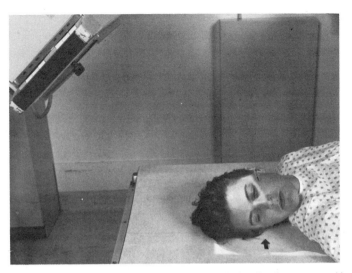

FIGURE 6–66. Semi-axial AP oblique (Owen's) projection for the petromastoid region.

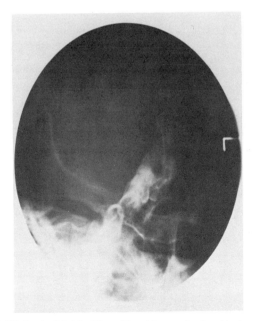

FIGURE 6–67. Semi-axial AP oblique (Owen's) x-ray for the side down. Use 30-degree obliquity of MSP from the table

MASTOIDS: AXIOLATERALS (LAW'S)[46] OR LATERAL TRANSCRANIAL (LAW'S)[47]

| 8 x 10 in. | 8 x 10 in. | 8 x 10 in. |
| 20 x 24 cm | 20 x 24 cm | 20 x 24 cm |

FILM: Table Bucky. Collimate to the area of interest or use a cone.

CR: A 15-degree caudal angle entering 2 inches (1 in. = 2.54 cm) posterior and 2 inches superior to the EAM of the side up.[50] Exit the EAM of the side down.

POSITION: The patient is semipronated upon the table or upright with the use of a Bucky or grid.

Remove hearing aids, eyeglasses, hairpins, earrings, necklaces, and clothing around neck. Ask the patient to remove dentures or dental bridges.

From the lateral position of the skull, rotate the skull 15 degrees toward the table or grid device (Fig. 6–68).

The IOML is parallel to the top of the film (transverse axis).

The IP remains perpendicular to the tabletop.

Both sides are taken for comparison.

Recheck all baselines before making an exposure.

NOTES:

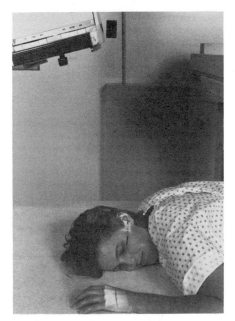

FIGURE 6–68. Axiolateral (Law's) position for the mastoid.

NOTES:

STRUCTURES DEMONSTRATED: The mastoid air cells of the side down (Fig. 6–69).

With an increased technique, this projection is also used for bilateral, open, and closed mouth studies of the TMJs (Fig. 6–70). Side down side seen.

COMMON ERROR: The incorrect rotation or obliquity. Use a 24-degree obliquity of the MSP for a brachycephalic skull. Use a 15-degree obliquity of the MSP for a mesocephalic skull. Use a 10-degree obliquity of the MSP for a dolichocephalic skull.[51]

TECHNIQUE

KV _____ MA _____ SECS _____ MAS _____ CALIPER _____ cm

_____ :1 GRID / B / none SCREEN: RE / High / Par / Detail / None

SID: _____ Rm _____ ADULT / CHILD age: _____ mos. / yrs.

HABITUS: Hyper / s / hypo / a   XS   S   M   L   XL   XXL

NOTES:

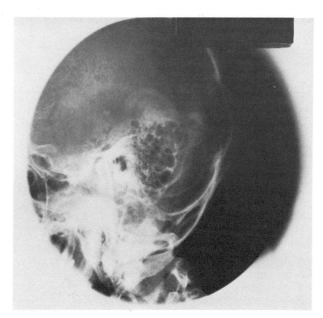

FIGURE 6–69. Axiolateral (Law's) x-ray for the mastoid of the side down.

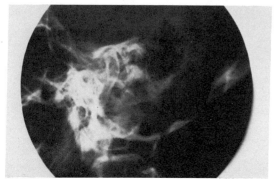

FIGURE 6–70. Axiolateral (Law's) x-ray for the closed TMJ of the side down. Use increased technique over that of mastoid area.

Abdomen and Contrast Studies

ABDOMEN: AP (KUB)

14 x 17 in.
35 x 43 cm

14 x 17 in.
35 x 43 cm

FILM: Collimate to or slightly less than the size of the film depending upon the patient's size. Table Bucky.

CR: Perpendicular to the midpoint of the film when the bottom of the film is at the level of the symphysis pubis.

POSITION: The patient is supinated (Fig. 7–1).

Center the patient's midsagittal plane (MSP) to the center of the table or grid cassette.

Place a sponge under the knees to take the pressure off of the patient's lower back.

Have the patient place the hands upon the chest with elbows resting at the side or the arms down by the side, away from the body if for an acute abdominal series.

Make sure the pelvis is flat and the patient is not favoring one side or the other. Use gonadal shielding for male patients.

Make the exposure at the end of full expiration for a survey film or have the patient stop breathing (or inhale a small breath) in order to include the diaphragm on the film.

NOTE: The PA projection for a scout film is utilized when kidneys are of less importance. The PA projection will also reduce the radiation dose to the gonads (as compared with the AP projection).

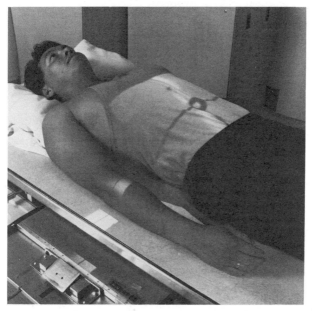

FIGURE 7–1. AP projection of the abdomen (KUB).

STRUCTURES DEMONSTRATED: The kidneys, ureters, and bladder (KUB) areas are seen in their entirety (Fig. 7–2). For an acute abdominal series, sometimes the bottom of the film is placed at the level of the ASIS in order to include the diaphragms.

The ilia will be bisymmetrical while seen in an obliqued position.

The soft tissue of the lateral abdominal walls and properitoneal fat layers should be visualized.

The psoas muscles are demonstrated.

The inferior border of the liver is seen on the right side of the patient.

The vertebral column is seen centered on the film.

Gastrointestinal patterns are demonstrated, as are intra-abdominal calcifications and abdominal masses, if present.

COMMON ERRORS: (1) The symphysis pubis is not included due to the divergence of the x-ray beam or centering too high. Use the "T" method to find the end of the femoral neck, or palpate the greater trochanter to find the level of the symphysis pubis in order to include it on the film. (See Chapter 1 on body landmarks for further instruction on these methods.) (2) There is intestinal motion on the film. For other than an acute abdominal series, make sure you hesitate a second or two to make the exposure after instructing the patient to exhale completely. This allows the contents of the intestinal tract to come to a rest before making the exposure. (3) Overpenetration. The film must have an adequate technique in order to visualize soft tissue as well as bony structures.

TECHNIQUE

KV _____ MA _____ SECS _____ MAS _____ CALIPER _____ cm
_____ :1 GRID / B / none SCREEN: RE / High / Par / Detail / None
SID: _____ Rm _____ ADULT / CHILD age: _____ mos. / yrs.
HABITUS: Hyper / s / hypo / a XS S M L XL XXL

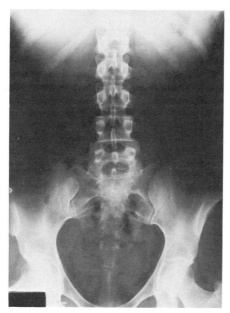

FIGURE 7–2. KUB x-ray.

NOTES:

ACUTE ABDOMINAL SERIES: PA CHEST

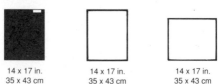

| 14 x 17 in. | 14 x 17 in. | 14 x 17 in. |
| 35 x 43 cm | 35 x 43 cm | 35 x 43 cm |

FILM: Collimate to or slightly less than the size of the film, depending upon the patient's size.

CR: Perpendicular at the MSP at the level of T-6. (Use T2-3 at the level of the suprasternal or jugular notch to locate T-6.)

Collimate to the size of the film or smaller.

POSITION: Patient should be upright (orthostatic). The patient may be seated if necessary.

A chest stand or chest film holder usually without a grid (72 inches or 183 cm SID*) or with an air gap† (120 inches or 305 cm SID) is used.

The anterior chest is touching the film or film holder.

Weight should be evenly balanced on each foot.

Place the patient's chin upon the chin rest.

Have the patient bend the arms to place the hands on hips.

Roll the shoulders forward and slightly downward to remove the scapulae from superimposing the lung fields (Fig. 7–3). The shoulders should be level.

Make sure that the shoulders are touching the film. If the patient cannot touch the film with the shoulders, turn the hands internally so that the dorsal surfaces of the hands lie against the hips. Position each shoulder as close as possible and at the same distance from the film.

The top of the film should be placed 2 inches (5 cm) higher than the shoulders. An exception to this is the hypersthenic patient, who requires that the top of the crosswise film be placed *at* the upper level of the shoulders (the soft tissue mass of the upper torso is greater and therefore uses the 2 inches of distance routinely allowed).

Check the inferior, lateral rib margins with the borders of the film by placing your hands on the patient's sides. Now, extend your fingers, so that the tips touch the film or film holder (see Fig. 1–10). You can ensure that the lateral lung fields are included on

---

*Source-to-image distance. For most radiography procedures, this distance is usually 40 inches or approximately 100 cm. Chest radiography is usually taken at 72 inches or 183 (rounded to 200) cm SID.

†Air gap is usually performed with a 10-inch or 15-cm space between the patient and in front of the film in order to allow the dissipation of scattered x-rays. This serves much as a grid functions but without the disadvantages of a grid, namely, grid lines on the finished radiograph.

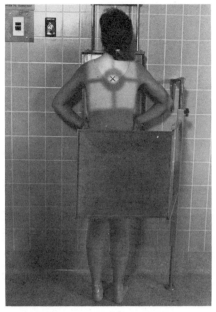

FIGURE 7–3. PA projection of the chest.

the film by assessing your fingertip position relative to the film borders (see Fig. 1–10). Allow a sufficient border of ½ to 1 inch (1.25 to 2.54 cm) of film space on each side of your fingertips in order to allow for rib expansion upon full inspiration of the patient.

Have the patient take a deep breath without straining and make the exposure.

STRUCTURES DEMONSTRATED: The cardiac shadow with both lung fields and diaphragm in their entirety (Fig. 7–4).

The lungs should be aerated up to the ninth or tenth rib.

Both right and left hemidiaphragms in their entirety in order to demonstrate free air in the peritoneum entrapped under the diaphragm. Because the amount of free air is frequently small (1 to 3 cc), the PA chest technique will best demonstrate this free air by its usual underpenetration of the upper abdomen. Frequently, the abdomen film technique will overpenetrate and thus obscure this small amount of free air.

The sternal or proximal aspects of the clavicles should be equidistant from the thoracic spine. The unequal distances of the proximal clavicles from the MSP indicate patient rotation.

NOTE: The source-to-image distance (SID) for chest radiographs usually is 72 inches (183 cm) or 10 feet (305 cm) for air-gap techniques. This increased SID over other exams (usually 40 inches or 102 cm SID) decreases magnification of the cardiac shadow and results in a more accurate measurement of the cardiac shadow.

COMMON ERRORS: (1) Insufficient aeration of the lungs. (2) Technique either too light or too dark. A commonly used technique assessment is to be able to barely see the thoracic spine through the cardiac shadow. Use a high kVp, low mAs technique. (3) Not including all of the diaphragm.

TECHNIQUE

KV _____ MA _____ SECS _____ MAS _____ CALIPER _____ cm

_____ :1 GRID / B / none SCREEN: RE / High / Par / Detail / None

SID: _____ Rm _____ ADULT / CHILD age: _____ mos. / yrs.

HABITUS: Hyper / s / hypo / a XS S M L XL XXL

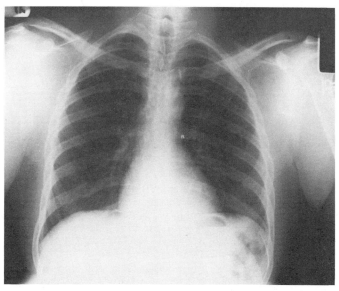

FIGURE 7–4. PA chest x-ray to specifically include the area under the diaphragm.

ACUTE ABDOMINAL SERIES: AP UPRIGHT

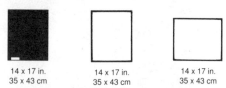

14 x 17 in.
35 x 43 cm

14 x 17 in.
35 x 43 cm

14 x 17 in.
35 x 43 cm

FILM: Collimate to or slightly less than the size of the film depending upon the patient's size. Table Bucky.

CR: Perpendicular, while using a horizontal CR, to the midpoint of the film. (1) When including the diaphragm, place the top of the film at the level of the inferior angle of the patient's scapula (Fig. 7–5). *Or,* (2) when centering for a KUB, place the bottom of the film at the level of the symphysis pubis.

Position the patient sitting up or, if not able to be seated, in the semi-erect recumbent position for 5 to 10 minutes in order to allow migration of free air and redistribution of air-fluid levels.

POSITION: Secure the footboard on the table and test before using. Make sure the locks are engaged correctly. Lock the Bucky tray so it does not migrate when the table is moved toward the upright position. The patient's hands should not be placed near the Bucky tray track during table movement. If moving the table from the supine position, stop halfway to assess the patient. Have the patient move the feet slightly forward for better balance at vertical.

The patient is upright and in the anatomical position. Patients who are acutely ill must be monitored continuously, and they must not remain in the upright position. *If a semi-erect position is used, the central ray must remain horizontal to depict air-fluid levels.*[52] If the patient cannot stand, use the lateral decubitus position (see next position).

Center the patient's MSP to the center of the table or grid cassette.

Make sure the pelvis is level and the patient is not favoring one side or the other.

Make the exposure having the patient simply stop breathing or take in a slight breath when including the diaphragm. Make the exposure at the end of full expiration if positioning for a KUB.

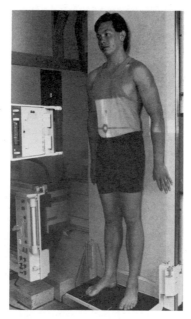

FIGURE 7–5. Upright AP projection of the abdomen to include the diaphragm.

STRUCTURES DEMONSTRATED: (1) The diaphragm in its entirety. Free air within the peritoneum will be collected under the diaphragm (Fig. 7–6). *Or* (2) the kidneys, ureters, and bladder areas are seen in their entirety with the symphysis pubis included on the film when the diaphragm is not of importance.

Air-fluid levels of the abdominal contents.

The soft tissue of the lateral abdominal walls and properitoneal fat layers should be visualized.

The psoas muscles are demonstrated.

The inferior border of the liver is seen on the right.

The vertebral column is centered on the film.

COMMON ERRORS: (1) The diaphragm is not included in its entirety. (2) Underpenetration. An increase in technique is needed because of the increased density of the abdominal contents due to gravity. Your technique will need to be increased proportionately as the patient's abdominal size and mobility increase. (3) There is intestinal motion on the film. Make sure you hesitate a second or two to make the exposure after giving the patient respiratory instructions. This allows the contents of the intestinal tract to come to rest before making the exposure. (4) On the KUB film, the symphysis pubis is not included due to the divergence of the x-ray beam or centering too high. Center 2 inches (5 cm) above the iliac crest at midline or use the "T" method to find the end of the femoral neck, or palpate the greater trochanter to find the level of the symphysis pubis in order to include it on the film. (See Chapter 1 on body landmarks for further instruction on these methods.)

TECHNIQUE

KV _____ MA _____ SECS _____ MAS _____ CALIPER _____ cm

_____ :1 GRID / B / none SCREEN: RE / High / Par / Detail / None

SID: _____ Rm _____ ADULT / CHILD age: _____ mos. / yrs.

HABITUS: Hyper / s / hypo / a   XS   S   M   L   XL   XXL

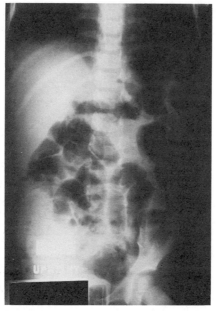

FIGURE 7–6. Abdomen x-ray to include the diaphragm.

ACUTE ABDOMINAL SERIES: LEFT LATERAL DECUBITUS

14 x 17 in.
35 x 43 cm

14 x 17 in.
35 x 43 cm

FILM: Collimate to or slightly less than the size of the film, depending upon the patient's size. Use a grid. A table Bucky may be used when the patient is placed upon a gurney in front of the upright table.

CR: With a horizontal beam, perpendicular to the midpoint of the film. To include the diaphragm, place the top of the film (and grid) at the level of the inferior angle of the patient's scapula.

Position the patient on the side for 5 to 10 minutes before making an exposure in order to allow migration of free air and redistribution of air-fluid levels.

POSITION: When moving the patient from the supine, have the patient lie on the left side with the film and grid against the abdomen for a PA projection (Fig. 7–7). If the patient has a large abdomen, when you are transferring him or her from wheelchair, bed, or gurney to the x-ray table, place the head at the right side of the x-ray table. Now have the patient turn on the left side for an AP projection. Both methods produce a left lateral decubitus position (Fig. 7–8).

NOTE: If the patient has multiple trauma or is postoperative on the left side, an opposite lateral decubitus or alternate decubitus position may be used.

Position the patient's arms over the head, with both knees equal and slightly flexed for balance.

The film and grid should be as close to the body as possible without tilting.

To include the diaphragm on the film, the top of the film and grid should be at the level of the scapula's inferior angle. Make sure the film's ID blocker is down so as to not obscure the area of interest.

If the entire diaphragm is desired on the film, take the right lateral decubitus position as well, or if possible, use a radiolucent pad underneath the patient's thorax for the left lateral decubitus position.

Mark at the waist with a *right* marker and a marker indicating the direction up (an arrow, "up," etc.). Avoid confusion by not using the title of the position (left lateral decubitus) on the film unless you place it on the patient's left side so that it is also anatomically correct.

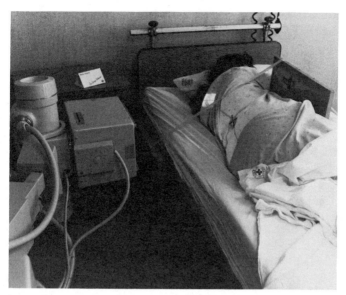

FIGURE 7–7. Left lateral decubitus position (PA projection) with horizontal beam.

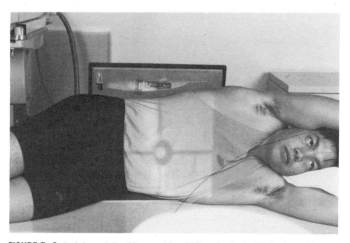

FIGURE 7–8. Left lateral decubitus position (AP projection) with horizontal beam.

STRUCTURES DEMONSTRATED: The left hemidiaphragm in its entirety and part of the right hemidiaphragm. Free air within the peritoneum will most commonly be collected at this site.

Air-fluid levels of the abdominal contents down to the ASIS (Fig. 7–9).

The soft tissue of the lateral abdominal walls and properitoneal fat layers should be visualized.

The vertebrae are barely penetrated.

COMMON ERRORS: (1) Overpenetration. Bony anatomy is less important when looking for free air in the abdominal cavity or for air-fluid levels. (2) There is intestinal motion on the film. Make sure you hesitate a second or two to make the exposure after giving the patient respiratory instructions. This allows the contents of the intestinal tract to come to rest before making the exposure.

TECHNIQUE

KV _____ MA _____ SECS _____ MAS _____ CALIPER _____ cm

_____ :1 GRID / B / none SCREEN: RE / High / Par / Detail / None

SID: _____ Rm _____ ADULT / CHILD age: _____ mos. / yrs.

HABITUS: Hyper / s / hypo / a   XS   S   M   L   XL   XXL

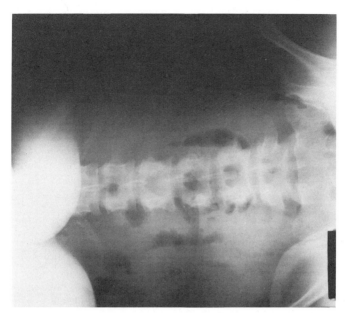

FIGURE 7–9. Left lateral decubitus x-ray for air-fluid levels. Slightly overpenetrated for upper soft tissue area of thorax.

IVP: AP or PA SCOUT (EXCRETORY UROGRAM)

14 x 17 in.   14 x 17 in.
35 x 43 cm   35 x 43 cm

FILM: Collimate to or slightly less than the size of the film depending upon the patient's size. Table Bucky.

CR: Perpendicular at MSP at level of or 1 inch (2.54 cm) above iliac crest.

POSITION: The patient is supinated for the AP (Fig. 7–10).

Place a sponge under the knees to take the pressure off of the lower back of the patient.

Have the patient place the hands upon the chest with elbows resting at the side or down by side but away from the body.

The patient is pronated for the PA (Fig. 7–11).

Center the patient's MSP to the center of the table or grid cassette.

Make sure the pelvis is flat and the patient is not favoring one side or the other. Use gonadal shielding for male patients.

Make the exposure at the end of full expiration.

NOTES:

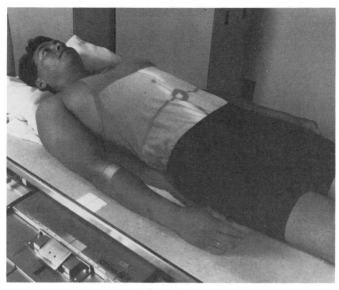

FIGURE 7–10. AP projection of the abdomen.

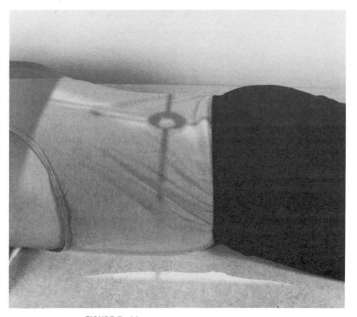

FIGURE 7–11. PA projection of the abdomen.

STRUCTURES DEMONSTRATED: The assessment of the effectiveness of the patient prep.

Survey film of the abdomen and abdominal contents in the AP projection (Fig. 7–12) and PA projection (Fig. 7–13).
COMMON ERROR: Clipping the upper poles of the kidneys off of the film.

TECHNIQUE

KV _____ MA _____ SECS _____ MAS _____ CALIPER _____ cm

_____ :1 GRID / B / none SCREEN: RE / High / Par / Detail / None

SID: _____ Rm _____ ADULT / CHILD age: _____ mos. / yrs.

HABITUS: Hyper / s / hypo / a   XS   S   M   L   XL   XXL

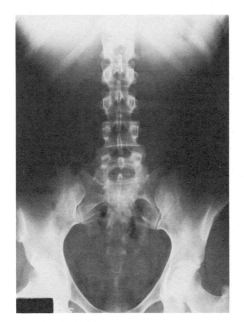

FIGURE 7–12. AP abdomen scout x-ray.

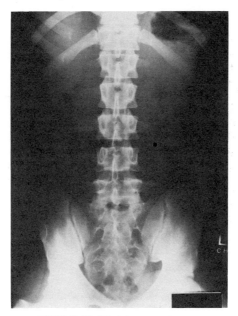

FIGURE 7–13. PA abdomen scout x-ray.

413

IVP: AP 1, 2, 3, 4, 5, 6, OR 7 MINUTES
(EXCRETORY UROGRAM)

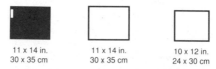

| 11 x 14 in. | 11 x 14 in. | 10 x 12 in. |
| 30 x 35 cm | 30 x 35 cm | 24 x 30 cm |

FILM: Collimate to or slightly less than the size of the film depending upon the patient's size. Table Bucky.

CR: Perpendicular at MSP at level of or 1 inch (2.54 cm) above iliac crest for 14 × 17 inch (35 × 43 cm) lengthwise film. For 11 × 14 inches (28 × 43 cm) crosswise, center at MSP at end of ribs (or place the bottom of the film at the level of the iliac crest and then center to the center of the film). *Use the scout to make sure that the upper poles of the kidneys are included using these methods of centering.*

POSITION: The patient is supinated.

Center the patient's MSP to the center of the table or grid cassette.

Place a sponge under the knees to take the pressure off of the lower back of the patient.

Have the patient place the hands upon the chest with elbows resting at his or her side (Fig. 7–14).

Make sure the pelvis is flat and the patient is not favoring one side or the other. Use gonadal shielding.

Make the exposure at the end of full expiration.

STRUCTURES DEMONSTRATED: The 1-, 2-, and 3-minute films (nephrograms) represent a study of hypertensive kidney function.

The time sequencing will profile the contrast in the collecting tubules, the renal parenchyma, and later, with the use of a large film, the ureters and urinary bladder (Fig. 7–15).

COMMON ERROR: Clipping the upper poles of the kidneys off of the film if using a 14 × 17 inch (35 × 43 cm) film lengthwise with the bottom of the film placed at the level of the symphysis pubis. Long-waisted patients need to have the film placement elevated slightly to include the upper poles.

TECHNIQUE

KV _____ MA _____ SECS _____ MAS _____ CALIPER _____ cm
_____ :1 GRID / B / none SCREEN: RE / High / Par / Detail / None
SID: _____ Rm _____ ADULT / CHILD age: _____ mos. / yrs.
HABITUS: Hyper / s / hypo / a   XS   S   M   L   XL   XXL

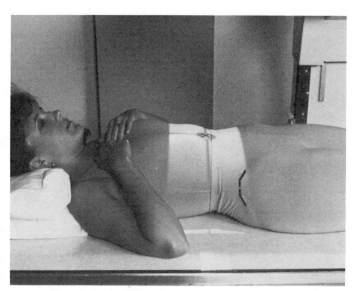

FIGURE 7–14. Position for the IVP (excretory urogram) 1-minute film of the kidney region.

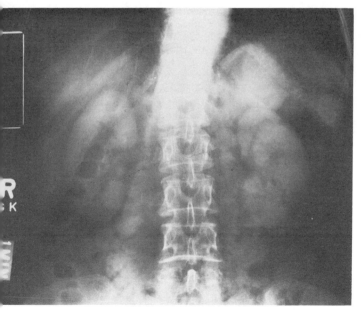

FIGURE 7–15. One minute x-ray of the kidneys (hypertensive study).

IVP: AP OR PA OBLIQUES (EXCRETORY UROGRAM)

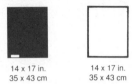

14 x 17 in.   14 x 17 in.
35 x 43 cm   35 x 43 cm

FILM: Collimate to or slightly less than the size of the film, depending upon the patient's size. Table Bucky.

CR: Perpendicularly to the midpoint of the film, when the bottom of the film is placed at the level of the greater trochanter or symphysis pubis (see Fig. 1–17). *Use the scout to make sure the upper poles of the kidneys are included with this method of centering.*

POSITION: The patient should be semisupinated for the AP oblique projections (either the RPO [Fig. 7–16] or the LPO position).

The patient should be semipronated for the PA oblique projections (RAO/LAO positions). Flex the knee of the side up for stability.

Use a 30-degree obliquity of the patient with the entire body obliqued as a unit.

For AP obliques, center the imaginary *surface*—the coronal plane that intersects the ASIS—to the center of the table. If the patient is hypersthenic or has a large abdomen, measure the width of the obliqued abdominal area right costal margin to left relative to its position on the table; find the center of this distance. Now center this point to the center of the x-ray table.

For PA obliques (RAO and LAO positions) palpate the lumbar spinous processes in order to center 2 inches (5 cm) anterior from the spinous processes, that is, the midline of the obliqued lumbar spine, to the center of the x-ray table. If the patient is hypersthenic or has a large abdomen, measure the width of the obliqued abdominal area left to right; find the center of this distance. Now center this point to the center of the x-ray table.

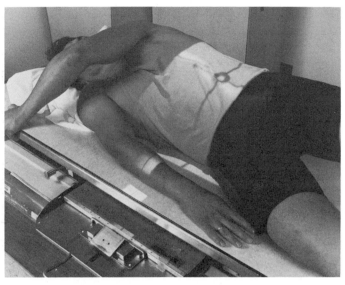

FIGURE 7–16. IVP (excretory urogram) RPO position.

STRUCTURES DEMONSTRATED: For AP obliques, the kidney closer to the film will be projected through its transverse medial to lateral aspect (Fig. 7–17). The kidney farther from the film will be seen in its full, anterior profile.

For PA obliques, the kidney closer to the film will be seen in its full, anterior profile. The kidney farther from the film will be projected on its lateral to medial transverse axis.

The ureters in their entirety.

The partially filled urinary bladder.

COMMON ERROR: Clipping the upper poles of the kidneys. See comment under CR above.

TECHNIQUE

KV _____ MA _____ SECS _____ MAS _____ CALIPER _____ cm
_____ :1 GRID / B / none SCREEN: RE / High / Par / Detail / None
SID: _____ Rm _____ ADULT / CHILD age: _____ mos. / yrs.
HABITUS: Hyper / s / hypo / a   XS   S   M   L   XL   XXL

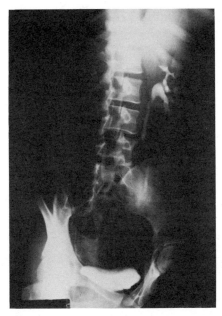

FIGURE 7–17. LPO x-ray for an IVP (excretory urogram).

IVP: AP UPRIGHT (EXCRETORY UROGRAM)

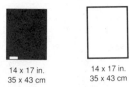

14 x 17 in.
35 x 43 cm

14 x 17 in.
35 x 43 cm

FILM: For a closely collimated projection of the bladder pre-void and/or post-void.

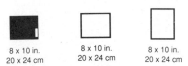

8 x 10 in.
20 x 24 cm

8 x 10 in.
20 x 24 cm

8 x 10 in.
20 x 24 cm

CR: Perpendicularly to the midpoint of the 14 × 17 inch (35 × 43 cm) film, when the bottom of the film is placed at the level of the greater trochanter or symphysis pubis (Fig. 7–18). *Use the scout to make sure the upper poles of the kidneys are included with this method of centering.*

For the smaller, 8 × 10 inch (20 × 24 cm) film, place the top of the film to include the ASIS and center to the MSP (Fig. 7–19).
POSITION: The patient is supinated.

Center the patient's MSP to the center of the table or grid cassette.

Have the patient place the arms at his or her side. Do not have the patient grasp the sides of the table as the movement of the Bucky tray may cause injury.

Make sure the pelvis is flat.

Make the exposure at the end of full expiration.

NOTE: Mark the bladder films accordingly when making a post-void film.

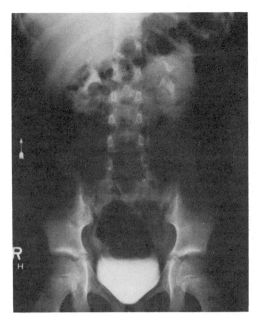

FIGURE 7–18. Upright abdomen for an IVP (excretory urogram).

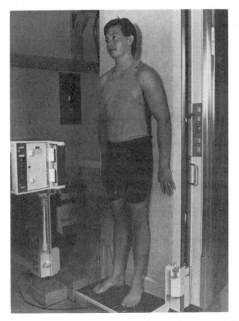

FIGURE 7–19. Upright bladder spot (pre-void or post-void).

STRUCTURES DEMONSTRATED: The upright abdomen to demonstrate any excursion of the kidneys and ureters.

The filled urinary bladder when pre-void. The partially emptied urinary bladder for the post-void (Fig. 7–20).

Post-void films will evaluate bladder retention or prolapse.

COMMON ERROR: Centering the film too low and clipping the kidneys off of the larger film.

TECHNIQUE

KV _____ MA _____ SECS _____ MAS _____ CALIPER _____ cm

_____ :1 GRID / B / none SCREEN: RE / High / Par / Detail / None

SID: _____ Rm _____ ADULT / CHILD age: _____ mos. / yrs.

HABITUS: Hyper / s / hypo / a XS S M L XL XXL

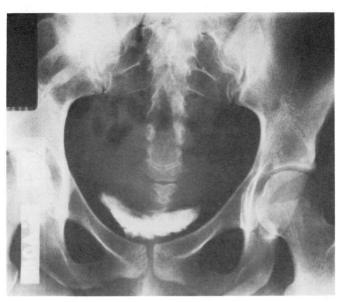

FIGURE 7–20. Upright, post-void bladder x-ray.

GALLBLADDER: AP or PA

| 14 x 17 in. | 14 x 17 in. | 10 x 12 in. | 10 x 12 in. | 8 x 10 in. |
| 35 x 43 cm | 35 x 43 cm | 24 x 30 cm | 24 x 30 cm | 20 x 24 cm |

FILM: Collimate to or slightly less than the size of the film depending upon the patient's size. Table Bucky.

CR: Perpendicular to the midpoint of the film when the bottom of the film is at the level of the symphysis pubis (Fig. 7–1) or center slightly above the level of the iliac crest (Fig. 7–21).

POSITION: The patient is supinated for the AP and pronated for the PA.

Center the patient's MSP to the center of the table or grid cassette.

For the AP, have the patient place the hands down by the side away from the body.

Center the MSP to the center of the film for the KUB area. Center the right side of the patient to the center of the table for the smaller, localized area (Fig. 7–21).

Make sure the pelvis is flat and the patient is not favoring one side or the other.

Make the exposure at the end of full expiration or just have the patient suspend respiration.

NOTE: Upright studies may be performed in the AP or PA projection. A smaller film, a spot film (usually an 8 × 10 in. or 20 × 24 cm film) is often used to increase detail. In addition, fluoroscopy is utilized for upright, well-collimated studies of the gallbladder (Fig. 7–22).

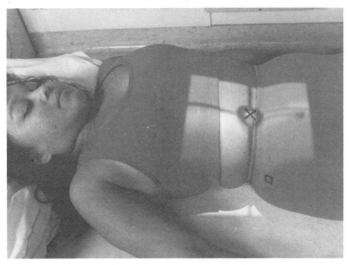

FIGURE 7–21. AP scout projection of the gallbladder. Iliac crest *(square)*.

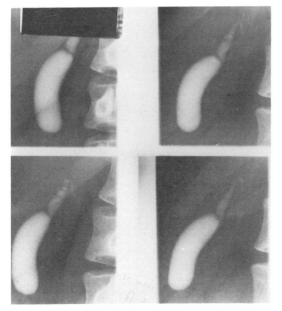

FIGURE 7–22. Upright, fluoroscopy gallbladder x-rays (i.e., spot films).

STRUCTURES DEMONSTRATED: Used for the assessment of the effectiveness of the patient prep and successful contrast medium uptake.

If a radiographic spot film is used, a closely collimated film detailing the contrast-filled gallbladder is seen (Fig. 7–23).

If a larger film is used, a survey of the abdomen and abdominal contents is seen, usually from the level of the ASIS on up. The soft tissue of the lateral abdominal walls and properitoneal fat layers should be visualized. The psoas muscles are demonstrated. The inferior border of the liver is seen on the right. The vertebral column is seen centered on the film. The contrast-filled gallbladder if present (Fig. 7–24).

COMMON ERROR: Intestinal motion on film. Have the patient exhale and wait 1 to 2 seconds before making the exposure. This allows the contents of the intestines to come to a rest.

TECHNIQUE

KV _____ MA _____ SECS _____ MAS _____ CALIPER _____ cm

_____ :1 GRID / B / none SCREEN: RE / High / Par / Detail / None

SID: _____ Rm _____ ADULT / CHILD age: _____ mos. / yrs.

HABITUS: Hyper / s / hypo / a XS S M L XL XXL

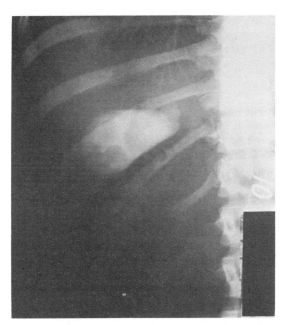

FIGURE 7–23. AP spot x-ray of the gallbladder.

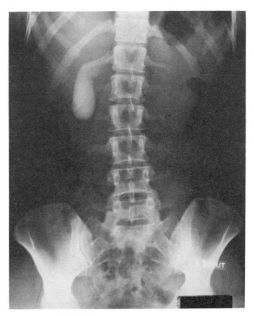

FIGURE 7–24. PA gallbladder scout x-ray.

GALLBLADDER: RPO

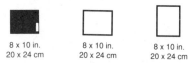

8 x 10 in.
20 x 24 cm

8 x 10 in.
20 x 24 cm

8 x 10 in.
20 x 24 cm

FILM: Collimate to or slightly less than the size of the film depending upon the patient's size. Table Bucky.

CR: Perpendicular at the gallbladder as located on the scout film.

POSITION: The patient is semisupinated with a 15- to 60-degree obliquity suitable to move the gallbladder away from the spine (Fig. 7–25). Check the scout film for this determination. The closer to the spine, the higher degree of obliquity needed.

Center the patient's right side to the center of the table. Place the patient's spine on the back margin (patient's posterior) of the film by comparing your palpation of the spinous processes to the posterior margin of collimation. (Remember that the collimation on the anterior surface of the patient's body is much smaller than that which will result on the film. Read the collimation values directly from the indications on the tube.)

Center the film to the gallbladder position as identified on the scout film.

NOTE: The LAO position may also be used to spot the gallbladder. Center over the posterior right side. The side of interest will be elevated.

STRUCTURES DEMONSTRATED: The gallbladder free from superimposition from the spine or bowel (Fig. 7–26). If the film is

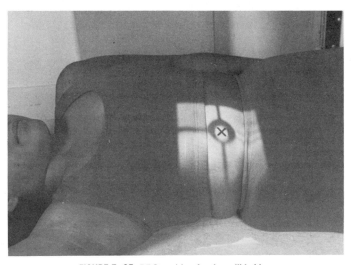

FIGURE 7-25. RPO position for the gallbladder.

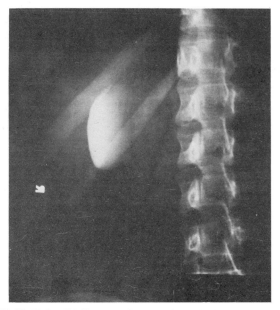

FIGURE 7-26. RPO gallbladder x-ray. Can you estimate the degree of obliquity from the position of the "Scottie dogs"? Answer: Since the transverse processes extend laterally outside of the bodies, the obliquity is less than 45 degrees.

unsuccessful, an upright study may be performed (Fig. 7–27) with the demonstration of fluid or calculi levels (Fig. 7–28). Make sure the film is marked up, upright or erect.

COMMON ERROR: Not enough obliquity to free the gallbladder from superimposition. Remember when increasing obliquity, you must move the patient back on the table in order to recenter over the gallbladder. The increased obliquity moves the gall-bladder away from the center of the table for the RPO.

TECHNIQUE

KV _____ MA _____ SECS _____ MAS _____ CALIPER _____ cm

_____ :1 GRID / B / none SCREEN: RE / High / Par / Detail / None

SID: _____ Rm _____ ADULT / CHILD age: _____ mos. / yrs.

HABITUS: Hyper / s / hypo / a XS S M L XL XXL

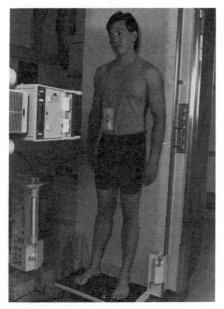

FIGURE 7–27. Upright, AP spot of the gallbladder.

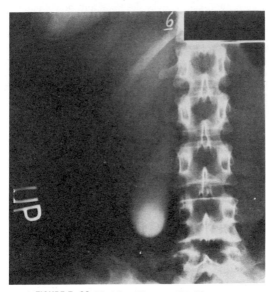

FIGURE 7–28. Upright, AP spot gallbladder x-ray.

GALLBLADDER: RIGHT LATERAL DECUBITUS

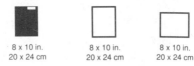

8 x 10 in.   8 x 10 in.   8 x 10 in.
20 x 24 cm   20 x 24 cm   20 x 24 cm

FILM: With a grid cassette. Collimate to or slightly less than the size of the film depending upon the patient's size. A table Bucky may be used when the patient is placed upon a gurney in front of the upright table. Use the length of the film to match the long axis of the gallbladder. Check the scout film.

CR: Using a horizontal beam, perpendicular to the midpoint of the film. Use the scout film to locate the longitudinal level of the gallbladder.

NOTE: Many technologists use a gurney to position the right lateral recumbent patient in front of the upright table. Another method is to use a stationary grid and film with the patient in the right lateral decubitus position (Fig. 7–29).

POSITION: Moving from the supine, have the patient lie on the right side with the film and grid against the gallbladder area for either an AP or PA projection depending if the patient is placed on the table with the head to the right (PA) or to the left (AP) (Fig. 7–29).

If you are using a gurney to take the decubitus projections, make sure all of the wheels are locked!

Have the patient's arms over the head and both knees equal and slightly flexed for balance.

The film and grid (or table Bucky) should be as close to the body as possible without tilting toward the spine.

Make sure the film's ID blocker is placed so that it is out of the way of the gallbladder.

Make the exposure at the end of full expiration or just have the patient suspend respiration.

STRUCTURES DEMONSTRATED: Fluid and calculi levels (if present) of the gallbladder (Fig. 7–30).

The decubitus position may be used in lieu of an upright study.

COMMON ERROR: Overpenetration. Use tight collimation to reduce scattered radiation.

TECHNIQUE

KV _____ MA _____ SECS _____ MAS _____ CALIPER _____ cm

_____ :1 GRID / B / none SCREEN: RE / High / Par / Detail / None

SID: _____ Rm _____ ADULT / CHILD age: _____ mos. / yrs.

HABITUS: Hyper / s / hypo / a   XS   S   M   L   XL   XXL

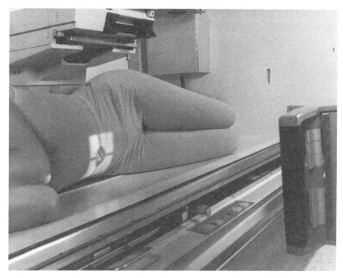

FIGURE 7–29. Right lateral decubitus position (AP projection) with horizontal beam.

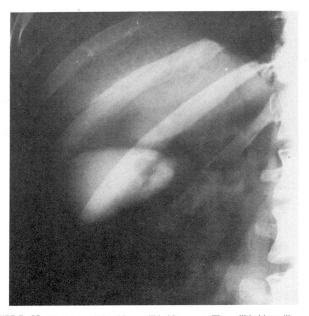

FIGURE 7–30. Right lateral decubitus gallbladder x-ray. The gallbladder will usually lie in the transverse plane due to gravity.

BARIUM SWALLOW: AP or PA ESOPHAGUS

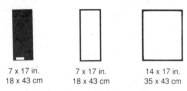

7 x 17 in.
18 x 43 cm

7 x 17 in.
18 x 43 cm

14 x 17 in.
35 x 43 cm

FILM: Collimate to the film or less than the size of the larger film depending upon the patient's size. Table Bucky.

CR: Perpendicular at the MSP at the level of T-6.

POSITION: The patient is supinated for the AP projection (Fig. 7–31).

The patient is pronated for the PA projection.

A cup of barium is provided. The patient is instructed to drink continuously while the exposure is made (Fig. 7–31). When a thick paste is used, the patient will hold the paste in the mouth until instructed to swallow, at which time the exposure is made.

STRUCTURES DEMONSTRATED. The entire barium-filled esophagus (Fig. 7–32). Include the fundus of the stomach for the esophageal–gastric junction.

COMMON ERROR: Underpenetration. Use a relatively higher technique to penetrate the thoracic spine as well as the barium-filled esophagus.

NOTE: Use a relatively high kVp technique when using barium products for x-ray studies.

TECHNIQUE

KV _____ MA _____ SECS _____ MAS _____ CALIPER _____ cm
_____ :1 GRID / B / none SCREEN: RE / High / Par / Detail / None
SID: _____ Rm _____ ADULT / CHILD age: _____ mos. / yrs.
HABITUS: Hyper / s / hypo / a   XS   S   M   L   XL   XXL

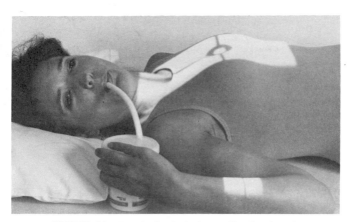

FIGURE 7–31. AP projection for barium swallow (esophagus).

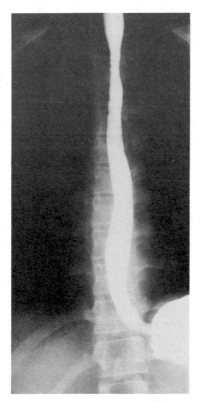

FIGURE 7–32. AP barium swallow (esophagus) x-ray. Although the neck area is not included here, if it is of radiographic importance usually fluoroscopy is utilized to achieve a dynamic assessment of function and structure.

BARIUM SWALLOW: RAO ESOPHAGUS

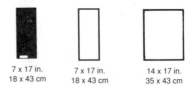

| 7 x 17 in. | 7 x 17 in. | 14 x 17 in. |
| 18 x 43 cm | 18 x 43 cm | 35 x 43 cm |

FILM: Collimate to the film or slightly less than the size of the larger film depending upon the patient's size. Table Bucky.

CR: Perpendicular at a point 4 to 5 inches (10 to 12 cm) anterior to the thoracic spinous processes at the level of T-6.

When using a 7 × 17 inch (18 × 43 cm) film cassette, center the patient so as to place the spinous process just off of the back edge of the film. Use the collimator light to assess this (remember it appears smaller on the elevated side of the patient than that on the film). If the patient is kyphotic, center the spinous process of T-3 and T-10 on the back edge of the film or use a larger film. Center to the longitudinal center of the film at the level of T-6.

POSITION: The recumbent patient is semipronated on the right side.

Place the patient's right arm down by the side, and the left up by the pillow. Flex the patient's left knee.

Oblique the patient about 30 to 40 degrees, or just enough to rotate the esophagus to the patient's left and in front of the thoracic spine (Fig. 7–33). The larger the patient the less the degree of obliquity used.

A cup of barium is provided. The patient is instructed to drink continuously while the exposure is made. When a thick paste is used, the patient will hold the paste in the mouth until instructed to swallow, at which time the exposure is made. Breathing instructions are not necessary.

STRUCTURES DEMONSTRATED: The entire, barium-filled esophagus (Fig. 7–34).

COMMON ERROR: Not enough barium filling the esophagus. A recumbent study or the use of thicker barium or a paste will have a relatively slower passage through the esophagus than an upright study or the use of thinner barium.

NOTE: Use a relatively high kVp technique when using barium products for x-ray studies.

TECHNIQUE

KV _____ MA _____ SECS _____ MAS _____ CALIPER _____ cm

_____ :1 GRID / B / none SCREEN: RE / High / Par / Detail / None

SID: _____ Rm _____ ADULT / CHILD age: _____ mos. / yrs.

HABITUS: Hyper / s / hypo / a   XS   S   M   L   XL   XXL

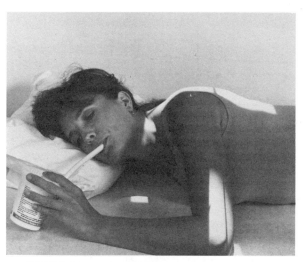

FIGURE 7–33. RAO position for barium swallow (esophagus).

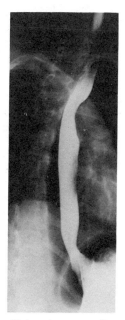

FIGURE 7–34. RAO barium-filled esophagus x-ray. Remember when viewed on the anatomical position, a PA oblique (RAO) will look similar to an AP oblique (LPO). See Chapter 10.

BARIUM SWALLOW: RIGHT LATERAL ESOPHAGUS

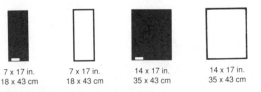

7 x 17 in.   7 x 17 in.   14 x 17 in.   14 x 17 in.
18 x 43 cm   18 x 43 cm   35 x 43 cm   35 x 43 cm

FILM: Collimate to the film or slightly less than the size of the larger film depending upon the patient's size. Table Bucky.

CR: Perpendicular at a point 3 to 4 inches (7 to 10 cm) anterior to the spinous processes at the level of T-6.

When using a 7 × 17 inch (18 × 43 cm) film cassette, center the patient so as to place the T-6 spinous process just off of the back edge of the film. If the patient is kyphotic, center the spinous process of T-3 on the back edge of the film (see Fig. 7–36) or use a larger film. Center to the longitudinal center of the film at the level of T-6.

POSITION: The patient is right lateral recumbent (Fig. 7–35) or upright.

A cup of barium is provided. The patient is instructed to drink continuously while the exposure is made. When a thick paste is used, the patient will hold the paste in the mouth until instructed to swallow, at which time the exposure is made. Breathing instructions are not necessary.

Center the patient in order to place the vertebral column at the back margin (patient's posterior) of the 7 × 17 sized collimation.

STRUCTURES DEMONSTRATED: The entire barium-filled esophagus (Fig. 7–36).

COMMON ERROR: Not enough barium filling the esophagus. A recumbent study or the use of thicker barium or a paste will have a relatively slower passage through the esophagus than an upright study or the use of thinner barium.

NOTE: Use a relatively high kVp technique when using barium products for x-ray studies.

TECHNIQUE

KV _____ MA _____ SECS _____ MAS _____ CALIPER _____ cm

_____ :1 GRID / B / none SCREEN: RE / High / Par / Detail / None

SID: _____ Rm _____ ADULT / CHILD age: _____ mos. / yrs.

HABITUS: Hyper / s / hypo / a   XS   S   M   L   XL   XXL

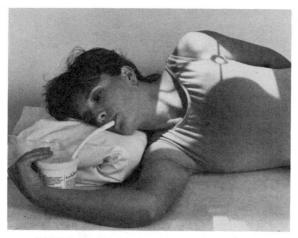

FIGURE 7–35. Right lateral barium swallow (esophagus).

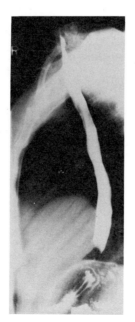

FIGURE 7–36. Right lateral barium-filled esophagus x-ray of a kyphotic patient.

UGI (STOMACH): AP

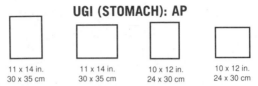

| 11 x 14 in. | 11 x 14 in. | 10 x 12 in. | 10 x 12 in. |
| 30 x 35 cm | 30 x 35 cm | 24 x 30 cm | 24 x 30 cm |

FILM: Collimate to the size of the film. Table Bucky.

CR: Perpendicular at the lesser curvature of the stomach. See recommendations below.

POSITION: The patient is supinated on the x-ray table.

Start by centering the left upper quadrant to the center of the table. Then adjust to body habitus.

(To perform accurate overhead radiographs after fluoroscopy of the stomach, it is advisable to simply observe the fluoroscopy procedure to locate the precise position of the patient's stomach. This is the most accurate method!)

For asthenic patients, place the bottom of the film to include the ASIS. Adjust your collimation to the size of the film. Place the patient's left side at the left-sided margin of collimation. This will maximize the duodenal area on the film. Center to the center of the film. The stomach will lie long and low.

For hypersthenic patients, use the cassette crosswise and just include the diaphragm on the top of the film. Center slightly left of midsagittal. The stomach will lie high and wide (transverse).

On sthenic and hyposthenic patients, always include the area that is 2 inches to the right of midsagittal in order to include the duodenal bulb (Fig. 7–37). Center the film at the level of the most anterior aspect of the *left*-sided seventh and eighth ribs (see Fig. 1–11, which shows how to palpate level on *right* side).

STRUCTURES DEMONSTRATED: The entire, partially barium-filled stomach. The fundus filled with barium (Fig. 7–38).

An air and barium mixture in the pyloric area producing a double-contrast study (air and barium).

An oblique view of the duodenal bulb.

COMMON ERROR: Clipping the stomach off of the film. If you do not have a closed-circuit television to watch the fluoroscopy, observe the location of the fluoroscopy unit when the radiologists takes spots. Better yet, ask the radiologist at the end of fluoroscopy to pinpoint the top of the fundus and the location of the duodenal bulb for you. It beats taking repeats!

NOTE: Use a relatively high kVp technique when using barium products for x-ray studies.

TECHNIQUE

KV _____ MA _____ SECS _____ MAS _____ CALIPER _____ cm

_____ :1 GRID / B / none SCREEN: RE / High / Par / Detail / None

SID: _____ Rm _____ ADULT / CHILD age: _____ mos. / yrs.

HABITUS: Hyper / s / hypo / a   XS   S   M   L   XL   XXL

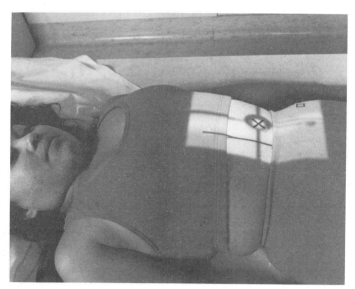

FIGURE 7–37. AP projection of the stomach. Iliac crest *(square)*. Long axis through duodenal bulb *(line)*.

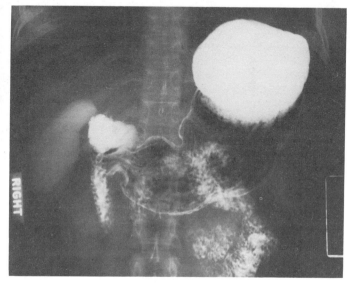

FIGURE 7–38. Barium-filled fundus, AP stomach x-ray of hyperesthenic patient.

UGI (STOMACH): LPO

| 11 x 14 in. | 11 x 14 in. | 10 x 12 in. | 10 x 12 in. |
| 30 x 35 cm | 30 x 35 cm | 24 x 30 cm | 24 x 30 cm |

FILM: Collimate to the size of the film. Table Bucky.

CR: Perpendicularly mid-left-sided at the level of the end of the ribs. Include the ASIS at the bottom of film for asthenic patients. Include the diaphragm at the top of the film for hypersthenic patients. Remember that the weight of the barium in the fundus may cause gravitational elevation in the customary position of the stomach.

POSITION: The patient is semisupinated on the left side (Fig. 7–39). Oblique the patient an average of 45 degrees. Place the patient's left side at the left-sided margin of collimation. This will maximize the duodenal area on the film.

STRUCTURES DEMONSTRATED: The entire, partially barium-filled stomach.

The barium-filled fundus (Fig. 7–40).

The double contrast of the lower body, pylorus, and duodenal bulb.

COMMON ERROR: Clipping the stomach off of the film. If you do not have a closed-circuit television to watch the fluoroscopy, observe the location of the fluoroscopy unit when the radiologists takes spots. Better yet, ask the radiologist at the end of fluoroscopy to pinpoint the top of the fundus and the location of the duodenal bulb for you. It beats taking repeats!

NOTE: Use a relatively high kVp technique when using barium products for x-ray studies.

TECHNIQUE

KV _____ MA _____ SECS _____ MAS _____ CALIPER _____ cm

_____ :1 GRID / B / none SCREEN: RE / High / Par / Detail / None

SID: _____ Rm _____ ADULT / CHILD age: _____ mos. / yrs.

HABITUS: Hyper / s / hypo / a   XS   S   M   L   XL   XXL

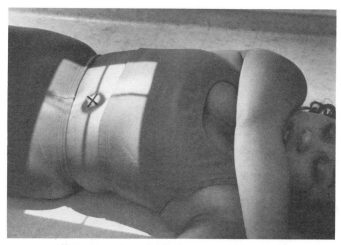

FIGURE 7–39. LPO position for the stomach of sthenic patient.

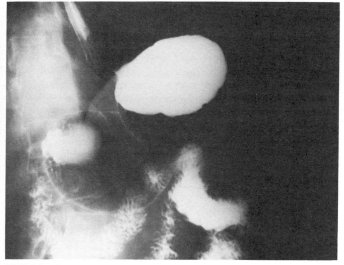

FIGURE 7–40. Barium-filled fundus of LPO stomach x-ray of hyperesthenic patient.

UGI (STOMACH): RAO

| 11 x 14 in. | 11 x 14 in. | 10 x 12 in. | 10 x 12 in. |
| 30 x 35 cm | 30 x 35 cm | 24 x 30 cm | 24 x 30 cm |

FILM: Collimate to the size of the film. Table Bucky.

CR: Centered perpendicularly to the film when the film is centered transversely 4 to 5 inches anterior to the spinous process of the lumbar vertebrae. Longitudinally center the film at the end of the ribs or lower, depending on body habitus (Fig. 7–41). Include the ASIS at the bottom of film for asthenic patients. Include the diaphragm at the top of the film for hypersthenic patients.

POSITION: The patient is semipronated on the right side.

Place the patient's right arm down by the side, and the left up by the pillow. Flex the patient's left knee.

Oblique the patient about 45 degrees. Use a greater obliquity for patients' stomachs that sharply hook or have the duodenal bulb superimposed over the pylorus (obviously you can assess this only for real-time observation during fluoroscopy or for repeat filming purposes).

STRUCTURES DEMONSTRATED: The entire, partially barium-filled stomach.

The body of the stomach is filled with barium.

The duodenal bulb and pylorus filled with barium and free from superimposition (Fig. 7–42).

Air or double contrast in the fundus of the stomach.

COMMON ERROR: Clipping the stomach off of the film. If you do not have a closed-circuit television to watch the fluoroscopy, observe the location of the fluoroscopy unit when the radiologist takes spots. Better yet, ask the radiologist at the end of fluoroscopy to pinpoint the top of the fundus and the location of the duodenal bulb for you. It beats taking repeats!

NOTE: Use a relatively high kVp technique when using barium products for x-ray studies.

TECHNIQUE

KV _____ MA _____ SECS _____ MAS _____ CALIPER _____ cm

_____ :1 GRID / B / none SCREEN: RE / High / Par / Detail / None

SID: _____ Rm _____ ADULT / CHILD age: _____ mos. / yrs.

HABITUS: Hyper / s / hypo / a   XS   S   M   L   XL   XXL

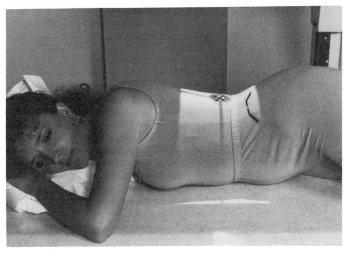

FIGURE 7–41. RAO position for the stomach of sthenic patient.

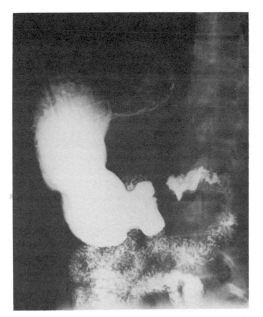

FIGURE 7–42. Barium-filled duodenal bulb, RAO stomach x-ray of sthenic patient. Make sure the spine is included on the back part of the film to include the duodenal bulb.

UGI (STOMACH): RIGHT LATERAL

11 x 14 in. 30 x 35 cm	11 x 14 in. 30 x 35 cm	10 x 12 in. 24 x 30 cm	10 x 12 in. 24 x 30 cm

FILM: Collimate to the size of the film. Table Bucky.

CR: Center perpendicularly at the end of the ribs longitudinally (Fig. 7–43). Adjust the longitudinal centering as to body habitus. Include the ASIS at the bottom of the film for asthenic patients. Include the diaphragm at the top of the film for hypersthenic patients.

POSITION: The patient is right lateral recumbent.

Open the collimation to the size of the film cassette.

Center the patient in order to place the vertebral column at the back (patient's right) margin of the collimation. The larger the patient's abdomen, the less of the vertebral column you want to include on the back part of the film. Hypersthenic right laterals should include only the anterior aspect of the vertebral column on the film (Fig. 7–44).

STRUCTURES DEMONSTRATED: The entire, partially barium-filled stomach.

The anterior and posterior borders of the stomach (Fig. 7–44).

Demonstration of the retrogastric space.

In hypersthenic patients, this position presents the best demonstration of the duodenal bulb.

COMMON ERROR: Clipping the stomach off of the film. If you do not have a closed-circuit television to watch the fluoroscopy, observe the location of the fluoroscopy unit when the radiologists takes spots. Better yet, ask the radiologist at the end of fluoroscopy to pinpoint the top of the fundus and the location of the duodenal bulb for you. It beats taking repeats!

NOTE: Use a relatively high kVp technique when using barium products for x-ray studies.

TECHNIQUE

KV _____ MA _____ SECS _____ MAS _____ CALIPER _____ cm

_____ :1 GRID / B / none SCREEN: RE / High / Par / Detail / None

SID: _____ Rm _____ ADULT / CHILD   age: _____ mos. / yrs.

HABITUS: Hyper / s / hypo / a   XS   S   M   L   XL   XXL

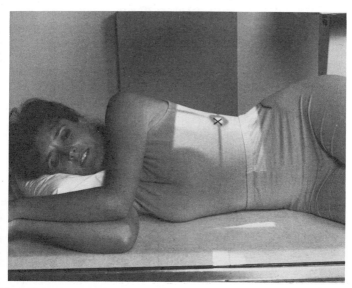

FIGURE 7–43. Right lateral position for the stomach of sthenic patient. Iliac crest (*curved line*).

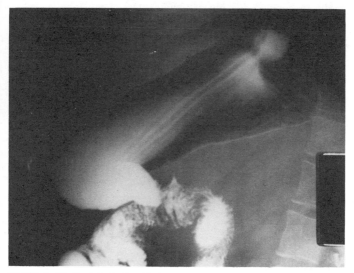

FIGURE 7–44. Partially barium-filled right lateral stomach x-ray of hypersthenic patient. Striations demonstrate gastric canal.

UGI (STOMACH): PA

11 x 14 in. 30 x 35 cm	11 x 14 in. 30 x 35 cm	10 x 12 in. 24 x 30 cm	10 x 12 in. 24 x 30 cm

FILM: Collimate to the size of the film. Table Bucky.

CR: Perpendicular to the center of the film when the film is centered at the level of the end of the ribs. Adjust accordingly for body habitus. Include the ASIS at the bottom of the film for asthenic patients. Include the diaphragm at the top of the film for hypersthenic patients.

POSITION: The patient is pronated on the table.

Center transversely the left upper or lower quadrant to the center of the table (Fig. 7–45).

Include the duodenal bulb at the point located 2 inches (5 cm) right from L2 within the collimation area.

STRUCTURES DEMONSTRATED: The entire, partially barium-filled stomach with air in the fundus (Fig. 7–46).

The body, pyloric antrum, and duodenal bulb filled with barium.

COMMON ERROR: Clipping the stomach off of the film. If you do not have a closed-circuit television to watch the fluoroscopy, observe the location of the fluoroscopy unit when the radiologist takes spots. Better yet, ask the radiologist at the end of fluoroscopy to pinpoint the top of the fundus and the location of the duodenal bulb for you. It beats taking repeats!

NOTE: Use a relatively high kVp technique when using barium products for x-ray studies.

TECHNIQUE

KV ____ MA ____ SECS ____ MAS ____ CALIPER ____ cm

____ :1 GRID / B / none SCREEN: RE / High / Par / Detail / None

SID: ____ Rm ____ ADULT / CHILD age: ____ mos. / yrs.

HABITUS: Hyper / s / hypo / a   XS   S   M   L   XL   XXL

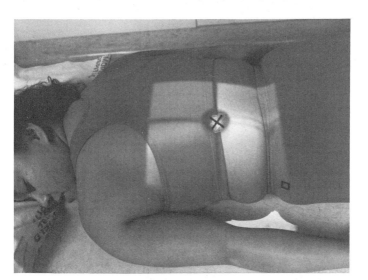

FIGURE 7–45. PA projection for the stomach. Notice patient is sthenic but short-waisted (you can include the iliac crest [*square*] and diaphragm easily on the film).

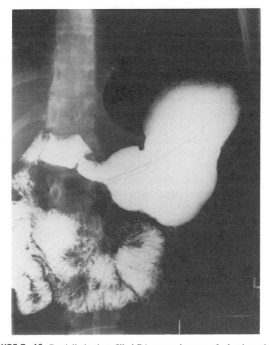

FIGURE 7–46. Partially barium-filled PA stomach x-ray of sthenic patient.

SMALL BOWEL SERIES: AP (KUB)

14 x 17 in.
35 x 43 cm

14 x 17 in.
35 x 43 cm

FILM: Collimate to the size of the film. Table Bucky.

CR: Perpendicular to the midpoint of the film when the bottom of the film is at the level of the symphysis pubis.

POSITION: The patient is supinated.

Center the patient's MSP to the center of the table or grid cassette (Fig. 7–47).

Have the patient place the hands upon the chest with elbows resting at the side (especially if covered with a blanket) or down by the side away from the body.

Make sure the pelvis is flat and the patient is not favoring one side or the other.

Mark the film as to the time from ingestion of barium. Check with your department supervisor or radiologist as to the appropriate time sequence to be performed (usually 15-, 30-, 45-, 60-, 90-minute films).

Make the exposure at the end of full expiration or just have the patient suspend respiration.

A fluoroscopy spot film with the use of compression is sometimes performed. The compression helps separate loops of small intestines from obscuring the ileocecal region. (*NOTE*: Some states require special certification or licensure of technologists in order to perform fluoroscopy spot filming.)

STRUCTURES DEMONSTRATED: The partially barium-filled small intestines over timed sequences in order to assess motility (Figs. 7–48 and 7–49). The study is terminated when barium reaches the ileocecal valve and enters the cecum.

The ilia will be symmetrical and seen in an obliqued position.

Gastrointestinal patterns are demonstrated as well as intra-abdominal calcifications and abdominal masses, if present.

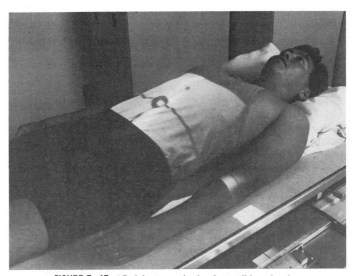

FIGURE 7-47. AP abdomen projection for small bowel series.

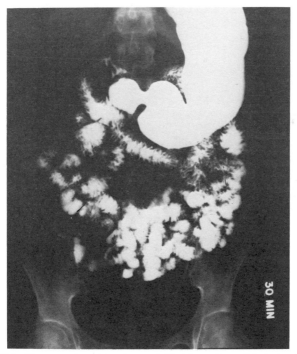

FIGURE 7-48. Thirty-minute delayed x-ray of AP abdomen for partially barium-filled small bowel showing maximum range of technique suitable for use.

451

COMMON ERRORS: (1) The symphysis pubis is not included due to the divergence of the x-ray beam or centering too high. Center 2 inches (5 cm) above the iliac crest at midline or use the "T" method to find the end of the femoral neck, or palpate the greater trochanter to find the level of the symphysis pubis in order to include it on the film. (See Chapter 1 on body landmarks for further instruction on these methods.) (2) There is intestinal motion on the film. Make sure you hesitate a second or two to make the exposure after instructing the patient to exhale completely. This allows the contents of the intestinal tract to come to a rest before making the exposure.

TECHNIQUE

KV _____ MA _____ SECS _____ MAS _____ CALIPER _____ cm

_____ :1 GRID / B / none SCREEN: RE / High / Par / Detail / None

SID: _____ Rm _____ ADULT / CHILD age: _____ mos. / yrs.

HABITUS: Hyper / s / hypo / a   XS   S   M   L   XL   XXL

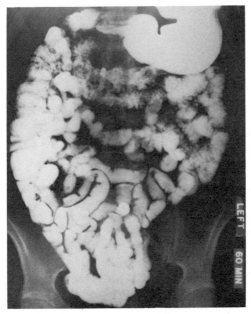

FIGURE 7—49. Sixty-minute delayed x-ray of AP abdomen for partially barium-filled small bowel showing minimum range of technique suitable for use.

BARIUM ENEMA: AP

14 x 17 in.
35 x 43 cm

14 x 17 in.
35 x 43 cm

FILM: Collimate to the size of the film. Table Bucky.

CR: Perpendicular to the midpoint of the film when the bottom of the film is at the level of the symphysis pubis.

POSITION: Be quick, but accurate.

The patient is supinated (Fig. 7–50). If the barium tip or retention catheter remains in place within the patient during the remainder of the study use the PA projection and be attentive to its transfer when the patient rotates positions.

Center the patient's MSP to the center of the table or grid cassette.

Have the patient place the hands upon the chest with elbows resting at the side or down by the side away from the body.

Make sure the pelvis is flat and the patient is not favoring one side or the other.

Make the exposure at the end of full expiration or have the patient suspend respiration.

NOTES:

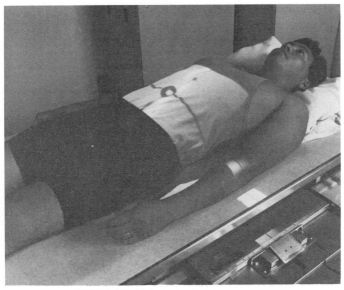

FIGURE 7–50. AP projection for a barium enema.

NOTES:

STRUCTURES DEMONSTRATED: The barium-filled large intestines for a single-contrast study (Fig. 7–51).

When a double-contrast study is performed, barium-coated, air-filled intestines with barium levels will be demonstrated. The coating action is produced by the many positional changes of the patient during the exam. In the AP projection, the air rises ventrally filling the transverse colon and sigmoid colon.[53] The remaining large intestinal structures will generally contain barium, depending on the amount used.

The vertebral column is seen centered on the film.

The vertebrae are well penetrated.

COMMON ERRORS: (1) There is intestinal motion on the film. Make sure you hesitate a second or two to make the exposure after instructing the patient to exhale completely. This allows the contents of the intestinal tract to come to a rest before making the exposure. (2) The flexures are not included on the film (clipped). You may want to use a crosswise film for the flexures on hypersthenic or elevated flexure patients. Usually the splenic flexure is higher than the hepatic flexure.

NOTE: Use a relatively high kVp technique when barium is used.

TECHNIQUE

KV _____ MA _____ SECS _____ MAS _____ CALIPER _____ cm

_____ :1 GRID / B / none SCREEN: RE / High / Par / Detail / None

SID: _____ Rm _____ ADULT / CHILD age: _____ mos. / yrs.

HABITUS: Hyper / s / hypo / a   XS   S   M   L   XL   XXL

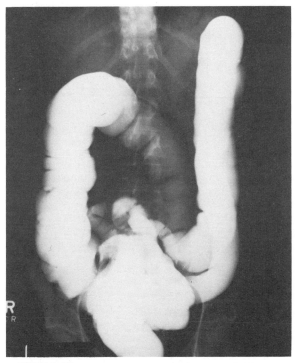

FIGURE 7–51. Single-contrast barium-filled large bowel AP x-ray.

BARIUM ENEMA: PA

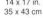

14 x 17 in.
35 x 43 cm

14 x 17 in.
35 x 43 cm

FILM: Collimate to the size of the film. Table Bucky.

CR: Perpendicular to the midpoint of the film when the bottom of the film is at the level of the symphysis pubis.

POSITION: Be quick, but accurate.

The patient is pronated (Fig. 7–52). If the barium tip or retention catheter remains in place within the patient during the remainder of the study, be attentive to its transfer when the patient rotates positions.

Center the patient's MSP to the center of the table.

Have the patient place the hands up by the pillow.

Make sure the pelvis is flat and the patient is not favoring one side or the other.

Make the exposure at the end of full expiration or have the patient suspend respiration.

STRUCTURES DEMONSTRATED: The barium-filled large intestines with a single-contrast study.

When a double-contrast study is performed (Fig. 7–53), barium-coated, air-filled intestines with barium levels will be demonstrated. The coating action is produced by the many positional changes of the patient during the exam. In the PA projection, the air rises dorsally, filling the right and left colon and rectum.[54] The remaining large intestinal structures (especially the transverse colon) will generally contain barium, depending on the amount used.

The vertebral column is seen centered on the film.

The vertebrae are well penetrated.

COMMON ERRORS: (1) There is intestinal motion on the film. Make sure you hesitate a second or two to make the exposure after instructing the patient to exhale completely. This allows the contents of the intestinal tract to come to a rest before making the exposure. (2) The flexures are not included on the film (clipped). You may want to use a crosswise film for the flexures on hypersthenic patients or for patients who have flexures that travel significantly when changing positions from upright to recumbent or side to side.

NOTE: Use a relatively high kVp technique when barium is used.

TECHNIQUE

KV _____ MA _____ SECS _____ MAS _____ CALIPER _____ cm

_____ :1 GRID / B / none SCREEN: RE / High / Par / Detail / None

SID: _____ Rm _____ ADULT / CHILD age: _____ mos. / yrs.

HABITUS: Hyper / s / hypo / a   XS   S   M   L   XL   XXL

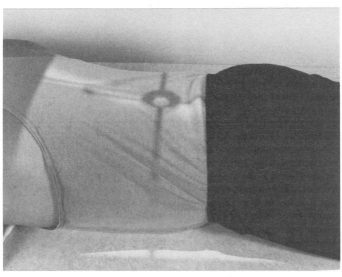

FIGURE 7–52. PA projection for a barium enema.

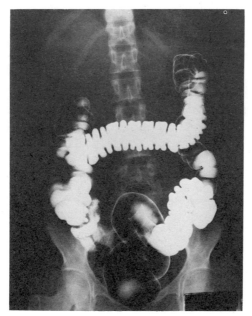

FIGURE 7–53. Double-contrast, barium- and air-filled large bowel PA x-ray.

BARIUM ENEMA: AP OR PA UPRIGHT

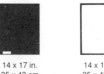

14 x 17 in.   14 x 17 in.
35 x 43 cm   35 x 43 cm

FILM: Collimate to the size of the film. Table Bucky.

CR: Perpendicular to the midpoint of the film. Place the bottom of the film at the level of the symphysis pubis *or* center 2 inches (5 cm) above the iliac crest at midline.

POSITION: Secure the footboard on the table and test before using. Make sure the locks are engaged correctly. Lock the Bucky tray so it does not migrate when the table is moved toward the upright position. If moving the table from the supine position, stop halfway to assess the patient. Have the patient move the feet slightly forward for better balance at vertical.

Be quick, but accurate.

The patient is upright and in the anatomical position for the AP projection (Fig. 7–54).

The patient is upright and facing the table for the PA projection. The PA projection will produce a lower gonadal dose than the AP projection.[55]

Center the patient's MSP to the center of the table or grid cassette.

Make sure the pelvis is level and the patient is not favoring one side or the other.

Make the exposure at the end of full expiration or just have the patient suspend respiration.

Patients who are acutely ill must be monitored continually, and not remain in the upright position. *If a semi-erect position is used, the central ray must remain horizontal to depict air/fluid levels.* If the patient cannot stand, use the lateral decubitus position (see next position).

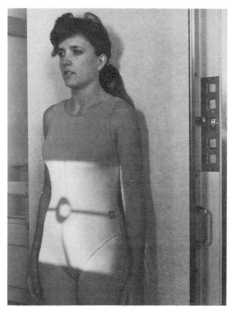

FIGURE 7–54. AP upright abdomen for a barium enema.

STRUCTURES DEMONSTRATED: Fluid and air levels.

The barium-coated large intestines will be demonstrated on their inferior aspect and air-filled large intestines will be shown on their elevated aspect (Fig. 7–55).

The vertebrae are well penetrated.

The vertebral column is centered on the film.

COMMON ERRORS: (1) Underpenetration. An increase in technique is needed because of the increased density of the abdominal contents due to gravity. Your technique will need to be increased proportionately as the patient's abdominal size and density increase due to gravitational compression. (2) There is intestinal motion on the film. Make sure you hesitate a second or two to make the exposure after giving the patient respiratory instructions. This allows the contents of the intestinal tract to come to rest before making the exposure. (3) Flexures are not included on the film (clipped). You may want to use a crosswise film for the flexures on hypersthenic patients or for patients who have flexures that travel significantly when changing positions from upright to recumbent or side to side.

NOTE: Use a relatively high kVp technique when barium is used.

TECHNIQUE

KV _____ MA _____ SECS _____ MAS _____ CALIPER _____ cm

_____ :1 GRID / B / none SCREEN: RE / High / Par / Detail / None

SID: _____ Rm _____ ADULT / CHILD age: _____ mos. / yrs.

HABITUS: Hyper / s / hypo / a   XS   S   M   L   XL   XXL

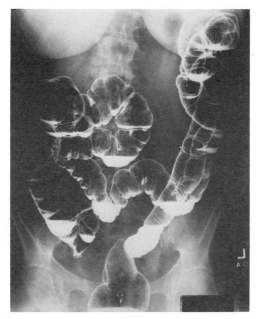

FIGURE 7—55. Double-contrast barium-filled and air-filled large bowel upright x-ray.

BARIUM ENEMA: LEFT AND RIGHT LATERAL DECUBITUS

14 x 17 in.
35 x 43 cm

14 x 17 in.
35 x 43 cm

14 x 17 in.
35 x 43 cm

FILM: Collimate to the size of the film. Use grid or the table Bucky when the patient is placed in front of the table on a gurney with the table upright.

CR: Using a horizontal beam, perpendicular to the midpoint of the film. Place the bottom of the film at the level of the greater trochanter or symphysis pubis.

POSITION: *NOTE:* Many technologists use a gurney to position the lateral recumbent patient in front of the upright table. Another method is to use a stationary grid and film with the patient in the lateral decubitus position (Fig. 7–56). *Whichever method you use— work expediently; sometimes the patient will not wait for you!*

When the patient's head is to your right, move the patient from the supine to lie on the right side with the film and grid against the abdomen for a PA projection (Fig. 7–56). Now have the patient turn over on the left side for an AP projection (Fig. 7–57). (Check with the radiologist if this is satisfactory; some like to keep both the projections consistently APs or both PAs. If they are to be consistent, the patient's head must be placed at one end of the table for one decubitus and then the other for the opposite decubitus study [see discussion of left lateral decubitus in Abdomen section and in Chapter 9]).

If you are using a gurney to take the decubitus projections, make sure all of the wheels are locked!

Position the patient's arms over the head and both knees equal and slightly flexed for balance.

The film and grid (or table Bucky) should be as close to the body as possible without tilting any part of the body.

Make sure the film's ID blocker is down so as not to obscure the right or left colonic flexures.

Make the exposure at the end of full expiration or just have the patient suspend respiration.

Be quick, but accurate.

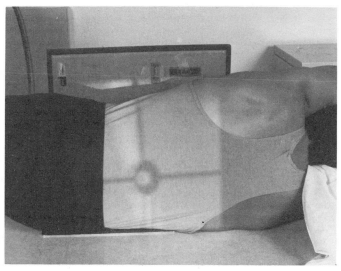

FIGURE 7–56. Right lateral decubitus position (PA projection) for a barium enema.

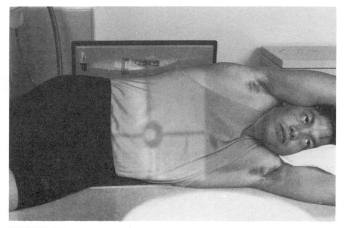

FIGURE 7–57. Left lateral decubitus position (AP projection) for a barium enema.

STRUCTURES DEMONSTRATED: Fluid and air levels (Fig. 7–58).

The air-filled large intestines will be visualized on the elevated side and the barium-filled large intestines on the lower side of the patient. That is, the barium-filled large intestines will be visualized on the side down.

The vertebrae are well penetrated.

COMMON ERROR: Clipping or missing the right or left colonic flexures (hepatic and splenic flexures). Make sure you watch the TV screen or check with the radiologist during fluoroscopy in order to identify severely elevated flexures, especially on hypersthenic patients.

NOTE: Use a relatively high kVp technique when barium is used.

TECHNIQUE

KV _____ MA _____ SECS _____ MAS _____ CALIPER _____ cm

_____ :1 GRID / B / none SCREEN: RE / High / Par / Detail / None

SID: _____ Rm _____ ADULT / CHILD age: _____ mos. / yrs.

HABITUS: Hyper / s / hypo / a   XS   S   M   L   XL   XXL

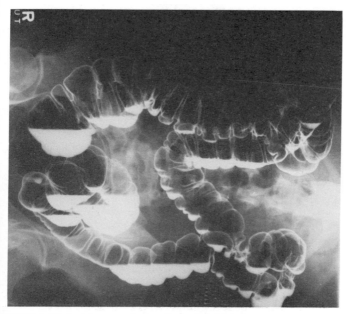

FIGURE 7–58. Double-contrast barium-filled and air-filled left lateral decubitus x-ray.

BARIUM ENEMA: LATERAL RECTUM

11 x 14 in.
30 x 35 cm

11 x 14 in.
30 x 35 cm

10 x 12 in.
24 x 30 cm

10 x 12 in.
24 x 30 cm

FILM: Use a grid for crosstable decubitus or the table Bucky with the patient recumbent. Collimate to the size of the film.

CR: Perpendicularly at the midcoronal plane longitudinally equidistant between the level of the greater trochanter and the iliac crest.

POSITION: Place the patient on the left side on the table with a pillow under the head (left lateral recumbent position, Fig. 7–59).

Flex the knees equally.

Lateralize the patient by adjusting the shoulders and hips to be directly superimposed.

Be quick, but accurate.

NOTE: Sometimes a ventral decubitus position with a horizontal beam is used to demonstrate the rectosigmoid area (Fig. 7–60). This position is described under myelography in Chapter 5. The centering of the central ray, however, is as indicated above.

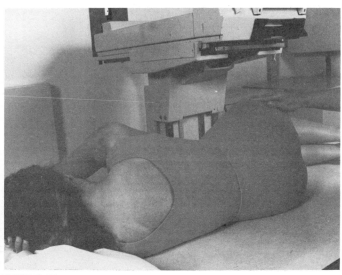

FIGURE 7–59. Lateral recumbent rectum position for a barium enema. Place the bottom of the film at the level of the greater trochanter (seen being palpated here).

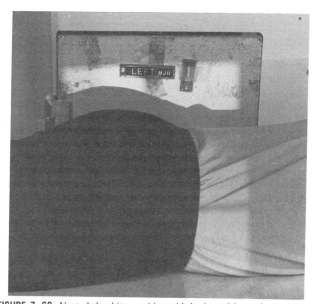

FIGURE 7–60. Ventral decubitus position with horizontal beam for barium enema rectum.

STRUCTURES DEMONSTRATED: The rectosigmoid area in its lateral aspect in a recumbent position (Fig. 7–61).

The double-contrast, barium-filled and air-filled rectosigmoid portion of the large bowel with the patient in a ventral decubitus position (Fig. 7–62).

COMMON ERROR: *Underpenetration. For manual techniques, remember that not only are you penetrating the lateral pelvis, but the presence of contrast necessitates an increased technique as well. A high-kVp technique is recommended.*

NOTE: Use a relatively high kVp technique when barium is used.

TECHNIQUE

KV _____ MA _____ SECS _____ MAS _____ CALIPER _____ cm

_____ :1 GRID / B / none SCREEN: RE / High / Par / Detail / None

SID: _____ Rm _____ ADULT / CHILD age: _____ mos. / yrs.

HABITUS: Hyper / s / hypo / a XS S M L XL XXL

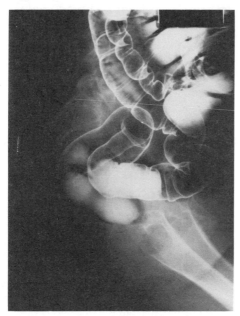

FIGURE 7–61. Double-contrast barium enema, lateral rectum x-ray with patient in recumbent position.

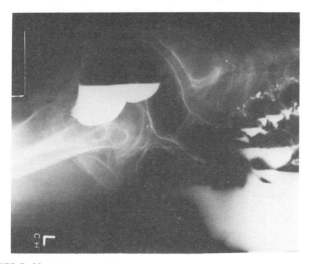

FIGURE 7–62. Double-contrast barium enema, lateral rectum x-ray in the ventral decubitus position with horizontal beam.

BARIUM ENEMA: ANGLED AP OR PA FOR RECTUM
(MODIFIED CHASSARD-LAPINE)

11 x 14 in. 30 x 35 cm	11 x 14 in. 30 x 35 cm	10 x 12 in. 24 x 30 cm	10 x 12 in. 24 x 30 cm

FILM: Collimate to the size of the film. Table Bucky.

CR: For the AP, a 30- to 40-degree cephalic angle exiting level of the ASIS (Fig. 7–63).

For the PA, a 30- to 40-degree caudal angle entering midsag at, or slightly above, the level of the iliac crest and exiting level of the ASIS (Fig. 7–64).

POSITION. Be quick, but accurate.

The patient is supinated for the angled AP projection. Some the LPO position is utilized in lieu of the AP.

The patient is pronated for the angled PA projection. Some the RAO position is used in lieu of the PA.

Center the MSP to the center of the table.

Make sure the pelvis is flat and the patient is not favorin side or the other.

Make the exposure at the end of full expiration.

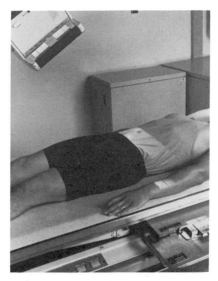

FIGURE 7–63. Angled AP (modified Chassard-Lapine) for barium enema rectum.

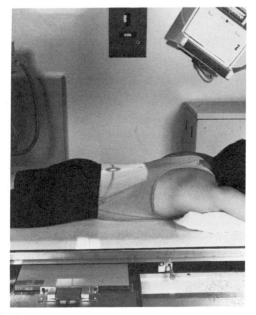

FIGURE 7–64. Angled PA (modified Chassard-Lapine) for barium enema rectum.

STRUCTURES DEMONSTRATED: An elongated rectosigmoid area (Fig. 7–65) with less superimposition than the unangled AP or PA projections.

COMMON ERROR: Centering is off. If too low, the film includes too much of the proximal femurs. The pubic bones should just be included at the lower aspect of the film. If the centering is too high, the inferior aspect of the rectum will be clipped.

NOTE: Use a relatively high kVp technique when barium is used.

TECHNIQUE

KV _____ MA _____ SECS _____ MAS _____ CALIPER _____ cm

_____ :1 GRID / B / none SCREEN: RE / High / Par / Detail / None

SID: _____ Rm _____ ADULT / CHILD age: _____ mos. / yrs.

HABITUS: Hyper / s / hypo / a   XS   S   M   L   XL   XXL

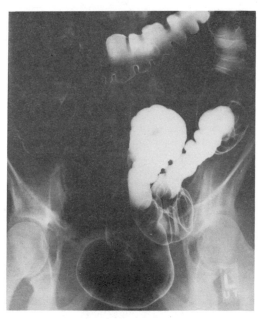

FIGURE 7–65. Angled AP x-ray for barium enema rectum. (Notice how elongated the obturator foramina are in this projection.)

BARIUM ENEMA: AP OR PA OBLIQUES

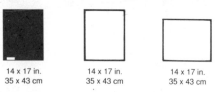

14 x 17 in.
35 x 43 cm

14 x 17 in.
35 x 43 cm

14 x 17 in.
35 x 43 cm

FILM: Collimate to the size of the film. Table Bucky.

CR: Perpendicularly to the midpoint of the film, when the bc of the film is placed at the level of the greater trochant symphysis pubis.

POSITION: The patient should be semisupinated for the oblique projections.

The patient should be semipronated for the PA oblique pr tions. Flex the knee of the side up for stability.

Use a 45-degree obliquity of the patient with the entire obliqued as a unit.

For AP obliques (LPO and RPO positions; Fig. 7–66), c the *surface,* coronal plane that intersects the side-up ASIS t center of the table. If the patient is hypersthenic or has a abdomen, measure the width of the obliqued abdominal area costal margin to left; find the center of this distance. Now c this point to the center of the x-ray table. Often, two cros films—one high and one low—may be taken for extremely patients. This will avoid clipping the flexures.

For PA obliques (RAO and LAO positions), palpate the lu spinous processes in order to center 2 to 3 inches (5 to 7 anterior from the spinous processes, that is, center the midli the obliqued lumbar spine to the center of the x-ray table (F 67). If the patient is hypersthenic or has a large abdomen, me the width of the obliqued abdominal area left costal marg right; find the center of this distance. Now center this point t center of the x-ray table. Often, two crosswise films—one higl one low—may be taken for extremely large patients. Thi avoid clipping the flexures or rectosigmoid area.

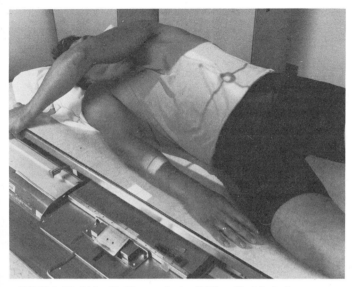

FIGURE 7–66. Right AP oblique projection (RPO position) for barium enema.

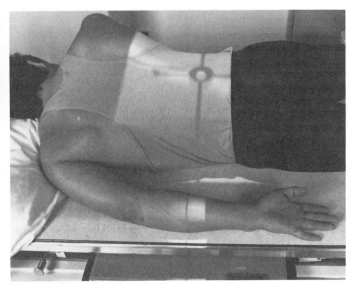

FIGURE 7–67. Left PA oblique projection (LAO position) for barium enema.

STRUCTURES DEMONSTRATED: The anterior oblique positions (RAO and LAO) will demonstrate the side down. The RAO will demonstrate the barium-filled ascending colon and the hepatic (right colonic) flexure. The LAO will demonstrate the barium-filled splenic or left colonic flexure and the descending colon (see Fig. 7–69).

The posterior oblique positions (LPO and RPO) will demonstrate the side up.

The LPO/RAO* will demonstrate the hepatic or right colonic flexure and ascending colon (Fig. 7–68). The RPO/LAO* will demonstrate the splenic or left colonic flexure and descending colon (Fig. 7–69).

COMMON ERROR: Clipping the flexures.

NOTE: Use a relatively high kVp technique when barium is used.

TECHNIQUE

KV _____ MA _____ SECS _____ MAS _____ CALIPER _____ cm

_____ :1 GRID / B / none SCREEN: RE / High / Par / Detail / None

SID: _____ Rm _____ ADULT / CHILD age: _____ mos. / yrs.

HABITUS: Hyper / s / hypo / a XS S M L XL XXL

See Chapter 9 for an explanation of complementary oblique positions or the 180 rule.

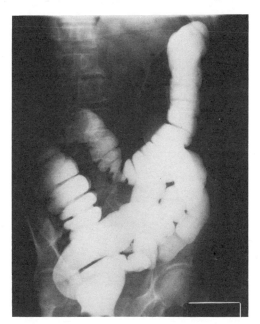

FIGURE 7–68. Single-contrast, RAO barium enema x-ray demonstrating the hepatic flexure.

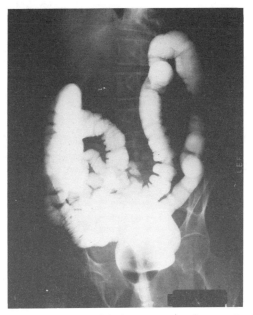

FIGURE 7–69. Single-contrast, LAO barium enema x-ray demonstrating the splenic flexure.

479

Portable Radiography

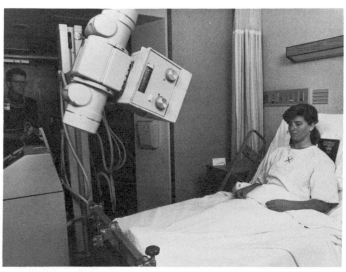

FIGURE 8–1. In the AP chest, notice that the film is padded with the bed pillow in order to place the film perpendicular to the CR. The technologist is wearing a lead apron and uses the length of the exposure cord to minimize his radiation exposure.

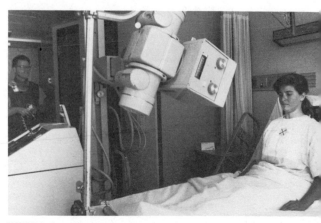

FIGURE 8–2. In the AP chest when traction bars are present, try to achieve a to 72-inch source-image distance (SID) as you are able. Notice here that t angle is not yet adjusted so that the CR is perpendicular to the film. If the t bars inhibit the use of a longer SID, adjust the head of the bed slightly to pl patient in a semierect position. When the cardiac shadow size accuracy is important, make sure you use a long SID. Check the patient's previous films o for history and continuing diagnosis.

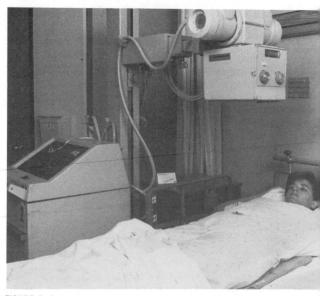

FIGURE 8–3. The abdomen film requires the use of a grid. Make sure the fil grid are level (they are not in this photo). Use rolled towels to adjust.

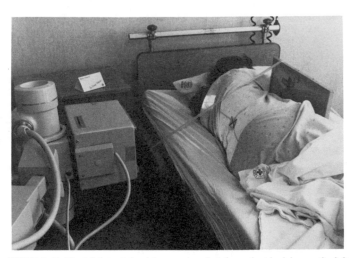

FIGURE 8–4. In this photo, notice that the film and grid are level. The pressure of the body against the bed mattress sometimes causes film angle. Use rolled towels to adjust.

FIGURE 8–5. The left lateral decubitus requires that the patient be lying on the left side in a lateral position. Either an AP or PA projection can be performed. The PA projection is common due to the prevailing design of some hospital rooms. In this case, the AP projection of the left lateral decubitus position would require that the patient be mobile enough to place the head at the opposite end of the bed or the portable be moved to the opposite side of the room. An AP will reduce object-image distance (OID) for a patient with a large abdomen.

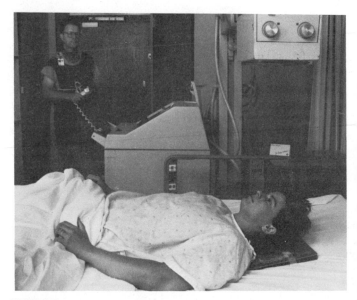

FIGURE 8–6. AP skull. The weight of the patient's shoulders can cause the film to be angled. The film's position produces a caudal angle with the infraorbitomeatal line (IOML). Use this film angle instead of moving the patient's head in order to adjust the orbitomeatal line (OML) or IOML for reverse Caldwell or reverse Waters' studies.

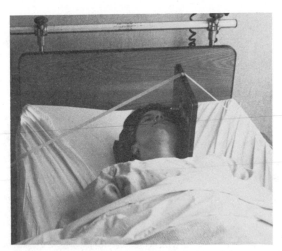

FIGURE 8–7. Lateral skull. Elevate the posterior skull with radiolucent sponges if the patient can tolerate the head movement and is not neck injured. This will avoid clipping the posterior skull. Use tape to secure the film and grid.

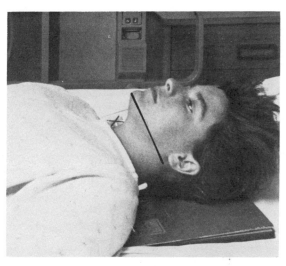

FIGURE 8–8. AP cervical spine. If the patient cannot be moved, take "as is" and match the plane (line) formed by the mentum and base of the skull (see Fig. 1–8) to the plane of the tube angle. This angle will maximize the upper cervical area on the film by superimposing the mentum and base of the skull on the radiograph. Tilting or elevating the top edge of the film and grid will produce a caudal angle, canceling some of the effect of the cephalic tube angle if it becomes too large.

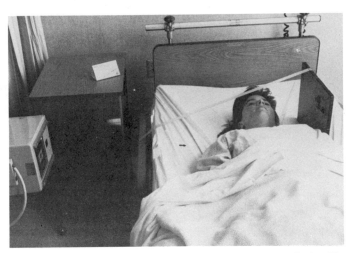

FIGURE 8–9. Lateral cervical spine. Use a longer SID to reduce magnification. The film needs to be placed at the shoulder in order to include C-7 on the film. The increased OID will serve as an "air gap," eliminating the need for a grid. Depress the shoulders by taking film on exhalation. Never apply traction or pressure on the shoulders without checking with a physician.

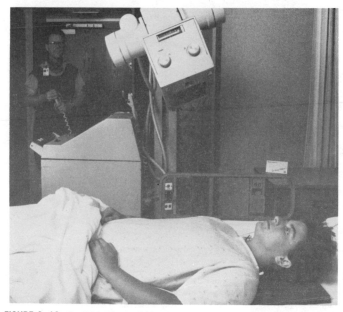

FIGURE 8–10. Double-angle cervical spine oblique for use when the patient cannot be moved from the anatomical position. Use a 45-degree transverse angle and a 20-degree cephalic angle. Results in an AP oblique projection (LPO) of the cervical spine demonstrating the intervertebral foramina of the side up. No grid.

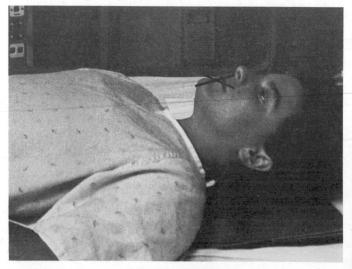

FIGURE 8–11. AP mandible.

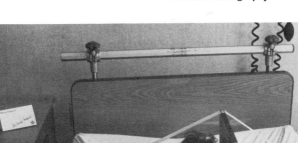

FIGURE 8–12. Axiolateral mandible. No grid. Have the patient extend the head and neck if there is no neck injury. (See p. 342.)

Projection Versus Position

Projection will always indicate an entrance side and an exit side of the patient. For the anteroposterior projection (AP), the entrance is the anterior aspect (A) and the exit is the posterior (P). For the posteroanterior projection (PA), the entrance side is posterior (P) and the exit side is anterior (A). The use of the term projection has been defined as the path of the central ray. Figure 9–1 demonstrates a PA projection.

The entrance side will be either the anterior (A) or the posterior (P). The exit side will then be the opposite of the first letter, either the "P" in A**P** or the "A" in P**A.** Obliqued positions (LAO, RAO, LPO, and RPO) truncate the use of the two letters describing projections and indicate only the exit side of the A**P** or P**A** projection. For example, the RPO position can also be described as a right, AP, oblique projection.

In the past, the exit side indicated what side was "viewed." The term "view" is no longer advocated for use in radiography. However, position is sometimes described as to how the film "sees" the patient's exit side. Knowing the exit side partially defines the patient's obliqued position, that is, R**A**O, L**A**O, R**P**O, and L**P**O. Another way to explain this is to relate the exit side to the side that is down on the x-ray table or film cassette. Therefore, the exit side, either "A" or "P," will be the center letter of the three initials of any position. A position that uses three initials describes a *unilateral* (right or left) *exit* side (A or P) of an *obliqued* patient. An RAO position is one that describes the **right** (R) side of the patient, the **anterior** (A) exit side or side on which the patient is resting, and the fact that they are **obliqued** (O).

Think of the patient lying on an x-ray table in the LPO position (Fig. 9–2). If you can imagine that you are the film and are looking up at the patient, you are looking at the patient's *left* side, the *posterior* aspect of that left side, and be seeing the patient in an *oblique* manner, hence L, P, and O. Reposition the patient to the RPO position and repeat the exercise (Fig. 9–3). Now change the patient to the RAO (Fig. 9–4) and LAO (Fig. 9–5), and repeat this exercise. Confirm your findings by referring to the figures indicated.

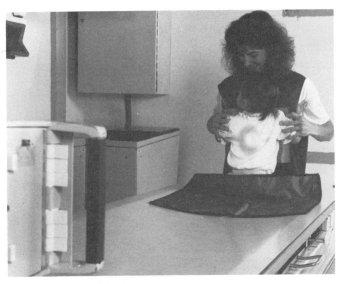

FIGURE 9–1. PA projection of the chest.

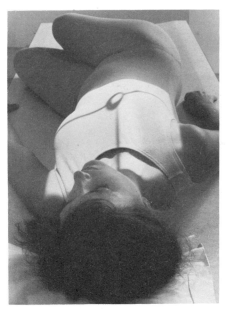

FIGURE 9–2. LPO position.

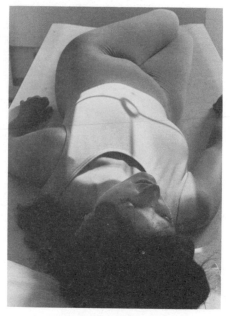

FIGURE 9–3. RPO position.

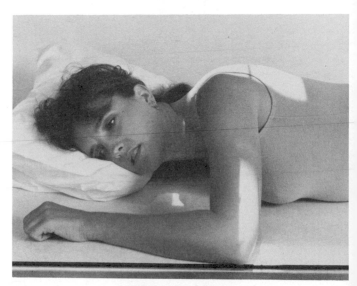

FIGURE 9–4. RAO position.

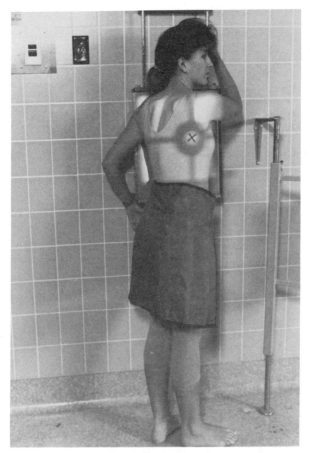

FIGURE 9–5. LAO upright position.

Another concept of oblique positioning is complementary positions, or what I call the 180 (degree) rule, that is, for example, that the RPO and the LAO positions (which are 180 degrees from each other) will be radiographically similar. If for instance, you have a patient at the chest board for a LAO position and reverse the location of the film and the tube 180 degrees while the patient remains in the same position, the x-ray will result in like-structure demonstration, i.e., the RPO. In essence we have changed only the tube and the film's location in order to change the orientation of the patient.

Now imagine the patient in the RAO position for upright rib obliques. The patient's right side along with the anterior aspect of the thorax is touching the film, and she is in an obliqued position (Fig. 9–6). Without moving the patient, mentally take the film (and film holder) away from the anterior surface and place it on the posterior. It will now touch the left side of the patient. Mentally switch the tube head to the other side as well. The patient's position relative to the film is now LPO. In this example, the 180-degree change ends with the patient in the same physical position— only the entrance and exit of the x-ray beam have been reversed. The 180 rule can be used with great success when dealing with patients who are debilitated or are in too much pain to achieve a particular obliquity—simply use the complementary obliquity. Thus, the RPO position for the gallbladder can be substituted with the complementary position, the LAO. The RAO position of the lumbar spine can be substituted with a LPO position. Knowing when to take the RAO over the LPO, or the LAO over the RPO is a function of variables such as identifying structures closest to the film for better detail, acceptable OID, patient condition, radiation safety, gravity, and air-fluid levels, to name just a few.

To review:

- A **projection** will always either be indicated by two initials, AP or PA.
- A **position** will be indicated by three initials, of which the first initial indicates unilateral aspect closest to film (right or left), the center initial is the exit side of the central ray or the side closest to the film, and the last initial always indicates that the position is an obliquity.
- The **180 rule** for obliques allows the RAO and LPO to be substituted for each other and the LAO and RPO to be substituted for each other under certain conditions (see Chap. 11).

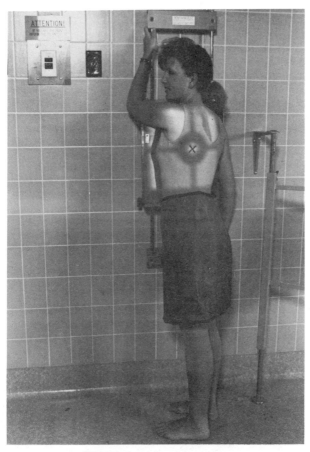

FIGURE 9-6. RAO upright position.

OTHER POSITIONS

Lateral positions are identified by the side closest to the film. Left side down or left side touching the film with the patient lateralized indicates that it is a left lateral position (Fig. 9–7).

Decubitus positions are always performed with a horizontal beam and always are described by the side that the patient is resting upon. A left lateral decubitus is a horizontal beam study with the patient lying on the left side in the lateral aspect (Fig. 9–8). Lateral decubitus positions can result in either an AP or PA projection. An example of a right lateral decubitus position resulting in an AP projection is given in Figure 9–9. An example of a right lateral

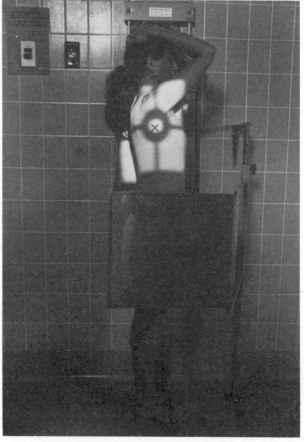

FIGURE 9–7. Left lateral upright position.

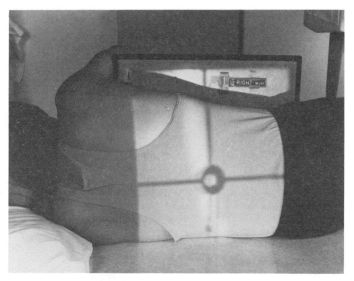

FIGURE 9–8. Left lateral decubitus position.

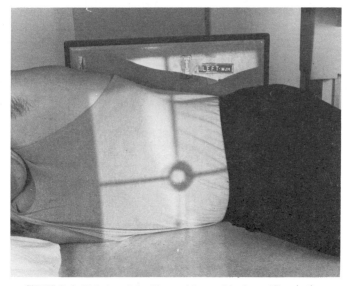

FIGURE 9–9. Right lateral decubitus position resulting in an AP projection.

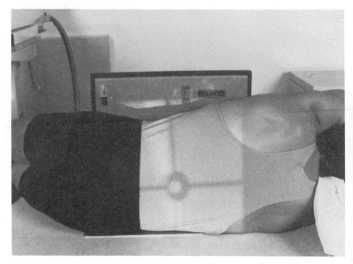

FIGURE 9–10. Right lateral decubitus position resulting in a PA projection.

decubitus position resulting in a PA projection is given in Figure 9–10. Referring to Figures 9–8 and 9–9, in which the patient is placed on the x-ray table head left, notice that in order to keep right and left decubitus positions the same projection, you must reverse the patient's position on the table for one of the two positions. (Keep this in mind when you are performing both decubitus positions in a barium enema study—it may be easier to take the right and left lateral decubitus positions with AP and PA projections rather than to have to move the enema-holding patient to the opposite end of the table!)

A ventral decubitus is a horizontal beam study with the patient resting upon the ventral or anterior aspect. In other words, the patient is pronated. This position always results in a lateral projection (Fig. 9–11). A dorsal decubitus position is one in which the patient is supinated using a horizontal x-ray beam. It, too, results in a lateral projection (Fig. 9–12).

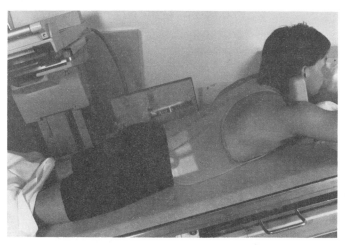

FIGURE 9–11. Ventral decubitus position (patient pronated).

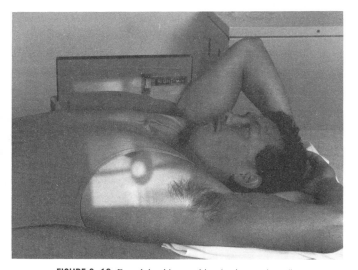

FIGURE 9–12. Dorsal decubitus position (patient supinated).

10

Orientation of Radiographs

Radiographic positioning should always be performed with fore-thought as to the placement of the patient ID blocker on the film cassette. Placement, however, is limited in range to four alternate positions: up, down, right, and left of the tube side only. Careful consideration should be given as to the blocker's final placement. If its placement is not considered, the blocker may obscure an anatomical area of interest. Many exams may be performed with cursory concern as to blocker placement. However, all film exposures of each exam must be preceded by blocker placement decisions with some degree of attention given to them. The use of blocker placement icons in this text and the ability to record blocker placement for each position address this process.

Many technologists adjust for blocker placement by mentally eliminating the entire transverse area of the film containing the blocker in assessments of area covered, thus making its placement a moot point. Other technologists use the blocker's neighboring film area "to get a little more information on the film." Inclusion of additional long bone is common. Sometimes the consistent, routine placement of the blocker will aid you when a left (or right) marker is omitted or misplaced. You can ascertain from the blocker position which side of the film is left or right and if AP or PA. The following step-by-step discussion of blocker placement pertains to that discovery. Remember, though, this method of identification of anatomical right and left and projection should *never* preclude the use of proper right or left markers on the x-ray film. You must mark your films accurately and consistently *before* they are devel-oped.

In Figure 10–1, a film cassette may be used lengthwise (vertically) with the blocker up. In this type of cassette, the blocker position will be in the upper right corner as you look at the front (tube side) of the cassette.

In Figure 10–2, a film cassette may be used lengthwise (vertically) with the blocker down. In this type of cassette, the blocker position will be in the lower left corner as you look at the front (tube side) of the cassette.

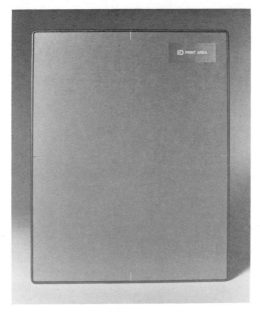

FIGURE 10–1. A lengthwise (vertical) film cassette with upper right blocker position.

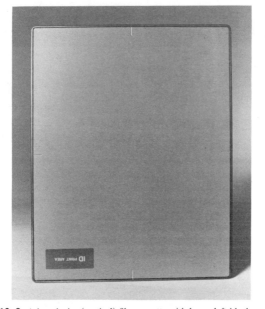

FIGURE 10–2. A lengthwise (vertical) film cassette with lower left blocker position.

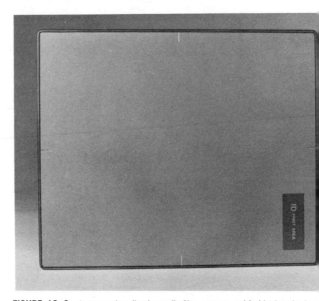

FIGURE 10–3. A crosswise (horizontal) film cassette with blocker in low position.

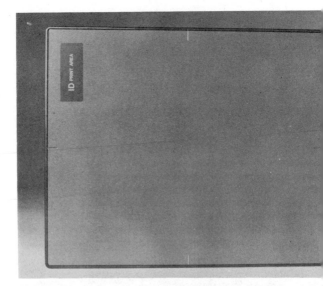

FIGURE 10–4. A crosswise (horizontal) film cassette with blocker in up position.

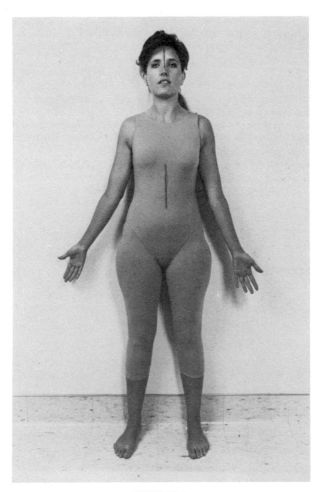

FIGURE 10–5

In Figure 10–3, a film cassette may be used crosswise (horizontally) with the blocker to the right.

In Figure 10–4, a film cassette may be used crosswise (horizontally) with the blocker to the left.

One of the guidelines for hanging radiographs is to hang them in the anatomical position. This means as you observe the person, your right will be the patient's left and that your left will be the patient's right. See Figure 10–5.

Because the only possible blocker positions are upper right and lower left when making a radiographic exposure (one cannot use the back side of the cassette toward the tube), you will be able to identify the projection from the blocker position. When performing radiographs that place the patient in a supine position (the anatomical position), one will always view the film with the blocker position in the lower left or upper right. In order for the film to be in the anatomical position on the viewbox, the right marker will be on your (the viewer's) left or the left marker will be on the viewer's right-hand side, where the blocker is lower left and the patient's right side is on your (the viewer's) left. Figure 10–6 is an example of an AP projection.

When performing pronated radiographic positions, one must turn over the finished radiograph in order to hang it in the anatomical position. Thus, all pronated positioned (PA) radiographs will have the blocker positions reversed from those of the AP projection. The blocker position for radiographs taken PA will have the blocker in the lower right or upper left.

Figure 10–7 is an example of a PA projection. The blocker relationships become very important if the film is not marked, or if there is some confusion as to the correct marking on the film.

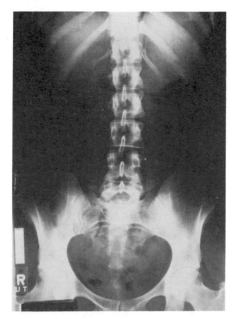

FIGURE 10–6

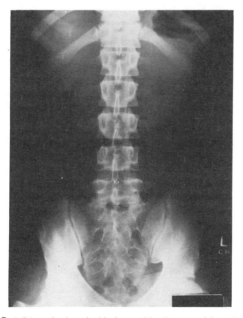

FIGURE 10–7. A PA projection; the blocker position is reversed from that of the AP because the film is flipped over when placed anatomically.

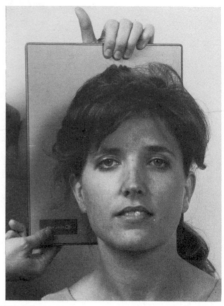

FIGURE 10–8. Demonstration of blocker position of AP skull.

If you forget to mark the film, knowing the projection tha
used will identify the correct manner in which to hang th
anatomically. For example, an unmarked film is placed c
viewbox, and it is known to be an AP skull. How would you
the film?

In Figure 10–8, know that the cassette's tube side demonst
the blocker position on an AP projection means that the b
can only be lower left (or upper right). The answer is to hav
film with the blocker lower left or upper right. Now, one of
positions will present the skull upside down, which obvio
not the correct orientation. If necessary, correct the vertic
entation.

In Figure 10–9, the PA skull projection will have op
blocker positions, lower right and upper left, when hung an
ically. But when the PA projection is placed on a viewbox
mounted in the anatomical position. In Figure 10–10, noti
blocker positions can be placed only in the lower right and
left when the PA is placed in the anatomical position.

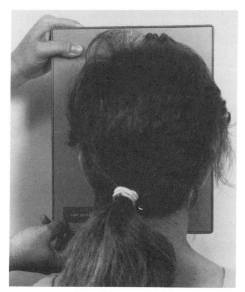

FIGURE 10–9. The orientation of the patient to the film cassette for the PA skull.

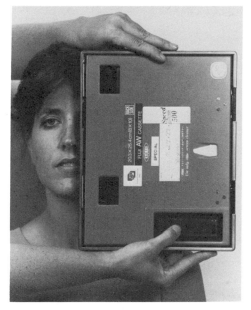

FIGURE 10–10. Demonstration of PA skull patient orientation in anatomical position.

How does this prove the patient's right side or left side? Knowing that the projection is an AP, with the blocker lower left or upper right, displays the film (or patient) anatomically. When the film is displayed anatomically, the patient's right will always be on your left. Thus, it is possible to identify right from left if you know the projection used for the radiograph. This, however, should not preclude the use of markers on radiographs. Look at the next film in Figure 10–11. You know that in your department, you always take PA chests. You have just developed a PA chest for someone else. You place it on the viewbox. The blocker should be in the lower right or upper left for a PA chest. Is it?

See Figure 10–11. The left marker should be on your right. Is it? You can see only a part of it. Yes, this is a PA projection and it is marked correctly. This exercise should be performed every time you check films in order to avoid marking errors affecting film interpretation. Avoid using anatomy to hang films because of random cases of situs inversus.

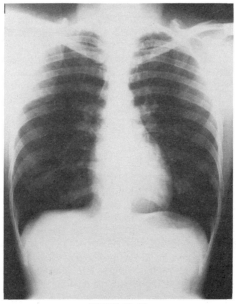

FIGURE 10–11

If the film is marked correctly and displayed in the anatomical position, and the blocker is on the lower left or upper right, is it an AP projection? Yes. Because you know now that the only way a patient can be oriented on the film with the blocker in the lower left or upper right is supine.

What happens if the film is marked incorrectly, or not at all? The only way to catch an error in this case is to mentally check the films for blocker placement when you hang them anatomically. You know what projections you routinely perform. Does the projection match with the blocker placement? Why is that blocker position in the PA position (lower right or upper left) when you know you performed an AP projection? Because it is marked incorrectly!

Here's a scenario common to us all.

You forgot to mark an angled PA mandible when you were on duty. The quality control technologist holds the films for you so that you can correctly indicate right from left. Picking up the film, you place the blocker in the lower right position on the viewbox. No, that's obviously not correct—it's upside down (Fig. 10–12).

Place the film right side up (Fig. 10–13). You know that you performed this x-ray in a PA projection. The blocker position represents that lower right or upper left configuration of the PA. The "patient" is now facing you in the anatomical position. You can now identify that the patient's right is on your left.

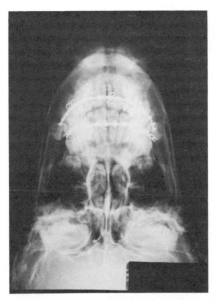

FIGURE 10–12. First step of identifying right or left on an unmarked film; hang as to pattern of projection.

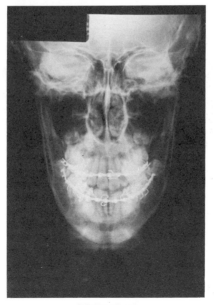

FIGURE 10–13

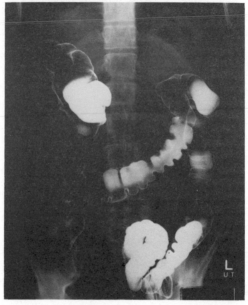

FIGURE 10–14. A PA barium enema projection. The blocker is lower right.

Study the radiographs in Figures 10–14 through 10–16. Assuming the markers are correct, identify the projections.

Always check that the films are placed in the anatomical position first by finding right or left markers on the film.

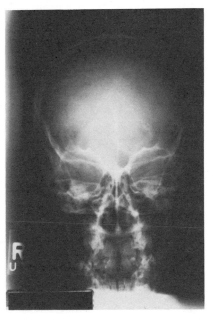

FIGURE 10–15. An AP skull projection. The blocker is lower left.

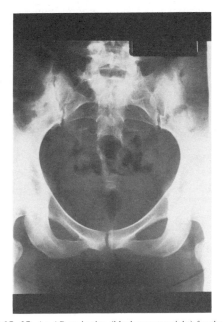

FIGURE 10–16. An AP projection (blocker upper right) for the coccyx.

TRANSVERSE FILMS

Transverse film placement can be assessed in much the same way but in very different orientations. PA projections will place the blockers transversely at the lower left or upper right. AP projections will place the blocker transversely at the lower right or upper left. This is the exact opposite of the longitudinal blocker orientations. What projection is the film in Figure 10–17?

BLOCKER VARIATIONS

There are some cassettes manufactured with alternate patient ID blockers, that is, in opposite positions other than those discussed above. The method described here is still valuable. If the patient ID blockers' positions vary, the cassette still only presents blocker placement in two positions when the patient is in the anatomical position. The AP projection will present blocker placement either up or down as you look at the cassette's tube side. The blockers can be right or left on the downside, or right or left on the upside as you observe the tube side. Whichever way that they present (right or left) as you look at the tube side of the upside and downside position of the ID blocker, that will be the blocker pattern of the AP projection. The PA projection of ID blocker will be the opposite of the AP. The transverse AP is opposite that of the AP vertical. The PA transverse position of the ID blocker will be the opposite of the PA vertical blocker position.

This method of identification of patient projection and anatomical right or left can be used only with rectangular, other than square, film cassettes.

Review of Blocker Orientation

Review of steps for identification of film orientation:

If you want to know the projection and the film is marked correctly:

1. Place the film in the anatomical position on the viewbox. A right marker will be on your left, a left marker on your right.
2. Recognize the blocker pattern. If the cassette is designed like the one discussed above, the blocker pattern for the AP is lower left, upper right. The blocker pattern for the PA is the opposite—lower right, upper left.

If you know the projection and the film is not marked (for the AP projection):

1. Place the film on the viewbox in the blocker pattern for the AP (if the cassette is designed like the one discussed above, the

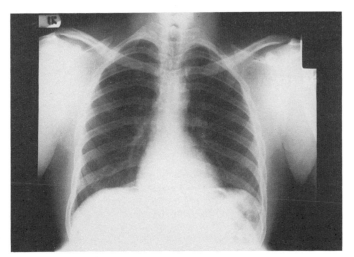

FIGURE 10–17. Assuming it is marked correctly, this is a PA chest.

pattern will be lower left or upper right). If the film is upside down, correct its vertical orientation by flipping it. The blocker pattern should remain consistent with either the lower left *or* upper right placement.
2. The film is in the anatomical position. The patient's right is now on your left and the patient's left is on your right.

If you know the projection and the film is not marked (for the PA projection):

1. Place the film on the viewbox in the blocker pattern for the PA (if the cassette is designed like the one discussed above, the pattern will be lower right or upper left). If the film is upside down, correct its vertical orientation by flipping it. The blocker pattern should remain consistent with either the lower right *or* upper left placement.
2. The film is in the anatomical position. The patient's right is now on your left and the patient's left is on your right.

Remember that you must establish the initial pattern of the blocker when the patient is supine for the particular type of film cassette at your own facility. They may differ from the type discussed here. Use this method only with rectangular, not square, film cassettes.

This assessment should never preclude the correct identification of "right" or "left" on radiographs or the permanent recording of "right" or "left" on radiographs.

11

Determining Side Best Demonstrated

If one had to follow a general guideline in choosing which projection or position to perform, it would be that which places the body part closest to the film. With ambulatory patients, this is a relatively simple decision and easily accomplished action. There are many occasions in the x-ray department and on portable studies when this guideline cannot be followed due to the varying physical constraints of the patients. So professional decisions must be made as to selection of the position that will give the best information, that which will minimize patient discomfort while not aggravating the patient's condition or lessening the quality of examination, and that which reduces the patient's radiation dose.

As you will see from the following outline, technologists have many choices using obliquities in order to demonstrate the right or left side of a body part. Use this summary as a study guide for your Boards and/or use it with the realization that just because we perform lumbar spine obliques in the PA oblique projection (RAO or LAO positions) or knees in the AP oblique projections (RPO or LPO positions), it doesn't necessarily mean that it is the best method for all patients all of the time. Frequently, technologists end up doing routines in the same manner day-after-day-after-day either because of the large number of patients that some facilities handle, because radiology staff can handle more volume with fewer procedure variations, or because a sense of "it works, why change?" comes over us. The good part about fewer variations is that one does acquire greater skills with repetition and along with these increased skills, our film repeat rates remain low. The other side of this argument is that as professionals, we start to get tunnel vision, "one way for all." Certainly this should not be true and is not a very professional viewpoint.

To avoid the performance trap of repetitive x-ray procedures, take the time and effort to relearn or review unfamiliar but not uncommon positions. Do you know the best reasons to perform either anterior oblique projections (RAO/LAO) or posterior oblique projections (RPO/LPO) for each routine? Talk to other staff members. Compare notes. Grow in your knowledge of how fellow technologists make decisions as to how and, equally impor-

TABLE 11–1. AP OBLIQUES (RPO/LPO POSITIONS) SIDE BEST DEMONSTRATED

Anatomical Area	RPO	LPO	Structure Demonstrated
Cervical spine	Side up—left	Side up—right	Intervertebral foramina
Lungs	Side up—left	Side up—right	Lung field
Thoracic spine	Side up—left	Side up—right	Apophyses
Lumbar spine	Side down—right	Side down—left	Apophyses
Sacroiliac joints	Side up—left	Side up—right	Joint spaces
Ribs	Side down—right	Side down—left	Axillary ribs
Colon	Side up—left	Side up—right	Left = descending colon Right = ascending colon
Skull			
AP semi-axial Arcelin	Side up—left	Side up—right	IAC, petrous pyramid, mastoid tip
AP semi-axial Mayer's	Side down—right	Side down—left	Tympanic cavity, ossicles

tant, when to perform certain oblique x-ray positions rather than others. Who has the reputation for precision skull work, spine obliques, that L5-S1 spot? It could be you!

Start here. Review which oblique demonstrates what. Cover up a portion of Table 11–1 and see how you do.

For those student technologists studying for the Boards, notice that only three anatomical parts—lumbar spine, ribs and AP semi-axial oblique skull–Mayer's—differ from the rest of the anatomy listed in Table 11–1. (An easier way to memorize large amounts of data is to remember the differing factors rather than to try to remember the whole list.) Therefore, for the anatomy listed in Table 11–1 in the AP oblique projections (RPO/LPO positions), lumbar spine, Mayer's skull, and ribs show the side down while everything else listed demonstrates the side up. It makes a much smaller table (Table 11–2) to memorize.

Another fact to consider is that recumbent patients having a unilateral rib exam (side down, side seen) must lie *on* the injury—not a pleasant situation and a very good reason to perform them with an upright PA obliquity (side up, side seen).

TABLE 11–2. AP OBLIQUES (RPO/LPO POSITIONS)

Lumbar spine:	Side down, side seen
Ribs:	Side down, side seen
Skull (Mayer's):	Side down, side seen

TABLE 11-3. AP OBLIQUES—EXTREMITIES (SIDE BEST DEMONSTRATED)

Anatomical Area	AP Lateral Oblique	AP Medial Oblique
Ankle		Side up—lateral malleolus
Elbow	Side down—radial head/capitulum	Side down—coronoid process/trochlea
Knee	Side up—medial condyle	Side up—lateral condyle, tibiofibular articulation
	External Rotation	**Internal Rotation**
Shoulder	Greater tuberosity on lateral aspect (anatomical position)	Lesser tuberosity on medial aspect

TABLE 11-4. PA OBLIQUES (RAO/LAO POSITIONS) SIDE BEST DEMONSTRATED

Anatomical Area	RAO	LAO
Cervical spine	Side down—right	Side down—left
Lungs	Side down—right	Side down—left
Thoracic spine	Side down—right	Side down—left
Lumbar spine	Side up—left	Side up—right
Sacroiliac joints	Side down—right	Side down—left
Ribs	Side up—left	Side up—right
Colon	Side down—right	Side down—left
Skull		
PA semi-axial Stenver's (IAC, petrous pyramid, mastoid tip)	Side down—right	Side down—left
Law's axiolateral (mastoids)	Side down—right	Side down—left

TABLE 11-5. PA OBLIQUES—EXTREMITIES (SIDE BEST DEMONSTRATED)

Anatomical Area	PA Lateral Oblique	PA Medial Oblique
Knee	Side down—medial condyles	Side down—lateral condyles/proximal tibiofibular articulations
Wrist	Side up—lateral carpals	

In case you are wondering why kidneys and ureters (intravenous pyelograms or excretory urograms) are not included in this list, it is because they represent a bilateral study. That is, one particular oblique will best demonstrate anatomy on both its right and left aspects. For instance, a RPO position will show the *right* kidney on its full medial-to-lateral or transverse axis (in side profile), demonstrate a magnified *left* ureter, as well as the ureterovesical junction where the ureter joins the *left* posterolateral aspect of the bladder. So the anatomy demonstrated is both side up and side down.

The terms used for RAO, LAO, RPO, or LPO positions are not customarily used for extremities. Instead, the direction of rotation from the aspect of the anatomical position is used to describe the AP oblique or PA oblique. For instance, the PA medial oblique of the knee rotates the leg so that the toes are in, and the AP medial oblique of the knee rotates the toes as well. Pronated or supinated, the motion is expressed from the anterior surface movement. Specific anatomical structures that are best demonstrated are indicated in Tables 11–3 through 11–5.

Cranial Radiography Summaries

SUMMARY OF CRANIAL BASELINES AND TUBE ANGLES

Baselines (other than the midsagittal plane [MSP]) and tube angles used with the positions or projections listed:

ORBITOMEATAL LINE (RADIOGRAPHIC)

Towne's	30° caudal
Haas PA	25° cephalic
PA Caldwell	15° caudal
Waters'	37° from perp.
Modified Waters'	perp. to film

INFRAORBITOMEATAL LINE (REID'S)

Towne's	37° caudal
Towne's	37° caudal (post.* clinoids–sella turcica)
Towne's	30° caudal (ant.* clinoids–sella turcica)
Schuller's (SMV)	CR perp. to IOML
Reverse Waters'	30° cephalic
Tangential (May's)	CR perp. to IOML
Lateral facial bones	perp. to film
Lateral skull	perp. to film
Stenver's	12° cephalic
Arcelin's	10°–12° caudal

INTERPUPILLARY LINE

Mayer's	45° caudal . . . Mayer's semi-axial oblique

ACANTHOMEATAL LINE

Modified lateral (Law's)	15° caudal . . . Modified lateral (Law's)
Rhese PA oblique	perp. to film
Axiolateral	25° cephalic

Lat. facial bones	CR perp.
Lat. nasal bones	CR perp.
Lat. sella turcica	CR perp.
Lat. skull	CR perp.

GLABELLOMEATAL LINE

PA Caldwell	23° caudal

MENTOMEATAL LINE

Waters'	perp. to film

*Key: perp., perpendicular; post., posterior; ant., anterior; Lat., lateral.

CRANIAL TUBE ANGLES AND POSITIONING SUMMARY

The amount of tube angle used is specified first; supination (S) or pronation (P) or lateralization (L) is indicated second; and position of the head or position of planes used for the positions or projections listed is third *(the MSP is perpendicular (perp.) to the film unless otherwise stated)*:

Arcelin's .... 10°–12° caudal / S /45° rotation MSP away from side of interest and IOML perp. to film

Axiolateral (mandible) ..... 25° cephalic / L / IP and AML perp. and MSP parallel to film

Haas, PA semi-axial .... 25° cephalic / P / OML perp. to film

Lateral facial bones .... CR perp. / L / IP and IOML perp. and MSP parallel to film

Lateral nasal bones .... CR perp. / L / IP and IOML perp. and MSP parallel to film

Lateral skull .... CR perp. / L / IP and IOML perp. and MSP parallel to film

Modified lateral (Law's) .... 15° caudal / L / 15° MSP to film, IP and AML parallel to transverse film axis

Mayer's .... 45° caudal / S / 45° rotation MSP toward side of interest IP perp.

Modified Waters' .... CR perp. / P / OML and film 55°

PA .... CR perp. / P / OML perp. to film

PA Caldwell .... 15° caudal / P / OML perp. to film

PA Caldwell .... 23° caudal / P / GML perp. to film

Reverse Waters' .... 30° cephalic / S / IOML perp. to film

Rhese PA oblique .... CR perp. / P / 53° MSP rotation from film (37° away from CR), AML perp.

Schuller's (SMV) .... CR perp. to IOML / S / hyperextended

Stenver's .... 12° cephalic / P / 45° rotation MSP toward side of interest

Tangential (VSM—May's) .. CR perp. to IOML / P / hyperextended, MSP 15°

Towne's .... 30° caudal / S / OML perp. to film

Towne's .... 37° caudal / S / IOML perp. to film

Towne's (ant. clinoids–sella turcica) .... 30° caudal / S / IOML perp. to film

Towne's (post. clinoids–sella turcica) .... 37° caudal / S / IOML perp. to film

Waters' .... CR perp. / P / MML perp. to film

Waters' .... CR perp. / P / OML and film 37°

References

1. Swallow RA, Naylor E (eds): Clark's Positioning in Radiography, 11th ed. Rockville, Md: Aspen, 1986, p 290.
2. Ballinger PW: Merrill's Atlas of Radiographic Positions and Radiologic Procedures, 7th ed. St Louis: CV Mosby, 1991, Vol I, pp 72–73.
3. Ballinger, Vol I, p 83.
4. Cullinan AM: Producing Quality Radiographs. Philadelphia: JB Lippincott, 1987, p 72.
5. Thompson TT: Cahoon's Formulating X-Ray Techniques, 9th ed. Durham, NC: Duke University Press, 1979, p 100.
6. Ballinger, Vol I, p 108.
7. Cullinan, p 72.
8. Thompson, p 100.
9. Curry TS III, Dowdy JE, Murry RC Jr: Christensen's Introduction to the Physics of Diagnostic Radiology, 3rd ed. Philadelphia: Lea & Febiger, 1984, p 86.
10. Swallow and Naylor, p 104.
11. Bontrager KL, Anthony BT: Textbook of Radiographic Positioning and Related Anatomy, 2nd ed. St Louis: CV Mosby, 1987, p 156.
12. Eisenberg RL, Dennis CA, May CR: Radiographic Positioning. Boston: Little, Brown and Co, 1989, p 115.
13. Bontrager and Anthony, p 171.
14. Ballinger, Vol I, p 214.
15. Cullinan, pp 82–83.
16. Ballinger, Vol I, pp 320–321.
17. Ballinger, Vol I, pp 318–319.
18. Ballinger, Vol I, p 314.
19. Drafke MW: Trauma and Mobile Radiography. Philadelphia: FA Davis, 1990, p 141.
20. Drafke, p 141.
21. Bontrager and Anthony, p 214.
22. Paris DQ: Craniographic Positioning with Comparison Studies. Philadelphia: FA Davis, 1983, p 68.
23. Eisenberg et al, p 283.
24. Bontrager and Anthony, p 216.
25. Ballinger, Vol II, p 228.
26. Ballinger, Vol II, p 296.
27. Bontrager and Anthony, p 235.
28. Drafke, p 146.
29. Eisenberg et al, p 298.
30. Swallow and Naylor, p 236.
31. American Registry of Radiologic Technologists: Skull Terminology. ARRT Newsletter, November 1991, p 3.

32. Ballinger, Vol II, p 302.
33. Paris, p 126.
34. Bontrager and Anthony, p 258.
35. Ballinger, Vol II, p 348.
36. Ballinger, Vol II, p 334.
37. Ballinger, Vol II, p 338.
38. Paris, p 148.
39. Ballinger, Vol II, p 316.
40. Bontrager and Anthony, p 258.
41. Eisenberg et al, p 288.
42. Ballinger, Vol II, p 384.
43. Ballinger, Vol II, p 423.
44. Paris, p 86.
45. Ballinger, Vol II, p 417.
46. Ballinger, Vol II, p 390.
47. Bontrager and Anthony, p 269.
48. Ballinger, Vol II, p 418.
49. Bontrager and Anthony, p 271.
50. Ballinger, Vol II, p 392.
51. Paris, p 90.
52. Cullinan, p 41.
53. Meschan I: Radiographic Positioning and Related Anatomy, 2nd ed. Philadelphia: WB Saunders, 1978, p 344.
54. Meschan, p 344.
55. Ballinger, Vol II, p 36

Bibliography

The American Registry of Radiologic Technologists. ARRT Newsletter, Mendota Heights, Minnesota, November, 1991.

Ballinger PW. Merrill's Atlas of Radiographic Positions and Radiologic Procedures. St Louis: CV Mosby, 1991.

Bushong SC. Radiation Physics. St Louis: CV Mosby, 1989.

Bontrager KL, Anthony BT. Textbook of Radiographic Positioning and Related Anatomy. St Louis: CV Mosby, 1987.

Cullinan AM. Producing Quality Radiographs. Philadelphia: JB Lippincott, 1987.

Curry TS III, Dowdy JE, Murry RC Jr. Christensen's Introduction to The Physics of Diagnostic Radiology. Philadelphia: Lea & Febiger, 1984.

Drafke MW. Trauma and Mobile Radiography. Philadelphia: FA Davis, 1990.

Eisenberg RL, Dennis CA, May CR. Radiographic Positioning. Boston: Little, Brown and Co, 1989.

Meschan I. Radiographic Positioning and Related Anatomy. Philadelphia: WB Saunders, 1978.

Miller B, Brackman Keane C. Encyclopedia and Dictionary of Medicine, Nursing, and Allied Health, 4th ed. Philadelphia: WB Saunders, 1987.

Paris DQ. Craniographic Positioning with Comparison Studies. Philadelphia: FA Davis, 1983.

Swallow RA, Naylor E. Clark's Positioning in Radiography. Rockville, Md: Aspen, 1986.

Thompson TT. Cahoon's Formulating X-Ray Techniques, Durham, NC: Duke University Press, 1979.

Milliampere/Seconds

Seconds*

mA	0.004 or 1/240	0.008 or 1/120	0.016 or 1/60	0.025 or 1/40	0.033 or 1/30	0.042 or 1/24	0.05 or 1/20	0.067 or 1/15	0.10 or 1/10
50	.21	.42	.84	1.2	1.7	2.1	2.5	3.3	5
100	.42	.83	1.7	2.5	3.3	4.2	5	6.7	10
150	.63	1.3	2.5	3.8	5	6.3	7.5	10	15
200	.83	1.7	3.3	5	6.7	8.3	10	13	20
300	1.3	2.5	5	7.5	10	12.5	15	20	30
400	1.7	3.3	6.7	10	13.3	16.7	20	27	40
500	2.1	4.2	8.3	13	16.7	21	25	33	50
600	2.5	5	10	15	20	25	30	40	60
800	3.3	6.7	13.3	20	27	33.3	40	53	80
1000	4.2	8.3	16.7	25	33.3	42	50	67	100

mA	.125 or 1/8	0.2 or 1/5	0.25 or 1/4	0.3 or 3/10	0.4 or 2/5	0.5 or 1/2	0.6 or 3/5	0.8 or 4/5	1
100	13	20	25	30	40	50	60	80	100
150	19	30	38	45	60	75	90	120	150
200	25	40	50	60	80	100	120	160	200
300	38	60	75	90	120	150	180	240	300
400	50	80	100	120	160	200	240	320	400
500	63	100	125	150	200	250	300	400	500
600	75	120	150	180	240	300	360	480	600
800	100	160	200	240	320	400	480	640	800
1000	125	200	250	300	400	500	600	800	1000

*Always check tube rating charts for maximum allowed usage.
Note: Decimal equivalents are rounded to thousandths and therefore will be slightly different from fraction computations (as reported above).

Add-On Positions and Projections

POSITION/PROJECTION

Circle or fill-in the appropriate conditions.

FILM: Tabletop, grid, or _____ Bucky.
Collimate to the area of interest or ____:_____.

CR: Perpendicular or angled _____ degrees
Cephalic/caudal to _____.
Enter _____.
Exit _____.

POSITION: Supinated/pronated.
AP or PA. RAO/LAO/RPO/LPO _____ degrees.
AP oblique or PA oblique _____ degrees.
LEFT OR RIGHT
Medio-lateral or Latero-medial.

**STRUCTURES
DEMONSTRATED:** Best demonstration of _____.

COMMON ERROR:

TECHNIQUE
KV _____ MA _____ SECS _____ MAS _____ CALIPER _____ cm
_____ :1 GRID / B / none SCREEN: RE / High / Par / Detail / None
SID: _____ Rm _____ ADULT / CHILD age: _____ mos. / yrs.
HABITUS: Hyper / s / hypo / a   XS   S   M   L   XL   XXL

Add-On Positions and Projections

POSITION/PROJECTION

Circle or fill-in the appropriate conditions.

FILM: Tabletop, grid, or _____ Bucky.
Collimate to the area of interest or _____.

CR: Perpendicular or angled _____ degrees
Cephalic/caudal to _____.
Enter _____.
Exit _____.

POSITION: Supinated/pronated.
AP or PA. RAO/LAO/RPO/LPO _____ degrees.
AP oblique or PA oblique _____ degrees.
LEFT OR RIGHT
Medio-lateral or Latero-medial.

STRUCTURES
DEMONSTRATED: Best demonstration of _____.

COMMON ERROR:

TECHNIQUE
KV _____ MA _____ SECS _____ MAS _____ CALIPER _____ cm
_____ :1 GRID / B / none SCREEN: RE / High / Par / Detail / None
SID: _____ Rm _____ ADULT / CHILD age: _____ mos. / yrs.
HABITUS: Hyper / s / hypo / a XS S M L XL XXL

Add-On Positions and Projections

POSITION/PROJECTION

Circle or fill-in the appropriate conditions.

FILM: Tabletop, grid, or _____ Bucky.
Collimate to the area of interest or _____.

CR: Perpendicular or angled _____ degrees.
Cephalic/caudal to _____.
Enter _____.
Exit _____.

POSITION: Supinated/pronated.
AP or PA. RAO/LAO/RPO/LPO _____ degrees.
AP oblique or PA oblique _____ degrees.
LEFT OR RIGHT.
Medio-lateral or Latero-medial.

**STRUCTURES
DEMONSTRATED:** Best demonstration of _____.

COMMON ERROR:

TECHNIQUE
KV _____ MA _____ SECS _____ MAS _____ CALIPER _____ cm
_____ :1 GRID / B / none SCREEN: RE / High / Par / Detail / None
SID: _____ Rm _____ ADULT / CHILD age: _____ mos. / yrs.
HABITUS: Hyper / s / hypo / a XS S M L XL XXL

Add-On Positions and Projections

POSITION/PROJECTION

Circle or fill-in the appropriate conditions.

FILM: Tabletop, grid, or _____ Bucky.
   Collimate to the area of interest or _____.

CR: Perpendicular or angled _____ degrees.
   Cephalic/caudal to _____.
   Enter _____.
   Exit _____.

POSITION: Supinated/pronated.
   AP or PA. RAO/LAO/RPO/LPO _____ degrees.
   AP oblique or PA oblique _____ degrees.
   LEFT OR RIGHT.
   Medio-lateral or Latero-medial.

STRUCTURES
   DEMONSTRATED: Best demonstration of _____.

COMMON ERROR:

TECHNIQUE
KV _____ MA _____ SECS _____ MAS _____ CALIPER _____ cm
_____ :1 GRID / B / none SCREEN: RE / High / Par / Detail / None
SID: _____ Rm _____ ADULT / CHILD   age: _____ mos. / yrs.
HABITUS: Hyper / s / hypo / a   XS   S   M   L   XL   XXL

Add-On Positions and Projections

POSITION/PROJECTION

Circle or fill-in the appropriate conditions.

FILM: Tabletop, grid, or _____ Bucky.
   Collimate to the area of interest or _____.

CR: Perpendicular or angled _____ degrees.
   Cephalic/caudal to _____.
   Enter _____.
   Exit _____.

POSITION: Supinated/pronated.
   AP or PA. RAO/LAO/RPO/LPO _____ degrees.
   AP oblique or PA oblique _____ degrees.
   LEFT OR RIGHT.
   Medio-lateral or Latero-medial.

STRUCTURES
   DEMONSTRATED: Best demonstration of _____.

COMMON ERROR:

TECHNIQUE
KV _____ MA _____ SECS _____ MAS _____ CALIPER _____ cm
_____ :1 GRID / B / none SCREEN: RE / High / Par / Detail / None
SID: _____ Rm _____ ADULT / CHILD age: _____ mos. / yrs.
HABITUS: Hyper / s / hypo / a   XS   S   M   L   XL   XXL

Add-On Positions and Projections

POSITION/PROJECTION

Circle or fill-in the appropriate conditions.

FILM: Tabletop, grid, or _____ Bucky.
Collimate to the area of interest or _____.

CR: Perpendicular or angled _____ degrees.
Cephalic/caudal to _____.
Enter _____.
Exit _____.

POSITION: Supinated/pronated.
AP or PA. RAO/LAO/RPO/LPO _____ degrees.
AP oblique or PA oblique _____ degrees.
LEFT OR RIGHT.
Medio-lateral or Latero-medial.

**STRUCTURES
DEMONSTRATED:** Best demonstration of _____.

COMMON ERROR:

TECHNIQUE
KV _____ MA _____ SECS _____ MAS _____ CALIPER _____ cm
_____ :1 GRID / B / none SCREEN: RE / High / Par / Detail / None
SID: _____ Rm _____ ADULT / CHILD age: _____ mos. / yrs.
HABITUS: Hyper / s / hypo / a   XS   S   M   L   XL   XXL

Add-On Positions and Projections

POSITION/PROJECTION

Circle or fill-in the appropriate conditions.

FILM: Tabletop, grid, or _____ Bucky.
Collimate to the area of interest or _____.

CR: Perpendicular or angled _____ degrees.
Cephalic/caudal to _____.
Enter _____.
Exit _____.

POSITION: Supinated/pronated.
AP or PA. RAO/LAO/RPO/LPO _____ degrees.
AP oblique or PA oblique _____ degrees.
LEFT OR RIGHT.
Medio-lateral or Latero-medial.

STRUCTURES
   DEMONSTRATED: Best demonstration of _____.

COMMON ERROR:

TECHNIQUE
KV _____ MA _____ SECS _____ MAS _____ CALIPER _____ cm
_____ :1 GRID / B / none SCREEN: RE / High / Par / Detail / None
SID: _____ Rm _____ ADULT / CHILD age: _____ mos. / yrs.
HABITUS: Hyper / s / hypo / a   XS   S   M   L   XL   XXL

Add-On Positions and Projections

POSITION/PROJECTION

Circle or fill-in the appropriate conditions.

FILM: Tabletop, grid, or _____ Bucky.
Collimate to the area of interest or _____.

CR: Perpendicular or angled _____ degrees.
Cephalic/caudal to _____.
Enter _____.
Exit _____.

POSITION: Supinated/pronated.
AP or PA. RAO/LAO/RPO/LPO _____ degrees.
AP oblique or PA oblique _____ degrees.
LEFT OR RIGHT.
Medio-lateral or Latero-medial.

STRUCTURES
DEMONSTRATED: Best demonstration of _____.

COMMON ERROR:

TECHNIQUE

KV _____ MA _____ SECS _____ MAS _____ CALIPER _____ cm
_____ :1 GRID / B / none SCREEN: RE / High / Par / Detail / None
SID: _____ Rm _____ ADULT / CHILD age: _____ mos. / yrs.
HABITUS: Hyper / s / hypo / a   XS   S   M   L   XL   XXL

Add-On Positions and Projections

POSITION/PROJECTION

Circle or fill-in the appropriate conditions.

FILM: Tabletop, grid, or _____ Bucky.
   Collimate to the area of interest or _____.

CR: Perpendicular or angled _____ degrees.
   Cephalic/caudal to _____.
   Enter _____.
   Exit _____.

POSITION: Supinated/pronated.
   AP or PA. RAO/LAO/RPO/LPO _____ degrees.
   AP oblique or PA oblique _____ degrees.
   LEFT OR RIGHT.
   Medio-lateral or Latero-medial.

STRUCTURES
   DEMONSTRATED: Best demonstration of _____.

COMMON ERROR:

TECHNIQUE
KV _____ MA _____ SECS _____ MAS _____ CALIPER _____ cm
_____ :1 GRID / B / none SCREEN: RE / High / Par / Detail / None
SID: _____ Rm _____ ADULT / CHILD age: _____ mos. / yrs.
HABITUS: Hyper / s / hypo / a   XS   S   M   L   XL   XXL

Add-On Positions and Projections

POSITION/PROJECTION

Circle or fill-in the appropriate conditions.

FILM: Tabletop, grid, or _____ Bucky.
Collimate to the area of interest or _____.

CR: Perpendicular or angled _____ degrees
Cephalic/caudal to _____.
Enter _____.
Exit _____.

POSITION: Supinated/pronated.
AP or PA. RAO/LAO/RPO/LPO _____ degrees.
AP oblique or PA oblique _____ degrees.
LEFT OR RIGHT.
Medio-lateral or Latero-medial.

STRUCTURES
DEMONSTRATED: Best demonstration of _____.

COMMON ERROR:

TECHNIQUE
KV _____ MA _____ SECS _____ MAS _____ CALIPER _____ cm
_____ :1 GRID / B / none SCREEN: RE / High / Par / Detail / None
SID: _____ Rm _____ ADULT / CHILD age: _____ mos. / yrs.
HABITUS: Hyper / s / hypo / a XS S M L XL XXL

Technique Records

CHEST AND BONY THORAX

_____ position/projection for _____
KV_____ MA_____ SECS_____ MAS_____ CALIPER_____cm
_____:1 GRID / B / none SCREEN: RE / High / Par / Detail / None
SID:_____ Rm_____ ADULT / CHILD age:_____mos. / yrs.
HABITUS: Hyper / s / hypo / a   XS   S   M   L   XL   XXL

_____ position/projection for _____
KV_____ MA_____ SECS_____ MAS_____ CALIPER_____cm
_____:1 GRID / B / none SCREEN: RE / High / Par / Detail / None
SID:_____ Rm_____ ADULT / CHILD age:_____mos. / yrs.
HABITUS: Hyper / s / hypo / a   XS   S   M   L   XL   XXL

_____ position/projection for _____
KV_____ MA_____ SECS_____ MAS_____ CALIPER_____cm
_____:1 GRID / B / none SCREEN: RE / High / Par / Detail / None
SID:_____ Rm_____ ADULT / CHILD age:_____mos. / yrs.
HABITUS: Hyper / s / hypo / a   XS   S   M   L   XL   XXL

_____ position/projection for _____
KV_____ MA_____ SECS_____ MAS_____ CALIPER_____cm
_____:1 GRID / B / none SCREEN: RE / High / Par / Detail / None
SID:_____ Rm_____ ADULT / CHILD age:_____mos. / yrs.
HABITUS: Hyper / s / hypo / a   XS   S   M   L   XL   XXL

_____ position/projection for _____
KV_____ MA_____ SECS_____ MAS_____ CALIPER_____cm
_____:1 GRID / B / none SCREEN: RE / High / Par / Detail / None
SID:_____ Rm_____ ADULT / CHILD age:_____mos. / yrs.
HABITUS: Hyper / s / hypo / a   XS   S   M   L   XL   XXL

_____ position/projection for _____
KV_____ MA_____ SECS_____ MAS_____ CALIPER_____cm
_____:1 GRID / B / none SCREEN: RE / High / Par / Detail / None
SID:_____ Rm_____ ADULT / CHILD age:_____mos. / yrs.
HABITUS: Hyper / s / hypo / a   XS   S   M   L   XL   XXL

Technique Records

CHEST AND BONY THORAX

_____ position/projection for _____
KV_____ MA_____ SECS_____ MAS_____ CALIPER_____cm
_____:1 GRID / B / none SCREEN: RE / High / Par / Detail / None
SID:_____ Rm_____ ADULT / CHILD age:_____mos. / yrs.
HABITUS: Hyper / s / hypo / a   XS   S   M   L   XL   XXL

_____ position/projection for _____
KV_____ MA_____ SECS_____ MAS_____ CALIPER_____cm
_____:1 GRID / B / none SCREEN: RE / High / Par / Detail / None
SID:_____ Rm_____ ADULT / CHILD age:_____mos. / yrs.
HABITUS: Hyper / s / hypo / a   XS   S   M   L   XL   XXL

_____ position/projection for _____
KV_____ MA_____ SECS_____ MAS_____ CALIPER_____cm
_____:1 GRID / B / none SCREEN: RE / High / Par / Detail / None
SID:_____ Rm_____ ADULT / CHILD age:_____mos. / yrs.
HABITUS: Hyper / s / hypo / a   XS   S   M   L   XL   XXL

_____ position/projection for _____
KV_____ MA_____ SECS_____ MAS_____ CALIPER_____cm
_____:1 GRID / B / none SCREEN: RE / High / Par / Detail / None
SID:_____ Rm_____ ADULT / CHILD age:_____mos. / yrs.
HABITUS: Hyper / s / hypo / a   XS   S   M   L   XL   XXL

_____ position/projection for _____
KV_____ MA_____ SECS_____ MAS_____ CALIPER_____cm
_____:1 GRID / B / none SCREEN: RE / High / Par / Detail / None
SID:_____ Rm_____ ADULT / CHILD age:_____mos. / yrs.
HABITUS: Hyper / s / hypo / a   XS   S   M   L   XL   XXL

_____ position/projection for _____
KV_____ MA_____ SECS_____ MAS_____ CALIPER_____cm
_____:1 GRID / B / none SCREEN: RE / High / Par / Detail / None
SID:_____ Rm_____ ADULT / CHILD age:_____mos. / yrs.
HABITUS: Hyper / s / hypo / a   XS   S   M   L   XL   XXL

Technique Records

CHEST AND BONY THORAX

_____ position/projection for _____
KV_____ MA_____ SECS_____ MAS_____ CALIPER_____cm
_____:1 GRID / B / none SCREEN: RE / High / Par / Detail / None
SID:_____ Rm_____ ADULT / CHILD age:_____mos. / yrs.
HABITUS: Hyper / s / hypo / a   XS   S   M   L   XL   XXL

_____ position/projection for _____
KV_____ MA_____ SECS_____ MAS_____ CALIPER_____cm
_____:1 GRID / B / none SCREEN: RE / High / Par / Detail / None
SID:_____ Rm_____ ADULT / CHILD age:_____mos. / yrs.
HABITUS: Hyper / s / hypo / a   XS   S   M   L   XL   XXL

_____ position/projection for _____
KV_____ MA_____ SECS_____ MAS_____ CALIPER_____cm
_____:1 GRID / B / none SCREEN: RE / High / Par / Detail / None
SID:_____ Rm_____ ADULT / CHILD age:_____mos. / yrs.
HABITUS: Hyper / s / hypo / a   XS   S   M   L   XL   XXL

_____ position/projection for _____
KV_____ MA_____ SECS_____ MAS_____ CALIPER_____cm
_____:1 GRID / B / none SCREEN: RE / High / Par / Detail / None
SID:_____ Rm_____ ADULT / CHILD age:_____mos. / yrs.
HABITUS: Hyper / s / hypo / a   XS   S   M   L   XL   XXL

_____ position/projection for _____
KV_____ MA_____ SECS_____ MAS_____ CALIPER_____cm
_____:1 GRID / B / none SCREEN: RE / High / Par / Detail / None
SID:_____ Rm_____ ADULT / CHILD age:_____mos. / yrs.
HABITUS: Hyper / s / hypo / a   XS   S   M   L   XL   XXL

_____ position/projection for _____
KV_____ MA_____ SECS_____ MAS_____ CALIPER_____cm
_____:1 GRID / B / none SCREEN: RE / High / Par / Detail / None
SID:_____ Rm_____ ADULT / CHILD age:_____mos. / yrs.
HABITUS: Hyper / s / hypo / a   XS   S   M   L   XL   XXL

Technique Records

CHEST AND BONY THORAX

_____ position/projection for _____
KV_____ MA_____ SECS_____ MAS_____ CALIPER_____cm
_____:1 GRID / B / none SCREEN: RE / High / Par / Detail / None
SID:_____ Rm_____ ADULT / CHILD age:_____mos. / yrs.
HABITUS: Hyper / s / hypo / a   XS   S   M   L   XL   XXL

_____ position/projection for _____
KV_____ MA_____ SECS_____ MAS_____ CALIPER_____cm
_____:1 GRID / B / none SCREEN: RE / High / Par / Detail / None
SID:_____ Rm_____ ADULT / CHILD age:_____mos. / yrs.
HABITUS: Hyper / s / hypo / a   XS   S   M   L   XL   XXL

_____ position/projection for _____
KV_____ MA_____ SECS_____ MAS_____ CALIPER_____cm
_____:1 GRID / B / none SCREEN: RE / High / Par / Detail / None
SID:_____ Rm_____ ADULT / CHILD age:_____mos. / yrs.
HABITUS: Hyper / s / hypo / a   XS   S   M   L   XL   XXL

_____ position/projection for _____
KV_____ MA_____ SECS_____ MAS_____ CALIPER_____cm
_____:1 GRID / B / none SCREEN: RE / High / Par / Detail / None
SID:_____ Rm_____ ADULT / CHILD age:_____mos. / yrs.
HABITUS: Hyper / s / hypo / a   XS   S   M   L   XL   XXL

_____ position/projection for _____
KV_____ MA_____ SECS_____ MAS_____ CALIPER_____cm
_____:1 GRID / B / none SCREEN: RE / High / Par / Detail / None
SID:_____ Rm_____ ADULT / CHILD age:_____mos. / yrs.
HABITUS: Hyper / s / hypo / a   XS   S   M   L   XL   XXL

_____ position/projection for _____
KV_____ MA_____ SECS_____ MAS_____ CALIPER_____cm
_____:1 GRID / B / none SCREEN: RE / High / Par / Detail / None
SID:_____ Rm_____ ADULT / CHILD age:_____mos. / yrs.
HABITUS: Hyper / s / hypo / a   XS   S   M   L   XL   XXL

Technique Records

UPPER EXTREMITIES

_____ position/projection for _____

KV_____ MA_____ SECS_____ MAS_____ CALIPER_____cm

_____:1 GRID / B / none SCREEN: RE / High / Par / Detail / None

SID:_____ Rm_____ ADULT / CHILD age:_____mos. / yrs.

HABITUS: Hyper / s / hypo / a   XS   S   M   L   XL   XXL

_____ position/projection for _____

KV_____ MA_____ SECS_____ MAS_____ CALIPER_____cm

_____:1 GRID / B / none SCREEN: RE / High / Par / Detail / None

SID:_____ Rm_____ ADULT / CHILD age:_____mos. / yrs.

HABITUS: Hyper / s / hypo / a   XS   S   M   L   XL   XXL

_____ position/projection for _____

KV_____ MA_____ SECS_____ MAS_____ CALIPER_____cm

_____:1 GRID / B / none SCREEN: RE / High / Par / Detail / None

SID:_____ Rm_____ ADULT / CHILD age:_____mos. / yrs.

HABITUS: Hyper / s / hypo / a   XS   S   M   L   XL   XXL

_____ position/projection for _____

KV_____ MA_____ SECS_____ MAS_____ CALIPER_____cm

_____:1 GRID / B / none SCREEN: RE / High / Par / Detail / None

SID:_____ Rm_____ ADULT / CHILD age:_____mos. / yrs.

HABITUS: Hyper / s / hypo / a   XS   S   M   L   XL   XXL

_____ position/projection for _____

KV_____ MA_____ SECS_____ MAS_____ CALIPER_____cm

_____:1 GRID / B / none SCREEN: RE / High / Par / Detail / None

SID:_____ Rm_____ ADULT / CHILD age:_____mos. / yrs.

HABITUS: Hyper / s / hypo / a   XS   S   M   L   XL   XXL

_____ position/projection for _____

KV_____ MA_____ SECS_____ MAS_____ CALIPER_____cm

_____:1 GRID / B / none SCREEN: RE / High / Par / Detail / None

SID:_____ Rm_____ ADULT / CHILD age:_____mos. / yrs.

HABITUS: Hyper / s / hypo / a   XS   S   M   L   XL   XXL

APPENDIX C

Technique Records

UPPER EXTREMITIES

_____ position/projection for _____

KV_____ MA_____ SECS_____ MAS_____ CALIPER_____cm

_____:1 GRID / B / none SCREEN: RE / High / Par / Detail / None

SID:_____ Rm_____ ADULT / CHILD age:_____mos. / yrs.

HABITUS: Hyper / s / hypo / a   XS   S   M   L   XL   XXL

_____ position/projection for _____

KV_____ MA_____ SECS_____ MAS_____ CALIPER_____cm

_____:1 GRID / B / none SCREEN: RE / High / Par / Detail / None

SID:_____ Rm_____ ADULT / CHILD age:_____mos. / yrs.

HABITUS: Hyper / s / hypo / a   XS   S   M   L   XL   XXL

_____ position/projection for _____

KV_____ MA_____ SECS_____ MAS_____ CALIPER_____cm

_____:1 GRID / B / none SCREEN: RE / High / Par / Detail / None

SID:_____ Rm_____ ADULT / CHILD age:_____mos. / yrs.

HABITUS: Hyper / s / hypo / a   XS   S   M   L   XL   XXL

_____ position/projection for _____

KV_____ MA_____ SECS_____ MAS_____ CALIPER_____cm

_____:1 GRID / B / none SCREEN: RE / High / Par / Detail / None

SID:_____ Rm_____ ADULT / CHILD age:_____mos. / yrs.

HABITUS: Hyper / s / hypo / a   XS   S   M   L   XL   XXL

_____ position/projection for _____

KV_____ MA_____ SECS_____ MAS_____ CALIPER_____cm

_____:1 GRID / B / none SCREEN: RE / High / Par / Detail / None

SID:_____ Rm_____ ADULT / CHILD age:_____mos. / yrs.

HABITUS: Hyper / s / hypo / a   XS   S   M   L   XL   XXL

_____ position/projection for _____

KV_____ MA_____ SECS_____ MAS_____ CALIPER_____cm

_____:1 GRID / B / none SCREEN: RE / High / Par / Detail / None

SID:_____ Rm_____ ADULT / CHILD age:_____mos. / yrs.

HABITUS: Hyper / s / hypo / a   XS   S   M   L   XL   XXL

Technique Records

UPPER EXTREMITIES

_____ position/projection for _____
KV____ MA____ SECS____ MAS____ CALIPER____cm
____:1 GRID / B / none SCREEN: RE / High / Par / Detail / None
SID:____ Rm____ ADULT / CHILD age:____mos. / yrs.
HABITUS: Hyper / s / hypo / a   XS   S   M   L   XL   XXL

_____ position/projection for _____
KV____ MA____ SECS____ MAS____ CALIPER____cm
____:1 GRID / B / none SCREEN: RE / High / Par / Detail / None
SID:____ Rm____ ADULT / CHILD age:____mos. / yrs.
HABITUS: Hyper / s / hypo / a   XS   S   M   L   XL   XXL

_____ position/projection for _____
KV____ MA____ SECS____ MAS____ CALIPER____cm
____:1 GRID / B / none SCREEN: RE / High / Par / Detail / None
SID:____ Rm____ ADULT / CHILD age:____mos. / yrs.
HABITUS: Hyper / s / hypo / a   XS   S   M   L   XL   XXL

_____ position/projection for _____
KV____ MA____ SECS__ __ MAS____ CALIPER____cm
____:1 GRID / B / none SCREEN: RE / High / Par / Detail / None
SID:____ Rm____ ADULT / CHILD age:____mos. / yrs.
HABITUS: Hyper / s / hypo / a   XS   S   M   L   XL   XXL

_____ position/projection for _____
KV____ MA____ SECS____ MAS____ CALIPER____cm
____:1 GRID / B / none SCREEN: RE / High / Par / Detail / None
SID:____ Rm____ ADULT / CHILD age:____mos. / yrs.
HABITUS: Hyper / s / hypo / a   XS   S   M   L   XL   XXL

_____ position/projection for _____
KV____ MA____ SECS____ MAS____ CALIPER____cm
____:1 GRID / B / none SCREEN: RE / High / Par / Detail / None
SID:____ Rm____ ADULT / CHILD age:____mos. / yrs.
HABITUS: Hyper / s / hypo / a   XS   S   M   L   XL   XXL

Technique Records

UPPER EXTREMITIES

_____ position/projection for _____
KV_____ MA_____ SECS_____ MAS_____ CALIPER_____cm
_____:1 GRID / B / none SCREEN: RE / High / Par / Detail / None
SID:_____ Rm_____ ADULT / CHILD age:_____mos. / yrs.
HABITUS: Hyper / s / hypo / a   XS   S   M   L   XL   XXL

_____ position/projection for _____
KV_____ MA_____ SECS_____ MAS_____ CALIPER_____cm
_____:1 GRID / B / none SCREEN: RE / High / Par / Detail / None
SID:_____ Rm_____ ADULT / CHILD age:_____mos. / yrs.
HABITUS: Hyper / s / hypo / a   XS   S   M   L   XL   XXL

_____ position/projection for _____
KV_____ MA_____ SECS_____ MAS_____ CALIPER_____cm
_____:1 GRID / B / none SCREEN: RE / High / Par / Detail / None
SID:_____ Rm_____ ADULT / CHILD age:_____mos. / yrs.
HABITUS: Hyper / s / hypo / a   XS   S   M   L   XL   XXL

_____ position/projection for _____
KV_____ MA_____ SECS_____ MAS_____ CALIPER_____cm
_____:1 GRID / B / none SCREEN: RE / High / Par / Detail / None
SID:_____ Rm_____ ADULT / CHILD age:_____mos. / yrs.
HABITUS: Hyper / s / hypo / a   XS   S   M   L   XL   XXL

_____ position/projection for _____
KV_____ MA_____ SECS_____ MAS_____ CALIPER_____cm
_____:1 GRID / B / none SCREEN: RE / High / Par / Detail / None
SID:_____ Rm_____ ADULT / CHILD age:_____mos. / yrs.
HABITUS: Hyper / s / hypo / a   XS   S   M   L   XL   XXL

_____ position/projection for _____
KV_____ MA_____ SECS_____ MAS_____ CALIPER_____cm
_____:1 GRID / B / none SCREEN: RE / High / Par / Detail / None
SID:_____ Rm_____ ADULT / CHILD age:_____mos. / yrs.
HABITUS: Hyper / s / hypo / a   XS   S   M   L   XL   XXL

Technique Records

LOWER EXTREMITIES

_____ position/projection for _____
KV_____ MA_____ SECS_____ MAS_____ CALIPER_____cm
_____:1 GRID / B / none SCREEN: RE / High / Par / Detail / None
SID:_____ Rm_____ ADULT / CHILD age:_____mos. / yrs.
HABITUS: Hyper / s / hypo / a   XS   S   M   L   XL   XXL

_____ position/projection for _____
KV_____ MA_____ SECS_____ MAS_____ CALIPER_____cm
_____:1 GRID / B / none SCREEN: RE / High / Par / Detail / None
SID:_____ Rm_____ ADULT / CHILD age:_____mos. / yrs.
HABITUS: Hyper / s / hypo / a   XS   S   M   L   XL   XXL

_____ position/projection for _____
KV_____ MA_____ SECS_____ MAS_____ CALIPER_____cm
_____:1 GRID / B / none SCREEN: RE / High / Par / Detail / None
SID:_____ Rm_____ ADULT / CHILD age:_____mos. / yrs.
HABITUS: Hyper / s / hypo / a   XS   S   M   L   XL   XXL

_____ position/projection for _____
KV_____ MA_____ SECS_____ MAS_____ CALIPER_____cm
_____:1 GRID / B / none SCREEN: RE / High / Par / Detail / None
SID:_____ Rm_____ ADULT / CHILD age:_____mos. / yrs.
HABITUS: Hyper / s / hypo / a   XS   S   M   L   XL   XXL

_____ position/projection for _____
KV_____ MA_____ SECS_____ MAS_____ CALIPER_____cm
_____:1 GRID / B / none SCREEN: RE / High / Par / Detail / None
SID:_____ Rm_____ ADULT / CHILD age:_____mos. / yrs.
HABITUS: Hyper / s / hypo / a   XS   S   M   L   XL   XXL

_____ position/projection for _____
KV_____ MA_____ SECS_____ MAS_____ CALIPER_____cm
_____:1 GRID / B / none SCREEN: RE / High / Par / Detail / None
SID:_____ Rm_____ ADULT / CHILD age:_____mos. / yrs.
HABITUS: Hyper / s / hypo / a   XS   S   M   L   XL   XXL

Technique Records

LOWER EXTREMITIES

_____ position/projection for _____
KV____ MA____ SECS____ MAS____ CALIPER____cm
____:1 GRID / B / none SCREEN: RE / High / Par / Detail / None
SID:____ Rm____ ADULT / CHILD age:____mos. / yrs.
HABITUS: Hyper / s / hypo / a   XS   S   M   L   XL   XXL

_____ position/projection for _____
KV____ MA____ SECS____ MAS____ CALIPER____cm
____:1 GRID / B / none SCREEN: RE / High / Par / Detail / None
SID:____ Rm____ ADULT / CHILD age:____mos. / yrs.
HABITUS: Hyper / s / hypo / a   XS   S   M   L   XL   XXL

_____ position/projection for _____
KV____ MA____ SECS____ MAS____ CALIPER____cm
____:1 GRID / B / none SCREEN: RE / High / Par / Detail / None
SID:____ Rm____ ADULT / CHILD age:____mos. / yrs.
HABITUS: Hyper / s / hypo / a   XS   S   M   L   XL   XXL

_____ position/projection for _____
KV____ MA____ SECS____ MAS____ CALIPER____cm
____:1 GRID / B / none SCREEN: RE / High / Par / Detail / None
SID:____ Rm____ ADULT / CHILD age:____mos. / yrs.
HABITUS: Hyper / s / hypo / a   XS   S   M   L   XL   XXL

_____ position/projection for _____
KV____ MA____ SECS____ MAS____ CALIPER____cm
____:1 GRID / B / none SCREEN: RE / High / Par / Detail / None
SID:____ Rm____ ADULT / CHILD age:____mos. / yrs.
HABITUS: Hyper / s / hypo / a   XS   S   M   L   XL   XXL

_____ position/projection for _____
KV____ MA____ SECS____ MAS____ CALIPER____cm
____:1 GRID / B / none SCREEN: RE / High / Par / Detail / None
SID:____ Rm____ ADULT / CHILD age:____mos. / yrs.
HABITUS: Hyper / s / hypo / a   XS   S   M   L   XL   XXL

Technique Records

LOWER EXTREMITIES

_____ position/projection for _____

KV_____ MA_____ SECS_____ MAS_____ CALIPER_____cm

_____:1 GRID / B / none SCREEN: RE / High / Par / Detail / None

SID:_____ Rm_____ ADULT / CHILD age:_____mos. / yrs.

HABITUS: Hyper / s / hypo / a   XS   S   M   L   XL   XXL

_____ position/projection for _____

KV_____ MA_____ SECS_____ MAS_____ CALIPER_____cm

_____:1 GRID / B / none SCREEN: RE / High / Par / Detail / None

SID:_____ Rm_____ ADULT / CHILD age:_____mos. / yrs.

HABITUS: Hyper / s / hypo / a   XS   S   M   L   XL   XXL

_____ position/projection for _____

KV_____ MA_____ SECS_____ MAS_____ CALIPER_____cm

_____:1 GRID / B / none SCREEN: RE / High / Par / Detail / None

SID:_____ Rm_____ ADULT / CHILD age:_____mos. / yrs.

HABITUS: Hyper / s / hypo / a   XS   S   M   L   XL   XXL

_____ position/projection for _____

KV_____ MA_____ SECS_____ MAS_____ CALIPER_____cm

_____:1 GRID / B / none SCREEN: RE / High / Par / Detail / None

SID:_____ Rm_____ ADULT / CHILD age:_____mos. / yrs.

HABITUS: Hyper / s / hypo / a   XS   S   M   L   XL   XXL

_____ position/projection for _____

KV_____ MA_____ SECS_____ MAS_____ CALIPER_____cm

_____:1 GRID / B / none SCREEN: RE / High / Par / Detail / None

SID:_____ Rm_____ ADULT / CHILD age:_____mos. / yrs.

HABITUS: Hyper / s / hypo / a   XS   S   M   L   XL   XXL

_____ position/projection for _____

KV_____ MA_____ SECS_____ MAS_____ CALIPER_____cm

_____:1 GRID / B / none SCREEN: RE / High / Par / Detail / None

SID:_____ Rm_____ ADULT / CHILD age:_____mos. / yrs.

HABITUS: Hyper / s / hypo / a   XS   S   M   L   XL   XXL

Technique Records

LOWER EXTREMITIES

_____ position/projection for _____
KV_____ MA_____ SECS_____ MAS_____ CALIPER_____cm
_____:1 GRID / B / none SCREEN: RE / High / Par / Detail / None
SID:_____ Rm_____ ADULT / CHILD age:_____mos. / yrs.
HABITUS: Hyper / s / hypo / a   XS   S   M   L   XL   XXL

_____ position/projection for _____
KV_____ MA_____ SECS_____ MAS_____ CALIPER_____cm
_____:1 GRID / B / none SCREEN: RE / High / Par / Detail / None
SID:_____ Rm_____ ADULT / CHILD age:_____mos. / yrs.
HABITUS: Hyper / s / hypo / a   XS   S   M   L   XL   XXL

_____ position/projection for _____
KV_____ MA_____ SECS_____ MAS_____ CALIPER_____cm
_____:1 GRID / B / none SCREEN: RE / High / Par / Detail / None
SID:_____ Rm_____ ADULT / CHILD age:_____mos. / yrs.
HABITUS: Hyper / s / hypo / a   XS   S   M   L   XL   XXL

_____ position/projection for _____
KV_____ MA_____ SECS_____ MAS_____ CALIPER_____cm
_____:1 GRID / B / none SCREEN: RE / High / Par / Detail / None
SID:_____ Rm_____ ADULT / CHILD age:_____mos. / yrs.
HABITUS: Hyper / s / hypo / a   XS   S   M   L   XL   XXL

_____ position/projection for _____
KV_____ MA_____ SECS_____ MAS_____ CALIPER_____cm
_____:1 GRID / B / none SCREEN: RE / High / Par / Detail / None
SID:_____ Rm_____ ADULT / CHILD age:_____mos. / yrs.
HABITUS: Hyper / s / hypo / a   XS   S   M   L   XL   XXL

_____ position/projection for _____
KV_____ MA_____ SECS_____ MAS_____ CALIPER_____cm
_____:1 GRID / B / none SCREEN: RE / High / Par / Detail / None
SID:_____ Rm_____ ADULT / CHILD age:_____mos. / yrs.
HABITUS: Hyper / s / hypo / a   XS   S   M   L   XL   XXL

Technique Records

LOWER EXTREMITIES

_____ position/projection for _____
KV_____ MA_____ SECS_____ MAS_____ CALIPER_____cm
_____:1 GRID / B / none SCREEN: RE / High / Par / Detail / None
SID:_____ Rm_____ ADULT / CHILD age:_____mos. / yrs.
HABITUS: Hyper / s / hypo / a   XS   S   M   L   XL   XXL

_____ position/projection for _____
KV_____ MA_____ SECS_____ MAS_____ CALIPER_____cm
_____:1 GRID / B / none SCREEN: RE / High / Par / Detail / None
SID:_____ Rm_____ ADULT / CHILD age:_____mos. / yrs.
HABITUS: Hyper / s / hypo / a   XS   S   M   L   XL   XXL

_____ position/projection for _____
KV_____ MA_____ SECS_____ MAS_____ CALIPER_____cm
_____:1 GRID / B / none SCREEN: RE / High / Par / Detail / None
SID:_____ Rm_____ ADULT / CHILD age:_____mos. / yrs.
HABITUS: Hyper / s / hypo / a   XS   S   M   L   XL   XXL

_____ position/projection for _____
KV_____ MA_____ SECS_____ MAS_____ CALIPER_____cm
_____:1 GRID / B / none SCREEN: RE / High / Par / Detail / None
SID:_____ Rm_____ ADULT / CHILD age:_____mos. / yrs.
HABITUS: Hyper / s / hypo / a   XS   S   M   L   XL   XXL

_____ position/projection for _____
KV_____ MA_____ SECS_____ MAS_____ CALIPER_____cm
_____:1 GRID / B / none SCREEN: RE / High / Par / Detail / None
SID:_____ Rm_____ ADULT / CHILD age:_____mos. / yrs.
HABITUS: Hyper / s / hypo / a   XS   S   M   L   XL   XXL

_____ position/projection for _____
KV_____ MA_____ SECS_____ MAS_____ CALIPER_____cm
_____:1 GRID / B / none SCREEN: RE / High / Par / Detail / None
SID:_____ Rm_____ ADULT / CHILD age:_____mos. / yrs.
HABITUS: Hyper / s / hypo / a   XS   S   M   L   XL   XXL

Technique Records

VERTEBRAL COLUMN

_____ position/projection for _____
KV_____ MA_____ SECS_____ MAS_____ CALIPER_____cm
_____:1 GRID / B / none SCREEN: RE / High / Par / Detail / None
SID:_____ Rm_____ ADULT / CHILD age:_____mos. / yrs.
HABITUS: Hyper / s / hypo / a   XS   S   M   L   XL   XXL

_____ position/projection for _____
KV_____ MA_____ SECS_____ MAS_____ CALIPER_____cm
_____:1 GRID / B / none SCREEN: RE / High / Par / Detail / None
SID:_____ Rm_____ ADULT / CHILD age:_____mos. / yrs.
HABITUS: Hyper / s / hypo / a   XS   S   M   L   XL   XXL

_____ position/projection for _____
KV_____ MA_____ SECS_____ MAS_____ CALIPER_____cm
_____:1 GRID / B / none SCREEN: RE / High / Par / Detail / None
SID:_____ Rm_____ ADULT / CHILD age:_____mos. / yrs.
HABITUS: Hyper / s / hypo / a   XS   S   M   L   XL   XXL

_____ position/projection for _____
KV_____ MA_____ SECS_____ MAS_____ CALIPER_____cm
_____:1 GRID / B / none SCREEN: RE / High / Par / Detail / None
SID:_____ Rm_____ ADULT / CHILD age:_____mos. / yrs.
HABITUS: Hyper / s / hypo / a   XS   S   M   L   XL   XXL

_____ position/projection for _____
KV_____ MA_____ SECS_____ MAS_____ CALIPER_____cm
_____:1 GRID / B / none SCREEN: RE / High / Par / Detail / None
SID:_____ Rm_____ ADULT / CHILD age:_____mos. / yrs.
HABITUS: Hyper / s / hypo / a   XS   S   M   L   XL   XXL

_____ position/projection for _____
KV_____ MA_____ SECS_____ MAS_____ CALIPER_____cm
_____:1 GRID / B / none SCREEN: RE / High / Par / Detail / None
SID:_____ Rm_____ ADULT / CHILD age:_____mos. / yrs.
HABITUS: Hyper / s / hypo / a   XS   S   M   L   XL   XXL

Technique Records

VERTEBRAL COLUMN

_____ position/projection for _____
KV_____ MA_____ SECS_____ MAS_____ CALIPER_____cm
_____:1 GRID / B / none SCREEN: RE / High / Par / Detail / None
SID:_____ Rm_____ ADULT / CHILD age:_____mos. / yrs.
HABITUS: Hyper / s / hypo / a   XS   S   M   L   XL   XXL

_____ position/projection for _____
KV_____ MA_____ SECS_____ MAS_____ CALIPER_____cm
_____:1 GRID / B / none SCREEN: RE / High / Par / Detail / None
SID:_____ Rm_____ ADULT / CHILD age:_____mos. / yrs.
HABITUS: Hyper / s / hypo / a   XS   S   M   L   XL   XXL

_____ position/projection for _____
KV_____ MA_____ SECS_____ MAS_____ CALIPER_____cm
_____:1 GRID / B / none SCREEN: RE / High / Par / Detail / None
SID:_____ Rm_____ ADULT / CHILD age:_____mos. / yrs.
HABITUS: Hyper / s / hypo / a   XS   S   M   L   XL   XXL

_____ position/projection for _____
KV_____ MA_____ SECS_____ MAS_____ CALIPER_____cm
_____:1 GRID / B / none SCREEN: RE / High / Par / Detail / None
SID:_____ Rm_____ ADULT / CHILD age:_____mos. / yrs.
HABITUS: Hyper / s / hypo / a   XS   S   M   L   XL   XXL

_____ position/projection for _____
KV_____ MA_____ SECS_____ MAS_____ CALIPER_____cm
_____:1 GRID / B / none SCREEN: RE / High / Par / Detail / None
SID:_____ Rm_____ ADULT / CHILD age:_____mos. / yrs.
HABITUS: Hyper / s / hypo / a   XS   S   M   L   XL   XXL

_____ position/projection for _____
KV_____ MA_____ SECS_____ MAS_____ CALIPER_____cm
_____:1 GRID / B / none SCREEN: RE / High / Par / Detail / None
SID:_____ Rm_____ ADULT / CHILD age:_____mos. / yrs.
HABITUS: Hyper / s / hypo / a   XS   S   M   L   XL   XXL

Technique Records

VERTEBRAL COLUMN

_____ position/projection for _____

KV_____ MA_____ SECS_____ MAS_____ CALIPER_____cm
_____:1 GRID / B / none SCREEN: RE / High / Par / Detail / None
SID:_____ Rm_____ ADULT / CHILD age:_____mos. / yrs.
HABITUS: Hyper / s / hypo / a XS S M L XL XXL

_____ position/projection for _____

KV_____ MA_____ SECS_____ MAS_____ CALIPER_____cm
_____:1 GRID / B / none SCREEN: RE / High / Par / Detail / None
SID:_____ Rm_____ ADULT / CHILD age:_____mos. / yrs.
HABITUS: Hyper / s / hypo / a XS S M L XL XXL

_____ position/projection for _____

KV_____ MA_____ SECS_____ MAS_____ CALIPER_____cm
_____:1 GRID / B / none SCREEN: RE / High / Par / Detail / None
SID:_____ Rm_____ ADULT / CHILD age:_____mos. / yrs.
HABITUS: Hyper / s / hypo / a XS S M L XL XXL

_____ position/projection for _____

KV_____ MA_____ SECS_____ MAS_____ CALIPER_____cm
_____:1 GRID / B / none SCREEN: RE / High / Par / Detail / None
SID:_____ Rm_____ ADULT / CHILD age:_____mos. / yrs.
HABITUS: Hyper / s / hypo / a XS S M L XL XXL

_____ position/projection for _____

KV_____ MA_____ SECS_____ MAS_____ CALIPER_____cm
_____:1 GRID / B / none SCREEN: RE / High / Par / Detail / None
SID:_____ Rm_____ ADULT / CHILD age:_____mos. / yrs.
HABITUS: Hyper / s / hypo / a XS S M L XL XXL

_____ position/projection for _____

KV_____ MA_____ SECS_____ MAS_____ CALIPER_____cm
_____:1 GRID / B / none SCREEN: RE / High / Par / Detail / None
SID:_____ Rm_____ ADULT / CHILD age:_____mos. / yrs.
HABITUS: Hyper / s / hypo / a XS S M L XL XXL

Technique Records

VERTEBRAL COLUMN

_____ position/projection for _____
KV_____ MA_____ SECS_____ MAS_____ CALIPER_____cm
_____:1 GRID / B / none SCREEN: RE / High / Par / Detail / None
SID:_____ Rm_____ ADULT / CHILD age:_____mos. / yrs.
HABITUS: Hyper / s / hypo / a   XS   S   M   L   XL   XXL

_____ position/projection for _____
KV_____ MA_____ SECS_____ MAS_____ CALIPER_____cm
_____:1 GRID / B / none SCREEN: RE / High / Par / Detail / None
SID:_____ Rm_____ ADULT / CHILD age:_____mos. / yrs.
HABITUS: Hyper / s / hypo / a   XS   S   M   L   XL   XXL

_____ position/projection for _____
KV_____ MA_____ SECS_____ MAS_____ CALIPER_____cm
_____:1 GRID / B / none SCREEN: RE / High / Par / Detail / None
SID:_____ Rm_____ ADULT / CHILD age:_____mos. / yrs.
HABITUS: Hyper / s / hypo / a   XS   S   M   L   XL   XXL

_____ position/projection for _____
KV_____ MA_____ SECS_____ MAS_____ CALIPER_____cm
_____:1 GRID / B / none SCREEN: RE / High / Par / Detail / None
SID:_____ Rm_____ ADULT / CHILD age:_____mos. / yrs.
HABITUS: Hyper / s / hypo / a   XS   S   M   L   XL   XXL

_____ position/projection for _____
KV_____ MA_____ SECS_____ MAS_____ CALIPER_____cm
_____:1 GRID / B / none SCREEN: RE / High / Par / Detail / None
SID:_____ Rm_____ ADULT / CHILD age:_____mos. / yrs.
HABITUS: Hyper / s / hypo / a   XS   S   M   L   XL   XXL

_____ position/projection for _____
KV_____ MA_____ SECS_____ MAS_____ CALIPER_____cm
_____:1 GRID / B / none SCREEN: RE / High / Par / Detail / None
SID:_____ Rm_____ ADULT / CHILD age:_____mos. / yrs.
HABITUS: Hyper / s / hypo / a   XS   S   M   L   XL   XXL

Technique Records

SKULL

_____ position/projection for _____
KV_____ MA_____ SECS_____ MAS_____ CALIPER_____cm
_____:1 GRID / B / none SCREEN: RE / High / Par / Detail / None
SID:_____ Rm_____ ADULT / CHILD age:_____mos. / yrs.
HABITUS: Hyper / s / hypo / a   XS   S   M   L   XL   XXL

_____ position/projection for _____
KV_____ MA_____ SECS_____ MAS_____ CALIPER_____cm
_____:1 GRID / B / none SCREEN: RE / High / Par / Detail / None
SID:_____ Rm_____ ADULT / CHILD age:_____mos. / yrs.
HABITUS: Hyper / s / hypo / a   XS   S   M   L   XL   XXL

_____ position/projection for _____
KV_____ MA_____ SECS_____ MAS_____ CALIPER_____cm
_____:1 GRID / B / none SCREEN: RE / High / Par / Detail / None
SID:_____ Rm_____ ADULT / CHILD age:_____mos. / yrs.
HABITUS: Hyper / s / hypo / a   XS   S   M   L   XL   XXL

_____ position/projection for _____
KV_____ MA_____ SECS_____ MAS_____ CALIPER_____cm
_____:1 GRID / B / none SCREEN: RE / High / Par / Detail / None
SID:_____ Rm_____ ADULT / CHILD age:_____mos. / yrs.
HABITUS: Hyper / s / hypo / a   XS   S   M   L   XL   XXL

_____ position/projection for _____
KV_____ MA_____ SECS_____ MAS_____ CALIPER_____cm
_____:1 GRID / B / none SCREEN: RE / High / Par / Detail / None
SID:_____ Rm_____ ADULT / CHILD age:_____mos. / yrs.
HABITUS: Hyper / s / hypo / a   XS   S   M   L   XL   XXL

_____ position/projection for _____
KV_____ MA_____ SECS_____ MAS_____ CALIPER_____cm
_____:1 GRID / B / none SCREEN: RE / High / Par / Detail / None
SID:_____ Rm_____ ADULT / CHILD age:_____mos. / yrs.
HABITUS: Hyper / s / hypo / a   XS   S   M   L   XL   XXL

Technique Records

SKULL

_____ position/projection for _____

KV_____ MA_____ SECS_____ MAS_____ CALIPER_____cm

_____:1 GRID / B / none SCREEN: RE / High / Par / Detail / None

SID:_____ Rm_____ ADULT / CHILD age:_____mos. / yrs.

HABITUS: Hyper / s / hypo / a   XS   S   M   L   XL   XXL

_____ position/projection for _____

KV_____ MA_____ SECS_____ MAS_____ CALIPER_____cm

_____:1 GRID / B / none SCREEN: RE / High / Par / Detail / None

SID:_____ Rm_____ ADULT / CHILD age:_____mos. / yrs.

HABITUS: Hyper / s / hypo / a   XS   S   M   L   XL   XXL

_____ position/projection for _____

KV_____ MA_____ SECS_____ MAS_____ CALIPER_____cm

_____:1 GRID / B / none SCREEN: RE / High / Par / Detail / None

SID:_____ Rm_____ ADULT / CHILD age:_____mos. / yrs.

HABITUS: Hyper / s / hypo / a   XS   S   M   L   XL   XXL

_____ position/projection for _____

KV_____ MA_____ SECS_____ MAS_____ CALIPER_____cm

_____:1 GRID / B / none SCREEN: RE / High / Par / Detail / None

SID:_____ Rm_____ ADULT / CHILD age:_____mos. / yrs.

HABITUS: Hyper / s / hypo / a   XS   S   M   L   XL   XXL

_____ position/projection for _____

KV_____ MA_____ SECS_____ MAS_____ CALIPER_____cm

_____:1 GRID / B / none SCREEN: RE / High / Par / Detail / None

SID:_____ Rm_____ ADULT / CHILD age:_____mos. / yrs.

HABITUS: Hyper / s / hypo / a   XS   S   M   L   XL   XXL

_____ position/projection for _____

KV_____ MA_____ SECS_____ MAS_____ CALIPER_____cm

_____:1 GRID / B / none SCREEN: RE / High / Par / Detail / None

SID:_____ Rm_____ ADULT / CHILD age:_____mos. / yrs.

HABITUS: Hyper / s / hypo / a   XS   S   M   L   XL   XXL

Technique Records

SKULL

_____ position/projection for _____
KV_____ MA_____ SECS_____ MAS_____ CALIPER_____
_____:1 GRID / B / none SCREEN: RE / High / Par / Detail /]
SID:_____ Rm_____ ADULT / CHILD age:_____mos.
HABITUS: Hyper / s / hypo / a   XS   S   M   L   XL

_____ position/projection for _____
KV_____ MA_____ SECS_____ MAS_____ CALIPER_____
_____:1 GRID / B / none SCREEN: RE / High / Par / Detail /]
SID:_____ Rm_____ ADULT / CHILD age:_____mos.
HABITUS: Hyper / s / hypo / a   XS   S   M   L   XL

_____ position/projection for _____
KV_____ MA_____ SECS_____ MAS_____ CALIPER_____
_____:1 GRID / B / none SCREEN: RE / High / Par / Detail /]
SID:_____ Rm_____ ADULT / CHILD age:_____mos.
HABITUS: Hyper / s / hypo / a   XS   S   M   L   XL

_____ position/projection for _____
KV_____ MA_____ SECS_____ MAS_____ CALIPER_____
_____:1 GRID / B / none SCREEN: RE / High / Par / Detail /]
SID:_____ Rm_____ ADULT / CHILD age:_____mos.
HABITUS: Hyper / s / hypo / a   XS   S   M   L   XL

_____ position/projection for _____
KV_____ MA_____ SECS_____ MAS_____ CALIPER_____
_____:1 GRID / B / none SCREEN: RE / High / Par / Detail /]
SID:_____ Rm_____ ADULT / CHILD age:_____mos.
HABITUS: Hyper / s / hypo / a   XS   S   M   L   XL

_____ position/projection for _____
KV_____ MA_____ SECS_____ MAS_____ CALIPER_____
_____:1 GRID / B / none SCREEN: RE / High / Par / Detail /]
SID:_____ Rm_____ ADULT / CHILD age:_____mos.
HABITUS: Hyper / s / hypo / a   XS   S   M   L   XL

Technique Records

SKULL

_____ position/projection for _____

KV____ MA____ SECS____ MAS____ CALIPER____cm

____:1 GRID / B / none SCREEN: RE / High / Par / Detail / None

SID:____ Rm____ ADULT / CHILD age:____mos. / yrs.

HABITUS: Hyper / s / hypo / a   XS   S   M   L   XL   XXL

_____ position/projection for _____

KV____ MA____ SECS____ MAS____ CALIPER____cm

____:1 GRID / B / none SCREEN: RE / High / Par / Detail / None

SID:____ Rm____ ADULT / CHILD age:____mos. / yrs.

HABITUS: Hyper / s / hypo / a   XS   S   M   L   XL   XXL

_____ position/projection for _____

KV____ MA____ SECS____ MAS____ CALIPER____cm

____:1 GRID / B / none SCREEN: RE / High / Par / Detail / None

SID:____ Rm____ ADULT / CHILD age:____mos. / yrs.

HABITUS: Hyper / s / hypo / a   XS   S   M   L   XL   XXL

_____ position/projection for _____

KV____ MA____ SECS____ MAS____ CALIPER____cm

____:1 GRID / B / none SCREEN: RE / High / Par / Detail / None

SID:____ Rm____ ADULT / CHILD age:____mos. / yrs.

HABITUS: Hyper / s / hypo / a   XS   S   M   L   XL   XXL

_____ position/projection for _____

KV____ MA____ SECS____ MAS____ CALIPER____cm

____:1 GRID / B / none SCREEN: RE / High / Par / Detail / None

SID:____ Rm____ ADULT / CHILD age:____mos. / yrs.

HABITUS: Hyper / s / hypo / a   XS   S   M   L   XL   XXL

_____ position/projection for _____

KV____ MA____ SECS____ MAS____ CALIPER____cm

____:1 GRID / B / none SCREEN: RE / High / Par / Detail / None

SID:____ Rm____ ADULT / CHILD age:____mos. / yrs.

HABITUS: Hyper / s / hypo / a   XS   S   M   L   XL   XXL

Technique Records

ABDOMEN AND CONTRAST STUDIES

_____ position/projection for _____

KV_____ MA_____ SECS_____ MAS_____ CALIPER_____cm

_____:1 GRID / B / none SCREEN: RE / High / Par / Detail / None

SID:_____ Rm_____ ADULT / CHILD age:_____mos. / yrs.

HABITUS: Hyper / s / hypo / a   XS   S   M   L   XL   XXL

_____ position/projection for _____

KV_____ MA_____ SECS_____ MAS_____ CALIPER_____cm

_____:1 GRID / B / none SCREEN: RE / High / Par / Detail / None

SID:_____ Rm_____ ADULT / CHILD age:_____mos. / yrs.

HABITUS: Hyper / s / hypo / a   XS   S   M   L   XL   XXL

_____ position/projection for _____

KV_____ MA_____ SECS_____ MAS_____ CALIPER_____cm

_____:1 GRID / B / none SCREEN: RE / High / Par / Detail / None

SID:_____ Rm_____ ADULT / CHILD age:_____mos. / yrs.

HABITUS: Hyper / s / hypo / a   XS   S   M   L   XL   XXL

_____ position/projection for _____

KV_____ MA_____ SECS_____ MAS_____ CALIPER_____cm

_____:1 GRID / B / none SCREEN: RE / High / Par / Detail / None

SID:_____ Rm_____ ADULT / CHILD age:_____mos. / yrs.

HABITUS: Hyper / s / hypo / a   XS   S   M   L   XL   XXL

_____ position/projection for _____

KV_____ MA_____ SECS_____ MAS_____ CALIPER_____cm

_____:1 GRID / B / none SCREEN: RE / High / Par / Detail / None

SID:_____ Rm_____ ADULT / CHILD age:_____mos. / yrs.

HABITUS: Hyper / s / hypo / a   XS   S   M   L   XL   XXL

_____ position/projection for _____

KV_____ MA_____ SECS_____ MAS_____ CALIPER_____cm

_____:1 GRID / B / none SCREEN: RE / High / Par / Detail / None

SID:_____ Rm_____ ADULT / CHILD age:_____mos. / yrs.

HABITUS: Hyper / s / hypo / a   XS   S   M   L   XL   XXL

Technique Records

ABDOMEN AND CONTRAST STUDIES

_____ position/projection for _____
KV_____ MA_____ SECS_____ MAS_____ CALIPER_____cm
_____:1 GRID / B / none SCREEN: RE / High / Par / Detail / None
SID:_____ Rm_____ ADULT / CHILD age:_____mos. / yrs.
HABITUS: Hyper / s / hypo / a   XS   S   M   L   XL   XXL

_____ position/projection for _____
KV_____ MA_____ SECS_____ MAS_____ CALIPER_____cm
_____:1 GRID / B / none SCREEN: RE / High / Par / Detail / None
SID:_____ Rm_____ ADULT / CHILD age:_____mos. / yrs.
HABITUS: Hyper / s / hypo / a   XS   S   M   L   XL   XXL

_____ position/projection for _____
KV_____ MA_____ SECS_____ MAS_____ CALIPER_____cm
_____:1 GRID / B / none SCREEN: RE / High / Par / Detail / None
SID:_____ Rm_____ ADULT / CHILD age:_____mos. / yrs.
HABITUS: Hyper / s / hypo / a   XS   S   M   L   XL   XXL

_____ position/projection for _____
KV_____ MA_____ SECS_____ MAS_____ CALIPER_____cm
_____:1 GRID / B / none SCREEN: RE / High / Par / Detail / None
SID:_____ Rm_____ ADULT / CHILD age:_____mos. / yrs.
HABITUS: Hyper / s / hypo / a   XS   S   M   L   XL   XXL

_____ position/projection for _____
KV_____ MA_____ SECS_____ MAS_____ CALIPER_____cm
_____:1 GRID / B / none SCREEN: RE / High / Par / Detail / None
SID:_____ Rm_____ ADULT / CHILD age:_____mos. / yrs.
HABITUS: Hyper / s / hypo / a   XS   S   M   L   XL   XXL

_____ position/projection for _____
KV_____ MA_____ SECS_____ MAS_____ CALIPER_____cm
_____:1 GRID / B / none SCREEN: RE / High / Par / Detail / None
SID:_____ Rm_____ ADULT / CHILD age:_____mos. / yrs.
HABITUS: Hyper / s / hypo / a   XS   S   M   L   XL   XXL

Technique Records

ABDOMEN AND CONTRAST STUDIES

_____ position/projection for _____

KV_____ MA_____ SECS_____ MAS_____ CALIPER_____cm

_____:1 GRID / B / none SCREEN: RE / High / Par / Detail / None

SID:_____ Rm_____ ADULT / CHILD age:_____mos. / yrs.

HABITUS: Hyper / s / hypo / a   XS   S   M   L   XL   XXL

_____ position/projection for _____

KV_____ MA_____ SECS_____ MAS_____ CALIPER_____cm

_____:1 GRID / B / none SCREEN: RE / High / Par / Detail / None

SID:_____ Rm_____ ADULT / CHILD age:_____mos. / yrs.

HABITUS: Hyper / s / hypo / a   XS   S   M   L   XL   XXL

_____ position/projection for _____

KV_____ MA_____ SECS_____ MAS_____ CALIPER_____cm

_____:1 GRID / B / none SCREEN: RE / High / Par / Detail / None

SID:_____ Rm_____ ADULT / CHILD age:_____mos. / yrs.

HABITUS: Hyper / s / hypo / a   XS   S   M   L   XL   XXL

_____ position/projection for _____

KV_____ MA_____ SECS_____ MAS_____ CALIPER_____cm

_____:1 GRID / B / none SCREEN: RE / High / Par / Detail / None

SID:_____ Rm_____ ADULT / CHILD age:_____mos. / yrs.

HABITUS: Hyper / s / hypo / a   XS   S   M   L   XL   XXL

_____ position/projection for _____

KV_____ MA_____ SECS_____ MAS_____ CALIPER_____cm

_____:1 GRID / B / none SCREEN: RE / High / Par / Detail / None

SID:_____ Rm_____ ADULT / CHILD age:_____mos. / yrs.

HABITUS: Hyper / s / hypo / a   XS   S   M   L   XL   XXL

_____ position/projection for _____

KV_____ MA_____ SECS_____ MAS_____ CALIPER_____cm

_____:1 GRID / B / none SCREEN: RE / High / Par / Detail / None

SID:_____ Rm_____ ADULT / CHILD age:_____mos. / yrs.

HABITUS: Hyper / s / hypo / a   XS   S   M   L   XL   XXL

Technique Records

ABDOMEN AND CONTRAST STUDIES

_____ position/projection for _____
KV____ MA____ SECS____ MAS____ CALIPER____cm
____:1 GRID / B / none SCREEN: RE / High / Par / Detail / None
SID:____ Rm____ ADULT / CHILD age:____mos. / yrs.
HABITUS: Hyper / s / hypo / a   XS   S   M   L   XL   XXL

_____ position/projection for _____
KV____ MA____ SECS____ MAS____ CALIPER____cm
____:1 GRID / B / none SCREEN: RE / High / Par / Detail / None
SID:____ Rm____ ADULT / CHILD age:____mos. / yrs.
HABITUS: Hyper / s / hypo / a   XS   S   M   L   XL   XXL

_____ position/projection for _____
KV____ MA____ SECS____ MAS____ CALIPER____cm
____:1 GRID / B / none SCREEN: RE / High / Par / Detail / None
SID:____ Rm____ ADULT / CHILD age:____mos. / yrs.
HABITUS: Hyper / s / hypo / a   XS   S   M   L   XL   XXL

_____ position/projection for _____
KV____ MA____ SECS____ MAS____ CALIPER____cm
____:1 GRID / B / none SCREEN: RE / High / Par / Detail / None
SID:____ Rm____ ADULT / CHILD age:____mos. / yrs.
HABITUS: Hyper / s / hypo / a   XS   S   M   L   XL   XXL

_____ position/projection for _____
KV____ MA____ SECS____ MAS____ CALIPER____cm
____:1 GRID / B / none SCREEN: RE / High / Par / Detail / None
SID:____ Rm____ ADULT / CHILD age:____mos. / yrs.
HABITUS: Hyper / s / hypo / a   XS   S   M   L   XL   XXL

_____ position/projection for _____
KV____ MA____ SECS____ MAS____ CALIPER____cm
____:1 GRID / B / none SCREEN: RE / High / Par / Detail / None
SID:____ Rm____ ADULT / CHILD age:____mos. / yrs.
HABITUS: Hyper / s / hypo / a   XS   S   M   L   XL   XXL

Technique Records

PORTABLE RADIOGRAPHY

_____ position/projection for _____
KV_____ MA_____ SECS_____ MAS_____ CALIPER_____cm
_____:1 GRID / B / none SCREEN: RE / High / Par / Detail / None
SID:_____ Rm_____ ADULT / CHILD age:_____mos. / yrs.
HABITUS: Hyper / s / hypo / a   XS   S   M   L   XL   XXL

_____ position/projection for _____
KV_____ MA_____ SECS_____ MAS_____ CALIPER_____cm
_____:1 GRID / B / none SCREEN: RE / High / Par / Detail / None
SID:_____ Rm_____ ADULT / CHILD age:_____mos. / yrs.
HABITUS: Hyper / s / hypo / a   XS   S   M   L   XL   XXL

_____ position/projection for _____
KV_____ MA_____ SECS_____ MAS_____ CALIPER_____cm
_____:1 GRID / B / none SCREEN: RE / High / Par / Detail / None
SID:_____ Rm_____ ADULT / CHILD age:_____mos. / yrs.
HABITUS: Hyper / s / hypo / a   XS   S   M   L   XL   XXL

_____ position/projection for _____
KV_____ MA_____ SECS_____ MAS_____ CALIPER_____cm
_____:1 GRID / B / none SCREEN: RE / High / Par / Detail / None
SID:_____ Rm_____ ADULT / CHILD age:_____mos. / yrs.
HABITUS: Hyper / s / hypo / a   XS   S   M   L   XL   XXL

_____ position/projection for _____
KV_____ MA_____ SECS_____ MAS_____ CALIPER_____cm
_____:1 GRID / B / none SCREEN: RE / High / Par / Detail / None
SID:_____ Rm_____ ADULT / CHILD age:_____mos. / yrs.
HABITUS: Hyper / s / hypo / a   XS   S   M   L   XL   XXL

_____ position/projection for _____
KV_____ MA_____ SECS_____ MAS_____ CALIPER_____cm
_____:1 GRID / B / none SCREEN: RE / High / Par / Detail / None
SID:_____ Rm_____ ADULT / CHILD age:_____mos. / yrs.
HABITUS: Hyper / s / hypo / a   XS   S   M   L   XL   XXL

Technique Records

PORTABLE RADIOGRAPHY

_____ position/projection for _____
KV_____ MA_____ SECS_____ MAS_____ CALIPER_____cm
_____:1 GRID / B / none SCREEN: RE / High / Par / Detail / None
SID:_____ Rm_____ ADULT / CHILD age:_____mos. / yrs.
HABITUS: Hyper / s / hypo / a   XS   S   M   L   XL   XXL

_____ position/projection for _____
KV_____ MA_____ SECS_____ MAS_____ CALIPER_____cm
_____:1 GRID / B / none SCREEN: RE / High / Par / Detail / None
SID:_____ Rm_____ ADULT / CHILD age:_____mos. / yrs.
HABITUS: Hyper / s / hypo / a   XS   S   M   L   XL   XXL

_____ position/projection for _____
KV_____ MA_____ SECS_____ MAS_____ CALIPER_____cm
_____:1 GRID / B / none SCREEN: RE / High / Par / Detail / None
SID:_____ Rm_____ ADULT / CHILD age:_____mos. / yrs.
HABITUS: Hyper / s / hypo / a   XS   S   M   L   XL   XXL

_____ position/projection for _____
KV_____ MA_____ SECS_____ MAS_____ CALIPER_____cm
_____:1 GRID / B / none SCREEN: RE / High / Par / Detail / None
SID:_____ Rm_____ ADULT / CHILD age:_____mos. / yrs.
HABITUS: Hyper / s / hypo / a   XS   S   M   L   XL   XXL

_____ position/projection for _____
KV_____ MA_____ SECS_____ MAS_____ CALIPER_____cm
_____:1 GRID / B / none SCREEN: RE / High / Par / Detail / None
SID:_____ Rm_____ ADULT / CHILD age:_____mos. / yrs.
HABITUS: Hyper / s / hypo / a   XS   S   M   L   XL   XXL

_____ position/projection for _____
KV_____ MA_____ SECS_____ MAS_____ CALIPER_____cm
_____:1 GRID / B / none SCREEN: RE / High / Par / Detail / None
SID:_____ Rm_____ ADULT / CHILD age:_____mos. / yrs.
HABITUS: Hyper / s / hypo / a   XS   S   M   L   XL   XXL

APPENDIX C

Technique Records

PORTABLE RADIOGRAPHY

_____ position/projection for _____

KV_____ MA_____ SECS_____ MAS_____ CALIPER_____cm

_____:1 GRID / B / none SCREEN: RE / High / Par / Detail / None

SID:_____ Rm_____ ADULT / CHILD age:_____mos. / yrs.

HABITUS: Hyper / s / hypo / a   XS   S   M   L   XL   XXL

_____ position/projection for _____

KV_____ MA_____ SECS_____ MAS_____ CALIPER_____cm

_____:1 GRID / B / none SCREEN: RE / High / Par / Detail / None

SID:_____ Rm_____ ADULT / CHILD age:_____mos. / yrs.

HABITUS: Hyper / s / hypo / a   XS   S   M   L   XL   XXL

_____ position/projection for _____

KV_____ MA_____ SECS_____ MAS_____ CALIPER_____cm

_____:1 GRID / B / none SCREEN: RE / High / Par / Detail / None

SID:_____ Rm_____ ADULT / CHILD age:_____mos. / yrs.

HABITUS: Hyper / s / hypo / a   XS   S   M   L   XL   XXL

_____ position/projection for _____

KV_____ MA_____ SECS_____ MAS_____ CALIPER_____cm

_____:1 GRID / B / none SCREEN: RE / High / Par / Detail / None

SID:_____ Rm_____ ADULT / CHILD age:_____mos. / yrs.

HABITUS: Hyper / s / hypo / a   XS   S   M   L   XL   XXL

_____ position/projection for _____

KV_____ MA_____ SECS_____ MAS_____ CALIPER_____cm

_____:1 GRID / B / none SCREEN: RE / High / Par / Detail / None

SID:_____ Rm_____ ADULT / CHILD age:_____mos. / yrs.

HABITUS: Hyper / s / hypo / a   XS   S   M   L   XL   XXL

_____ position/projection for _____

KV_____ MA_____ SECS_____ MAS_____ CALIPER_____cm

_____:1 GRID / B / none SCREEN: RE / High / Par / Detail / None

SID:_____ Rm_____ ADULT / CHILD age:_____mos. / yrs.

HABITUS: Hyper / s / hypo / a   XS   S   M   L   XL   XXL

Technique Records

PORTABLE RADIOGRAPHY

_____ position/projection for _____
KV_____ MA_____ SECS_____ MAS_____ CALIPER_____cm
_____:1 GRID / B / none SCREEN: RE / High / Par / Detail / None
SID:_____ Rm_____ ADULT / CHILD age:_____mos. / yrs.
HABITUS: Hyper / s / hypo / a   XS   S   M   L   XL   XXL

_____ position/projection for _____
KV_____ MA_____ SECS_____ MAS_____ CALIPER_____cm
_____:1 GRID / B / none SCREEN: RE / High / Par / Detail / None
SID:_____ Rm_____ ADULT / CHILD age:_____mos. / yrs.
HABITUS: Hyper / s / hypo / a   XS   S   M   L   XL   XXL

_____ position/projection for _____
KV_____ MA_____ SECS_____ MAS_____ CALIPER_____cm
_____:1 GRID / B / none SCREEN: RE / High / Par / Detail / None
SID:_____ Rm_____ ADULT / CHILD age:_____mos. / yrs.
HABITUS: Hyper / s / hypo / a   XS   S   M   L   XL   XXL

_____ position/projection for _____
KV_____ MA_____ SECS_____ MAS_____ CALIPER_____cm
_____:1 GRID / B / none SCREEN: RE / High / Par / Detail / None
SID:_____ Rm_____ ADULT / CHILD age:_____mos. / yrs.
HABITUS: Hyper / s / hypo / a   XS   S   M   L   XL   XXL

_____ position/projection for _____
KV_____ MA_____ SECS_____ MAS_____ CALIPER_____cm
_____:1 GRID / B / none SCREEN: RE / High / Par / Detail / None
SID:_____ Rm_____ ADULT / CHILD age:_____mos. / yrs.
HABITUS: Hyper / s / hypo / a   XS   S   M   L   XL   XXL

_____ position/projection for _____
KV_____ MA_____ SECS_____ MAS_____ CALIPER_____cm
_____:1 GRID / B / none SCREEN: RE / High / Par / Detail / None
SID:_____ Rm_____ ADULT / CHILD age:_____mos. / yrs.
HABITUS: Hyper / s / hypo / a   XS   S   M   L   XL   XXL

Index

A

Abdomen, 394–397
  acute series for, 398–409
    AP upright in, 402–405
    left lateral decubitus position for, 406–409
    PA chest in, 398–401
  AP of, 394–397
  portable radiography of, 482–483
  technique records for, 558–561
Acanthion, on lateral position of nasal bones, 354
Acanthomeatal line (AML), 4
  tube angles and positions/projections for, 518
Acetabulum, on AP of hip, 220
Acoustic meatus, external, 3
  on semi-axial oblique of petromastoids, 388
  internal, on semi-axial AP of petromastoids, 386
  on semi-axial PA of petromastoids, 382
Acoustic ossicles, on semi-axial AP oblique of petromastoids, 388
Acromioclavicular joints, of shoulder, 134–137
Acromion process, on lateral position of scapula, 141, 144
Air-fluid levels, of abdomen, AP upright, 402–405
  on left lateral decubitus positions, 408
Anatomical position, 1
Ankle, AP medial (internal) oblique of, 178–179

Ankle *(Continued)*
  AP of, 174–177
  lateral position of, 180–181
Ankle mortise, 178–179
Anterior superior iliac spine (ASIS), in lateralized patients, 12
  in localizing femoral head and neck, 15–17
  in recumbent patients, 10
  in supinated patients, 12
Antrum, on semi-axial AP oblique of petromastoids, 388
Apical lung fields, on AP lordotic chest, 30
Arcelin projection, of petromastoids, 384–387
Arthritis, rheumatoid, ballcatcher's position for hand in diagnosis of, 80
Articular pillars, on vertebral arch study, 258
Articular processes, on AP of cervical spine, 236
  on AP/PA obliques of lumbar spine, 276
  on extension lateral position of cervical spine, 252
  on vertebral arch study, 258
Articulations. See *Joint(s)*.
Atlantooccipital area, on AP dens of vertical spine, 238
Attic, on semi-axial AP oblique of petromastoids, 388
Auditory meatus. See *Acoustic meatus.*
Auditus, on semi-axial AP oblique of petromastoids, 388

ISBN 0-7216-3981-X

90053

9 780721 639819